ONE WEEK LOAN
UNIVERSITY OF GLAMORGAN
TREFOREST LEARNING RESOURCES CENTRE
Pontypridd, CF37 1DL
Telephone: (01443) 482626
Books are to be returned on or before the last date below

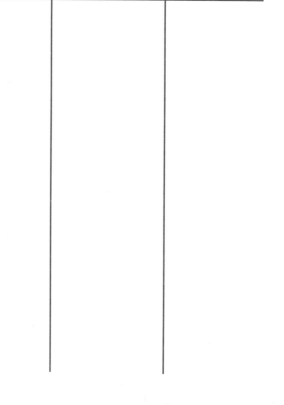

Quantitative Methods
in Population Health

Quantitative Methods in Population Health

Extensions of Ordinary Regression

Mari Palta

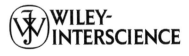
WILEY-INTERSCIENCE

A JOHN WILEY & SONS, INC., PUBLICATION

For general information on our other products and services please contact our Customer Care Department within the U.S. at 877-762-2974, outside the U.S. at 317-572-3993 or fax 317-572-4002.

Wiley also publishes its books in a variety of electronic formats. Some content that appears in print, however, may not be available in electronic format.

For ordering and customer service, call 1-800-CALL-WILEY.

Library of Congress Cataloging-in-Publication Data:

Palta, Mari, 1948–
    Quantitative methods in population health: extensions of ordinary regression / Mari Palta.
        p. cm.
    Includes bibliographical references and index.
    ISBN 0-471-45505-9 (cloth)
     1. Medical statistics. 2. Regression analysis. 3. Population–Health aspects–Statistical methods. 4. Health surveys–Statistical methods. I. Title.

RA409.P34 2003
614.4'2'0727—dc21

2003050087

List of Figures

List of Tables

Contents

Preface

This text arose from my many years working with several long-term population-based observational studies. As I was asked to put together a third-semester statistics course for our new Ph.D. program in Population Health, I decided to assemble the information I had seen investigators and students need most often, and I also decided to answer as many questions as possible out of those I had typically been asked. The resulting mix of topics is guided by this experience. I have attempted to pull in and deal with the aberrations of observational data such as confounding and selection bias. Some traditional topics regarding small sample inference, analysis of variance, and experimental design are deemphasized, as I have found that they confuse rather than help population health researchers. I am using data sets from my own research and collaborations as examples to ensure that subject matter interpretations are meaningful, and that the reader becomes familiar with the "non-textbook" appearance of real data.

While keeping the material immediately applicable by providing detailed instructions for how to run and interpret procedures in SAS, I find it irresponsible to do so without creating some "common sense" about the methods and their assumptions. The beginning chapters lay the mathematical groundwork necessary for topics in later chapters. Whenever possible, I have made a point of inserting practical issues that are answered by specific mathematical derivations.

In addition, each topic starts with an explanation of the theoretical background necessary to allow reasonable judgment as to when the technique is applicable and to facilitate future learning of related methods and software. In the process the reader is exposed to some of the underpinnings of statistics that are often omitted from applied texts and courses. While the text is anchored in the terminology of the biostatistical tradition, I point to some important connections to techniques and terminology used in econometrics and psychometrics. Because of the historic emphasis of biostatistics on experiments and randomization, I have often found that econometric approaches provide further insight in the observational framework.

For progress in addressing current population health issues, it is necessary for researchers in epidemiology and health services to understand and apply regression analysis with weights to deal with unequal variance and correlated and longitudinal outcomes by mixed effects, generalized linear models, and generalized estimating equations. In addition, many data sets in these areas include survey weights. Increasingly, investigators are also called upon to examine the possible impact on their results of missing observations. I suggest straightforward methodology that can be implemented with standard software. The material is presented on a level that will make it accessible to epidemiologists and health services researchers, as well as to applied statisticians. This corresponds roughly to a third-semester applied statistics sequence for statistics non-majors. It is assumed that the reader is already well acquainted with ordinary and logistic regression analysis and has at least rudimentary knowledge of the SAS package.

The explanations are designed to assume as little background in mathematics and statistical theory as possible, except that some knowledge of calculus is necessary for certain parts, such as in understanding maximum likelihood and generalized linear models. The reader may wish to review the rules and uses of derivatives, which are not covered here. On the other hand, all relevant aspects of linear algebra and statistical theory are explained within the text. Important formulas are derived, but with an eye to avoiding excessive algebra.

SAS commands are provided for applying the methods. The SAS procedures emphasized are PROC REG, PROC MIXED, and PROC GENMOD, with occasional references to others. Useful data manipulation commands are introduced as needed to illustrate the techniques in the specific data sets, and the SAS ODS system is briefly introduced to accomplish viewing random effects from mixed models. However, basic commands used to read in data sets and annotate them are considered well known and are not always provided in the text.

Mari Palta

Madison, Wisconsin

Acknowledgments

I have been fortunate to collaborate with wonderful investigators in epidemiology and health services research. They have continually inspired me to look into new statistical issues and have provided me with the insights needed to link the statistics to the subject matter. My longest and closest collaborations have been with Mona Sadek-Badawi in research on the outcomes of very-low-birth-weight neonates, with Kit Allen in diabetes research, and with Terry Young in research in sleep disorders. We have together tackled many challenges that arise in long-term subject follow-up, such as the difficulty in locating subjects and the effects of some participants skipping samples or questionnaires. The research has also interested me, among many other things, in latent variables and in examining between and within individual effects. Many other individuals working on these projects, including Tammy LeCaire and Laurel Finn, have helped me obtain the data for the examples.

Many of the specifics addressed in this book arose from the research of Paul Peppard on the association of sleep apnea with blood pressure. These data form a core example that is traced through the various analytic techniques. I appreciate the many discussions and penetrating questions raised by Paul. Among health services researchers, Maureen Smith has perked my interest in econometric and other social science techniques and has lent me many books. Dennis Fryback shared his data and questions on health care cost analyses.

The book could not have been pulled together without the help of Lin Wang, a Ph.D. student in Statistics who critically reviewed the text, served as a sounding board for methodology, and helped with the formatting of the text. Other former statistics Ph.D. students whose research contributed to the methodology are T.-Y. Yao, Chin-Yu Lin, Wei-Hsiung Chao, Soomin Park, Lei Shen and Liang Li. Many students who have taken the class Quantitative Methods in Population Health, for which this text was initially drafted, have challenged me to explain statistics more clearly and have forced me to consider how different techniques relate to each other and why we do statistics the way we do.

Last but not least, I owe a lot to all the people who have supported me personally and who have pitched in when and wherever needed. My family has been wonderfully accommodating to my obsession with this book. I could not have completed this task without their love and support. In addition, everyone working on the Newborn Lung Project, including Aggie Albanese, Kathleen Madden, and Hana Said and the staff of the Diabetes Registry, make my immediate work environment fun and rewarding.

New methodological developments underlying certain parts of the book were supported by grant CA53786 from the National Cancer Institute and by grant P01 HL42242 from the National Heart Lung and Blood Institute.

M. P.

Acronyms

ANOVA	Analysis of variance
BLUE	Best linear unbiased estimator
GHb	Glycosylated hemoglobin
ML	Maximum likelihood
NICU	Neonatal intensive care unit
NHANES	National health and nutrition examination survey
REML	Restricted maximum likelihood
SAS	Statistical Analysis System®
SBP	Systolic blood pressure
se	standard error
VLBW	Very low birth weight

Introduction

Some Data Sets Used as Examples in This Text

In this book, we focus on extending ordinary regression analysis by considering situations where some of the usual assumptions are violated. As we discuss in more detail in future chapters, violations of assumptions are common in population health data sets. For example, when we want to model presence versus absence of a disease the outcome variable is binary. Because ordinary regression is designed for normally distributed outcomes, the presence of binary outcomes leads to the extension of ordinary regression to logistic regression. We discuss this extension and others that apply to non-normally distributed outcomes in later chapters. With normally distributed outcomes, we encounter situations with violation of equal variance and independence assumptions. For example, subjects may be followed longitudinally, which leads to correlated residuals. The fitting of models and inference in such cases is the topic of the earlier chapters. Throughout, we illustrate with the use of data sets that have accrued from population health research. The purpose of this introduction is to briefly describe these data sets. All analyses were run in SAS 8.2 [1] for Solaris. For graphics we occasionally used SAS 8.2 for Windows.

I.1 NEWBORN LUNG PROJECT

The Newborn Lung Project enrolled a cohort that included all very-low-birth-weight admissions to six neonatal intensive care units in Wisconsin and Iowa during 8/1/88–6/30/91. There were 1040 admissions during this time period, and some baseline data were collected on all of them. Neonatal nurses collected medical record information on factors such as birth weight, supplemental oxygen use the first 24 hours, and hospital of birth without identifiers. Parents were approached as soon as possible for informed consent for interview and medical record abstracting. Due to human subjects concerns, parents were not approached after the neonate had died or if the neonate was in critical condition. A total of 810 infants survived the hospitalization, and the parents of 633 provided informed consent for abstracting. Recontract addresses were available only for the subgroup with informed consent. By age 5, six additional children had died. Among the 804 survivors, 438 were located, and a follow-up interview including health information and a functional assessment of 422 was performed. The parents of 345 children also gave informed consent for complete abstracting of medical records.

The original purpose of the study was to establish severity scores for neonatal lung disease and to find risk factors associated with it. Later, we described functional and respiratory outcomes at ages 5 and 8 years and their predictors. The record abstracting led to longitudinal data on number of hospitalizations and clinic visits during every year of life.

Examples used in the text arise from data collected during the initial hospitalization and from the follow-up. For example, we analyze functional outcome at age 5 and hospitalizations during the first five years of life as outcomes in regression analysis. We briefly illustrate principal component analysis of socioeconomic indicators collected by this study. We will also use this data set to show how to use the available data on those not followed to examine selection bias.

Some references that present data included in this text and that provide further background on the Newborn Lung Project are listed at the end of this Introduction.

I.2   WISCONSIN DIABETES REGISTRY

The Wisconsin Diabetes Registry targeted all individuals <30 years of age diagnosed with Type I diabetes in a 28-county area in southern Wisconsin 5/1/87–4/30/92. The primary mode of recruitment was by physician, diabetes educator, and self-referral. Also, all hospitals and most multipractice clinics were telephoned every 3 months to ascertain any unreferred cases. A total of 733 cases were found. Out of these, 597 gave informed consent for participation. Participants underwent a baseline interview, were requested to submit blood samples every 4 months, were sent a questionnaire inquiring about hospitalizations and other events every 6 months, and underwent physical examinations at 4, 7, and 9 years of duration. The blood samples were used to determine glycosylated hemoglobin (GHb), an important indicator of glycemic control. The purpose of the study is to map the acute and chronic outcomes of Type 1 diabetes from diagnosis and to consider risk factors such as GHb from the earliest stages of the disease onwards.

Examples used in this text arise from the longitudinal glycosylated hemoglobin measurements performed on the blood samples. Figure I.1 obtained by PROC CHART shows the number of participants with GHb data for 1 year, 2 years, and so on, up to 14 years of follow-up, at the time the data sets for this text were compiled. In most analysis here, we will for simplicity average all the GHb measures in a given year. The commands use to produce the number of years of GHb measurements for each individual were:

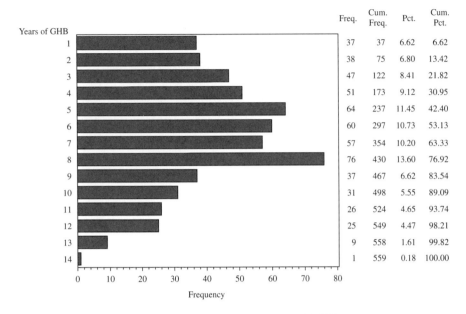

Years of GHB	Freq.	Cum. Freq.	Pct.	Cum. Pct.
1	37	37	6.62	6.62
2	38	75	6.80	13.42
3	47	122	8.41	21.82
4	51	173	9.12	30.95
5	64	237	11.45	42.40
6	60	297	10.73	53.13
7	57	354	10.20	63.33
8	76	430	13.60	76.92
9	37	467	6.62	83.54
10	31	498	5.55	89.09
11	26	524	4.65	93.74
12	25	549	4.47	98.21
13	9	558	1.61	99.82
14	1	559	0.18	100.00

Fig. I.1 The number of participants with GHb

```
PROC SORT; BY ID;
PROC MEANS NOPRINT; BY ID; VAR GHB;
OUTPUT OUT=MM N=NG;
DATA B; SET MM;
LABEL NG='YEARS OF GHB';
PROC CHART; HBAR NG;
```

Some references pertaining to GHb measurements in the Wisconsin Diabetes Registry Study are listed at the end of this Introduction.

I.3 WISCONSIN SLEEP COHORT STUDY

A survey questionnaire inquiring about sleep and sleep-related problems was sent to 6900 employees age 30–60 at four State of Wisconsin agencies. Completed surveys were received from 4927 respondents. A stratified random sample of the respondents was invited to spend the night in a completely equipped clinical sleep laboratory for overnight polysomnography and other tests. A total of 1370 individuals participated. Sleep studies were performed over an extended time period, resulting in some individuals being age 65 and older at the first visit. Blood pressure measurements were taken in the laboratory, and height and weight were measured. Subjects are reinvited for sleep studies every four years. The goals of the project are to identify risk factors and outcomes associated with sleep disorders.

Data used in this text are the longitudinal measures of systolic blood pressure and hypertension as associated with age, gender, and body mass index. Sample sizes in specific analyses vary slightly due to measurements sometimes being missing. For example, out of the 1370 total individuals, 5 had their first blood pressure measurement at the second visit. We also use data from a subproject on the cost of medical care for the cohort. A list of references from the study that involve these variables is provided below.

Suggested Reading

1. Palta M, Gabbert D, Weinstein MR, and Peters ME, Multivariate assessment of traditional risk factors for chronic lung disease in very low birth weight neonates, *Journal of Pediatrics,* **119:**285–292 (1991).
2. Palta M, Weinstein MR, McGuinness G, Gabbert D, Brady W, and Peters ME, A population study: Mortality and morbidity after availability of surfactant therapy, *Archives of Pediatrics and Adolescent Medicine,* **148:**1295–1301 (1994).
3. Palta M, Sadek M, Barnet JH, Evans M, Weinstein MR, McGuinness G, Peters ME, Gabbert D, Fryback D, and Farrell P, Evaluation of criteria for chronic lung disease in very low birth weight infants, *Journal of Pediatrics,* **132:**57–63 (1998).
4. Palta M, Sadek M, Evans M, Weinstein MR, and McGuinness G, Functional assessment of a multicenter VLBW cohort at age 5 years", *Archives of Pediatrics and Adolescent Medicine,* **154:**23–30 (2000).

Wisconsin Diabetes Registry

5. Allen C, Zaccaro D, Palta M, et al., Glycemic control in the first two years of insulin-dependent diabetes mellitus, *Diabetes Care,* **15:**980–987 (1992).
6. Palta M, Shen G, Allen C, Klein R, and D'Alessio D, Longitudinal glycosylated hemoglobin patterns from diagnosis in a population based cohort with IDDM, *American Journal of Epidemiology,* **114:**954–961 (1996).
7. Allen C, LeCaire T, Palta M, Daniels K, Meredith M, and D'Alessio D, Risk factors for frequent and severe hypoglycemia in Type I diabetes, *Diabetes Care,* **24:**1878–1881 (2001).

Wisconsin Sleep Cohort Study

8. Young T, Palta M, Dempsey J, Skatrud J, Weber S, and Badr S, Occurrence of sleep disordered breathing among middle-aged adults, *New England Journal of Medicine,* **328:**69–77 (1993).

9. Hla KM, Young TB, Bidwell T, Palta M, Skatrud J, and Dempsey J, Sleep apnea and hypertension—A population-based study, *Annals Internal Medicine*, **120:**382–388 (1994).

10. Young T, Finn L, Hla M, Morgan BJ, Palta M, Snoring as part of a dose–response relationship between sleep-disordered breathing and blood pressure, *Sleep*, **19** (supplement) (1996).

11. Peppard PE, Young T, Palta M, and Skatrud J, Association between sleep disordered breathing and hypertension, *New England Journal of Medicine*, **342:**1378–1384 (2000).

12. Young T, Peppard P, Palta M, Hla KM, Finn L, Morgan B, and Skatrud J, Population-based study of sleep disordered breathing as a risk factor for hypertension, *Archives of Internal Medicine*, **157:**1746–1752 (1997).

CHAPTER ONE

Review of Ordinary Linear Regression and Its Assumptions

1.1 THE ORDINARY LINEAR REGRESSION EQUATION AND ITS ASSUMPTIONS

A linear regression equation can be alternatively specified as

$$y_i = \beta_0 + \beta_1 x_i + \epsilon_i \quad \text{or}$$
$$\mu_{y|x} = \beta_0 + \beta_1 x \quad \text{or} \quad\quad (1.1)$$
$$E(y|x) = \beta_0 + \beta_1 x$$

to describe the quantitative relationship between a single predictor x and an outcome y. In the population health research projects described in the Introduction, y may be a measured GHb or the score of a very-low-birth-weight (VLBW) child on a test, or the systolic blood pressure (SBP) at a visit to the sleep clinic. In the first equation ϵ_i is a random regression error describing the deviation of a given value y_i from its mean. It can be viewed as capturing unmeasured influence on the outcome. In order to make both the first and the second equations of (1.1) correct, it is assumed that $E(\epsilon_i|x_i) = 0$. In other words, if the second equation is to describe the relationship of the mean y to x correctly, the random errors in the first equation must average to 0 for all x. This also implies that ϵ_i does not depend on x_i. The last two equations are just saying the same thing in different notation because the "expected value" $E(\cdot)$ of a variable is by definition the mean of that variable.

We assume that the reader is familiar with the "conditional on" notation implied by the "|". Conditioning on a variable means that the variable is (at that moment) considered a constant, so the parameters of the distribution of y may depend on x. In other words, when conditioning systolic blood pressure on a given age x, we are interested in the parameters of the distribution of blood pressure at that age. Estimation of the parameters of equations (1.1) usually proceeds by the method

Quantitative Methods in Population Health, by Mari Palta
ISBN 0-471-45505-9 Copyright © 2003 John Wiley & Sons, Inc.

of least squares. In dealing with the regression equation, forming estimators, and drawing inference, we commonly make a number of assumptions:

1.1.1 Straight-Line Relationship

Equation (1.1) implies that x and the mean of y are related in a straight-line fashion. This assumption can be alternatively stated as a constant difference in mean y between every pair of $x's$ that are separated by the same number of steps. For example, if y is systolic blood pressure from visit 1 in the Sleep Cohort Study and x is age, linearity implies that the difference in mean blood pressure between a 50-year-old and a 40-year-old is the same as that between a 40-year-old and a 30-year-old. Regardless of the level of x, $\mu_{y|x+1} - \mu_{y|x} = \beta_1$, so that the regression coefficient is the difference in mean with one step increase in x. Again, if y is systolic blood pressure and age x is recorded in years, β_1 is the increase in mean blood pressure every year. The linearity assumption is an inherent structural assumption, the validity of which is driven by the biological, sociological, and so on, mechanisms that relate y to x. When the linearity assumption holds, we are ahead statistically, because we need to estimate only two parameters β_0 and β_1 instead of a separate $\mu_{y|x}$ for every x.

Only in the situation that x is binary (e.g., designating two treatment groups) is the linearity assumption moot, or automatically satisfied. If y is systolic blood pressure and x is a 0–1 indicator of gender where 1 indicates male, then β_1 is the difference in mean blood pressure between males and females, and β_0 is the mean for females. In this situation, $\mu_{y|x}$ is simply a notation for representing the means of two groups (females and one-step difference involved). Since no assumptions are made on the mean structure, equations (1.1) estimate two parameters either way.

In other situations, the original x may just serve as a label for different groups, such as ethnic categories or treatments. The linearity assumption then makes little sense. However, we can expand (1.1) through the device of binary indicator variables, which bypass the linearity assumption, but again do not save us parameters as compared to estimating $\mu_{y|x}$ separately for each group. In the Wisconsin Sleep Cohort Study, we may wish to compare mean blood pressure between the four state agencies surveyed, by using three indicator variables. In SAS, indicator variables are created in many procedures by the CLASS statement [1].

In the simple cases presented in this chapter, we emphasize linearity of $\mu_{y|x}$ versus a single predictor. We can easily generalize equation (1.1) to more complicated cases by transforming y or x or by adding squared, cubic, and so on, terms in x. Note, however, that even when x or y is transformed or when polynomial terms are added, ordinary regression remains a linear expression of the regression parameters. This simplifies estimation. In Chapter 12, we will consider some situations when the regression equation for the mean is not linear in the parameters.

1.1.1.1 Example
OUTPUT PACKET I shows regression equations, plots of residuals versus predicted values, and mean plots for some variables from the data sets of interest. Later, we

will analyze some of these data sets longitudinally. However, for now we chose only one data point for each individual. Systolic blood pressure is analyzed from visit 1 to the sleep lab, and we selected GHb measured around 4 years diabetes duration. These variables are both regressed on age. To discern nonlinearity in the regression analysis, we look for any trend in the mean residual. Recall that the mean of the residual ϵ_i should be 0 at all levels of the predicted value $\mu_{y|x}$ and at all levels of x. Even a linear trend in the residual plot would indicate nonlinearity in the regression. (In contrast, we would look for curvature in a scatter plot, or a plot of means versus levels of x.) We see in the plot of GHb residuals on age that the residuals appear higher in the middle of the plot, at ages corresponding to the teenage years. It is known that adolescence is associated with poor glycemic control [2]. In the Sleep Cohort data set there is a hint of downturn of blood pressure residuals at the highest predicted values. We will see later that this may be due to some individuals with the highest levels of predicted systolic blood pressure taking blood-pressure-lowering medications. However, we see that all three residual plots display a great deal of variability in the data. This is typical of many epidemiologic and health services studies and can make it difficult to discern nonlinearity from such plots.

The regression analysis and residual plots can be generated by statements such as

PROC REG; MODEL SBP=AGE; PLOT RESIDUAL. *PREDICTED.;

However, to have residuals and predicted values available for further analysis, and especially for producing a histogram, we used statements

PROC REG; MODEL SBP=AGE; OUTPUT OUT=dataset R=RESID P=PRED;
PROC PLOT; PLOT RESID*PRED;
PROC UNIVARIATE PLOT: VAR RESID;

Here, residuals and predicted values are stored in the data set "dataset" together with the original variables. PROC UNIVARIATE provides a histogram of the residuals. PROC REG differs from most other SAS regression programs in its lack of ability to automatically create indicator variables and interactions. It has the advantage of being easy to run, and of accepting multiple model statements.

The plots of mean y_i were obtained by grouping x_i into intervals, so that $\overline{y}_{group}$ can be plotted against $\overline{x}_{group}$. To do so (except for the duration of diabetes, which was already an integer), we used statements

AGEGP=5*INT(AGE/5);
PROC SORT; BY AGEGP;
PROC MEANS NOPRINT; BY AGEGP; VAR SBP;
OUTPUT OUT=MM MEAN=SBPMEAN;
PROC PLOT; PLOT SBPMEAN*AGEGP;

Note how the integer function was applied to efficiently create 5-year age groups (e.g., 5*INT $(57/5) = 5$*INT(11.2) $= 5$*11 $= 55$, so that subjects age 55–59 are in age group 55). The over-65 group was pooled with the 60–64 group. There is a fairly linear relationship between age and systolic blood pressure at the time of the first visit to the sleep laboratory. On the other hand, the mean plot confirms that the relationship of mean GHb to age is far from linear. It appears that GHb rises rapidly until about age 14 or 15 and then declines.

1.1.1.2   Comment on Bias

If the linearity assumption does not hold in (1.1), the mean of ϵ_i is not 0 for all x_i, and (1.1) is not a good representation of $\mu_{y|x}$. The linearity assumption can also be phrased as lack of bias in representing, and later estimating, the mean $\mu_{y|x}$ by the regression equation. Lack of bias is often seen as the most important attribute of an estimator, making the linearity assumption of paramount importance in (1.1).

Technically, unbiasedness in an estimator is defined as the property of being "correct on average." As long as the linearity assumption holds, it can be shown (as we do later) that least-squares estimators of β_0 and β_1 are unbiased. This means that if studies producing estimators for (1.1) were done many, many times over, and the estimators $\hat{\beta}_0$ and $\hat{\beta}_1$ averaged across all these studies, the result would be the true β_0 and β_1. When $\hat{\beta}_0$ and $\hat{\beta}_1$ average to their correct values and (1.1) is a correct formulation, $\hat{\mu}_{y|x}$ is an unbiased estimator of the mean y at a given x.

As we will discuss in Chapter 7, bias can also be created by unequal probability sampling from the population. We will demonstrate there how to correct for such bias. A special case of selection bias occurs when subjects are chosen based on screening high on some risk factor [3].

1.1.1.3   Comment on Causal Interpretation

Even when there is technically no bias in equation (1.1) as stated conditionally on x, it is important to remember that β_1 may not have a causal interpretation. Consider a situation where the causal model conditional on both x and all confounders can be formulated:

$$y_i = \beta_0' + \beta_1' x_i + \beta_2\, w_i + \epsilon_i \tag{1.2}$$

where β_1' measures the causal effect of x on y and where w is a confounder. (Recall the definition of a confounder as a variable associated with both the outcome and risk factors.) If x and w are both normally distributed with correlation ρ_{xw} and variances σ_x^2 and σ_w^2, respectively, it can be shown that the formulation of (1.1), conditionally on only x, becomes

$$y_i = \beta_0 + \left(\beta_1' + \beta_2 \rho_{xw} \frac{\sigma_w}{\sigma_x} \right) x_i + \epsilon_i \tag{1.3}$$

with all assumptions of (1.1) satisfied. However, β_1 is confounded as

$$\beta_1 = \beta_1' + \beta_2 \rho_{xw} \frac{\sigma_w}{\sigma_x}$$

The above situation is known as confounding in epidemiology and as endogeneity in econometrics. Another way to describe endogeneity is that the unknown or error part $\beta_2 w_i + e_i$ in (1.2) does not have mean 0 for all x. However, we will not know that when we are fitting (1.1), unaware of the presence of w.

1.1.2 Equal Variance Assumption

The equal variance assumption can be written $\mathrm{Var}(\epsilon|x) = \sigma^2_{y|x}$, which implies that the variability of y around its mean is the same at every x. For example, the variability in systolic blood pressure is assumed to be the same at every age. The assumption enters in the formulation of the least-squares equations. Recall that in applying the least-squares principle, the expression $\sum(y_i - \hat{\mu}_{y_i|x_i})^2$ is minimized, where $\hat{\mu}_{y_i|x_i} = \hat{\beta}_0 + \hat{\beta}_1 x_i$. This expression treats all observation points equally. But, if $\mathrm{Var}(\epsilon_i|x_i)$ is not equal at all points, it would be sensible to give less weight to the points where this variability is greater. Where variability is wider, observations y_i tell us less about where the mean is. For example, at ages where GHb variability is the greatest, measurements are less informative about the location of the curve describing the mean. With biological measurements the variance often tends to increase with the size of the measurement, so if y is positively related to x, $\mathrm{Var}(\epsilon_i|x_i)$ is often higher when x_i is higher.

In addition to the above consideration, the estimate of the residual variance is difficult to interpret and cannot be assumed to yield valid significance tests when the true residual variance is not constant. We will see, in later chapters, how significance tests can be corrected to take unequal variance into account.

1.1.2.1 Example

In a plot of residuals versus predicted values, we assess the equal variance assumption by looking for whether the plot tends to fan out, usually to the right side. Some caution is in order, as there will be more spread among points in areas with many observations. In our residual plots, we see fanning out toward the high side of the predicted GHb. This corresponds to greater variability during the adolescent years when GHb peaks.

1.1.2.2 Comment on Efficiency

It is a general principle in statistics that weighting an observation by the inverse of its variance yields estimators with the smallest standard errors. Hence we foresee that similarly weighting observations in the least-squares estimator may be beneficial. However, we will need to provide mathematical justification for exactly how to do this weighting.

The property of smallest possible standard errors is referred to as *efficiency*. The word efficiency is used similarly when referring to an electrical device or engine: how well the input (i.e., the electricity/fuel or data) is utilized in producing the desired product (e.g., refrigeration/mileage or regression estimators). One familiar situation where the equal variance assumption is clearly violated is when y_i is a binary variable. Then $\mathrm{Var}(y_i)$ is $\pi_i(1 - \pi_i)$, which depends on the proportion of success π_i. When y_i is coded 0, 1 we have $\pi_i = \mu_{y|x_i}$, so the variance depends on the mean of y_i. We will see later how such relationships are taken into account. A common solution for binary outcome is to apply logistic regression, abandon the idea of least-squares estimation, and apply maximum likelihood. We will emphasize the link between the two approaches.

1.1.3 Normality Assumption

We usually assume that the distribution of the error term ϵ_i is normal. This assumption enters in forming inferences for the estimators. The normality assumption allows us use of the t-distribution to obtain tests and confidence intervals for individual coefficients and the validity of F-tests for the model as a whole. However, it can be shown that in large samples $\hat{\beta}_0$, $\hat{\beta}_1$, and their test statistics have approximately normal sampling distributions regardless of whether ϵ_i is normally distributed. The beauty of the t- and F-tests is that they are applicable even with small sample sizes as long as the normality assumption holds for the residuals. The reader is probably familiar with how, when we abandon the normality assumption, in logistic regression, we are "stuck with" χ^2-tests that yield correct inference only in large samples. It may be noted that for large sample sizes when the degrees of freedom for the estimator $s^2_{y|x}$ is large, so its random error vanishes, the t-distribution approaches the normal, t^2 approaches χ^2 (1), and the F distribution with m numerator degrees of freedom approaches $\chi^2(m)/m$.

Using maximum likelihood requires that a distributional assumption be made on ϵ_i. We will see later that the normality assumption leads to equality of least-squares and maximum likelihood estimators for model (1.1). However, even later we will see that the normal distribution is one example in a broader framework and that it is convenient to draw connections between maximum likelihood and least-squares estimation procedures for many common distributions.

1.1.3.1 Examples
The normality assumption can be assessed informally, but adequately, by looking at a histogram of the residuals. Our graph for the residuals of systolic blood pressure on age shows very slight skewness. This is rather typical. With a large data set, it is not of great concern, unless skewness is extreme. With a small data set, on the other hand, it may be difficult to assess normality.

Note that it is normality of the residuals that is required for t- and F-tests of regression coefficients to be valid in small samples, not normality of the outcome before taking x into account. It is not uncommon to see that normality improves when conditioning on x. The final example in OUTPUT PACKET I shows a regression analysis of number of days VLBW infants spend in the NICU on birth weight. We see that while the number of days has a rather skewed distribution, the skewness disappears when conditioning on the infant's birth weight.

1.1.3.2 Comment on Normality
Sometimes, a variable's distribution is fairly well known from previous studies to be normally distributed in populations that are unselected for the variable. Systolic blood pressure is an example of a measure that has been widely studied. It is

usually found to be very close to normally distributed, although some investigators have applied the transformation log(SBP-50) [4]. In our case this transformation reduced skewness only slightly, and the distribution became skewed in the opposite direction instead. It is interesting that designed variables such as IQ are typically scaled to have normal distributions in the population. Hence, the normality of such variables is "man-made," while the normality of biological variables is considered to be the result of many factors being added up, so that by the central limit theorem the end result is normally distributed. Recall that the central limit theorem states that means and sums of many independent variables tend toward normal distributions.

1.1.4 Independence Assumption

We usually assume that ϵ_i and $\epsilon_{i'}$ are independent for $i \neq i'$—that is, that the residuals for two different observations on y do not "travel together" once their corresponding x's are taken into account. We will see that the assumption enters when deriving the standard errors of regression coefficients. Intuitively, one can see that if ϵ_i and $\epsilon_{i'}$ are positively correlated, we really have less information than we presume, when we base our inference on thinking that all y's contribute a given piece. In other words, lack of independence implies that only part of the information about β_0 and β_1 imparted by $y_{i'}$ is new; the rest has already been gained from y_i.

Consider the data from the Wisconsin Diabetes Registry. Each individual provided a number of measurements on glycosylated hemoglobin across several years. Say we wish to examine how glycosylated hemoglobin (GHb) relates to the duration of diabetes. Obviously, much variability in GHb exists at each duration and is reflected in the ϵ. While it may be fairly reasonably assumed that ϵ from different individuals are independent, GHb of the same individual may tend to be uniformly on the high or low side, depending on the person's diet, diabetes care regimen, exercise level, and so on. We can usually not begin to hope that we have captured all these influences in the x's we have in the study. Hence ϵ on the same individual are not independent. Similarly, in the sleep study, having blood pressure data on 1251 measurements from three visits on 520 individuals does not convey the same information on, for example, gender differences as having 1251 measurements on 1251 different individuals.

Because there is less information in the data when residuals are positively correlated than when they are independent, standard errors can be underestimated. We will see that lack of independence can be dealt with either by maximum likelihood estimation where the joint distribution of the measurements is correctly modeled, or a modified least-squares approach.

1.1.4.1 Example

It is not easy to discern most cases of dependence in an overall scatter plot, or residual plot. One may target special cases of dependency that are expected in a given study. In OUTPUT PACKET I, we included only one GHb observation

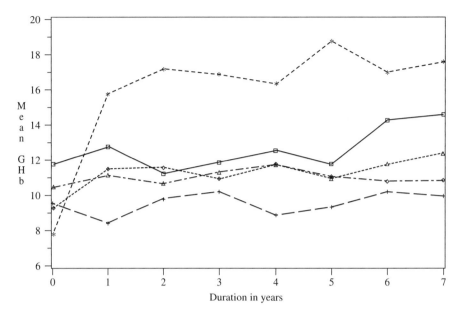

Fig. 1.1   Wisconsin Diabetes Registry Study GHb for the first five subjects

per individual, to improve independence of measurements. (Of course this is very wasteful, and one of our goals is to enable inclusion of all the data in the analysis). In Figure 1.1, GHb versus duration is shown for the first five individuals in the data set. We see that the values of a given individual tend to be on the high or low side. In fact, the average correlation among residuals from the same individual is 0.51. Systolic blood pressure residuals across visits in the sleep study correlate at 0.35 within person.

1.2   A NOTE ON HOW THE LEAST-SQUARES ESTIMATORS ARE OBTAINED

We need calculus to minimize the expression $\sum (y_i - \hat{\beta}_0 - \hat{\beta}_1 x_i)^2$ with respect to the estimators $\hat{\beta}_0, \hat{\beta}_1$. In this case, the two estimators constitute two "variables" in the calculus sense, and we take the derivatives of the least-squares expression, invoking the chain rule. Noting that

$$LS = \sum LS_i = \sum (y_i - \hat{\beta}_0 - \hat{\beta}_1 x_i)^2 = \sum \hat{\epsilon}_i^2$$

we have that

$$\frac{dLS_i}{d\hat{\epsilon}_i} = 2\hat{\epsilon}_i$$

so

$$\frac{\partial LS_i}{\partial \hat{\beta}_0} = 2\hat{\epsilon}_i \frac{\partial \hat{\epsilon}_i}{\partial \hat{\beta}_0} = 2(y_i - \hat{\beta}_0 - \hat{\beta}_1 x_i)(-1)$$

and

$$\frac{\partial LS_i}{\partial \hat{\beta}_1} = 2\hat{\epsilon}_i \frac{\partial \hat{\epsilon}_i}{\partial \hat{\beta}_1} = 2(y_i - \hat{\beta}_0 - \hat{\beta}_1 x_i)(-x_i)$$

We apply the rule that the derivative of a sum is the sum of derivatives. Then setting the final derivatives to 0 we obtain:

$$\frac{\partial LS}{\partial \hat{\beta}_0} = -2 \sum (y_i - \hat{\beta}_0 - \hat{\beta}_1 x_i) = 0$$

$$\frac{\partial LS}{\partial \hat{\beta}_1} = -2 \sum x_i (y_i - \hat{\beta}_0 - \hat{\beta}_1 x_i) = 0$$

(1.4)

Simultaneously solving these equations results in the usual estimators

$$\hat{\beta}_1 = \frac{\sum (x_i - \overline{x})(y_i - \overline{y})}{\sum (x_i - \overline{x})^2}$$

$$\hat{\beta}_0 = \overline{y} - \hat{\beta}_1 \overline{x}$$

OUTPUT PACKET I: EXAMPLES OF ORDINARY REGRESSION ANALYSES

I.1. Analysis of SBP Versus Age: Wisconsin Sleep Cohort Study

The REG Procedure

Model: MODEL1
Dependent Variable: SBP

Analysis of Variance

Source	DF	Sum of Squares	Mean Square	F Value	Pr > F
Model	1	11604	11604	56.43	<0.0001
Error	1363	280294	205.64520		
Corrected total	1364	291898			

Root MSE	14.34033	R-square	0.0398
Dependent mean	125.09145	Adjusted R-square	0.0390
Coefficient of variation	11.46388		

Parameter Estimates

Variable	DF	Parameter Estimate	Standard Error	t Value	$Pr > |t|$
Intercept	1	107.98092	2.31066	46.73	<0.0001
Age	1	0.36605	0.04873	7.51	<0.0001

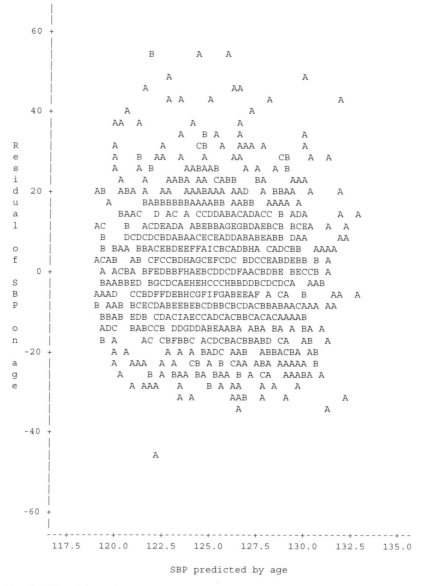

SBP predicted by age

Plot of resid*pred. Legend: A = 1 obs, B = 2 obs, and so on. *Note*: 13 obs had missing values.

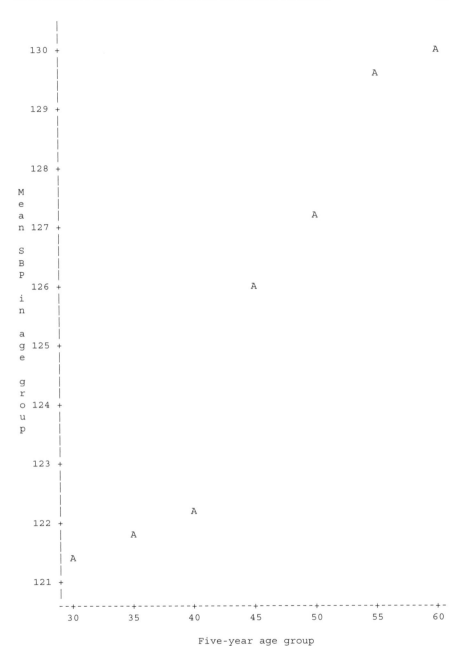

Plot of sbpmean*ageg. Legend: A = 1 obs, B = 2 obs, and so on.

The UNIVARIATE Procedure

Variable: resid (residual of SBP versus age)

Moments

N	1365	Sum weights	1365
Mean	0	Sum observations	0
Standard deviation	14.3350769	Variance	205.49443
Skewness	0.41763912	Kurtosis	0.61294189
Uncorrected SS	280294.403	Corrected SS	280294.403
Coefficient of variation		Standard error of mean	0.38800177

Basic Statistical Measures

Location		Variability	
Mean	0.00000	Standard deviation	14.33508
Median	−0.64707	Variance	205.49443
Mode	13.66973	Range	99.99362
		Interquartile range	18.47016

Tests for Location: Mu0 = 0

Test		Statistic		p Value
Student's t	t	0	Pr > $|t|$	1.0000
Sign	M	−23.5	Pr ≥ $|M|$	0.2131
Signed rank	S	−15323.5	Pr ≥ $|S|$	0.2930

Quantiles (Definition 5)

Quantile	Estimate
100% Max	55.669359
99%	41.669569
95%	24.621515
90%	17.771212
75% Q3	8.770605
50% Median	−0.647072
25% Q1	−9.699556
10%	−17.683597
5%	−22.715642
1%	−29.571613
0% Min	−44.324258

Extreme Observations

Lowest		Highest	
Value	Obs	Value	Obs
−44.3243	1167	47.8313	85
−35.4823	1080	53.4092	802
−33.3630	1190	54.6771	367
−32.3541	896	55.0596	1208
−32.0275	1194	55.6694	1322

Missing Values

	Percent of	
Missing Value Count	All Observations	Missing Obs
13	0.94	100.00

```
                   Histogram                          #        Boxplot
 57.5+*                                               2           0
    .*                                                2           0
 47.5+*                                               4           0
    .**                                               6           0
 37.5+**                                              8           0
    .****                                            18           |
 27.5+*****                                          24           |
    .********                                        45           |
 17.5+*************                                  65           |
    .*************************                      138           |
  7.5+********************************             157        +-----+
    .**************************************        190        |  +  |
 -2.5+******************************************** 198        *-----*
    .***********************************          177        +-----+
-12.5+****************************                137           |
    .******************                           92           |
-22.5+***********                                 54           |
    .********                                     36           |
-32.5+**                                          10           |
    .*                                             1           |
-42.5+*                                            1           0
     ----+----+----+----+----+----+----+
     *May represent up to 5 counts
```

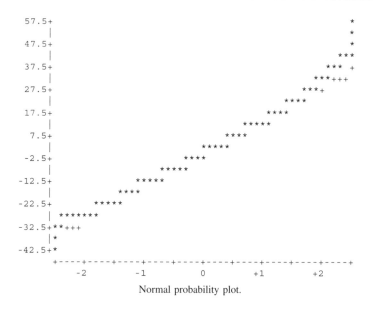

Normal probability plot.

I.2. Analysis of GHb Versus Age—Wisconsin Diabetes Registry

GHb Versus Age—Wisconsin Diabetes Registry
  The REG Procedure

Model: MODEL1
Dependent Variable: GHb

Analysis of Variance

Source	DF	Sum of Squares	Mean Square	F Value	Pr > F
Model	1	0.04566	0.04566	0.01	0.9381
Error	413	3119.52820	7.55334		
Corrected total	414	3119.57387			

Root MSE	2.74833	R-square	0.0000	
Dependent mean	11.28859	Adjusted R-square	−0.0024	
Coefficient of variation	24.34613			

Parameter Estimates

Variable	Label	DF	Parameter Estimate	Standard Error	t Value	Pr > |t|
Intercept	Intercept	1	11.26650	0.31444	35.83	<0.0001
Age	Age	1	0.00155	0.02000	0.08	0.9381

Residual Plot Versus Predicted Value

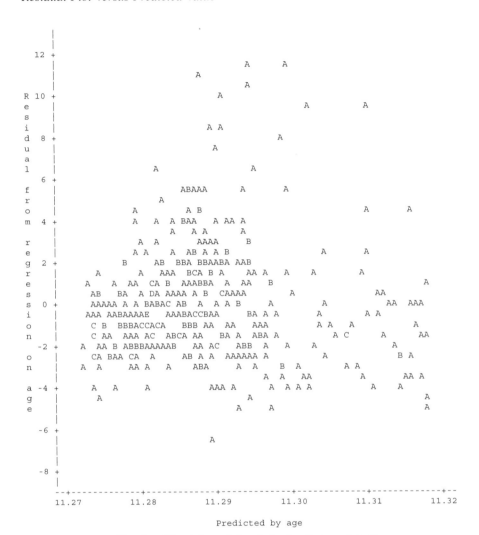

Plot of resid*pred. Legend: A = 1 obs, B = 2 obs, and so on.

Mean GHb by Four-Year Age Groups

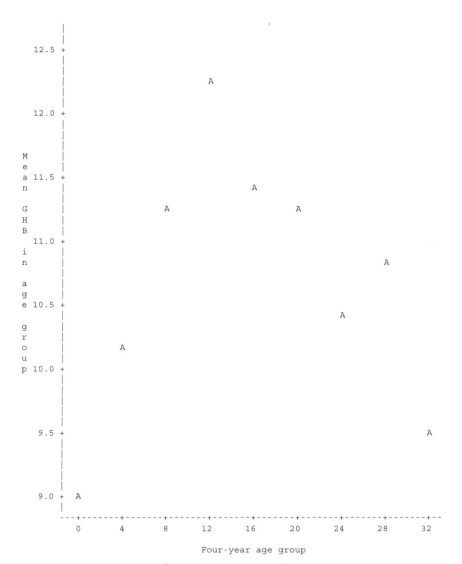

Plot of ghmean*iage. Legend: A = 1 obs, B = 2 obs, and so on.

Histogram of GHb Residuals
  The UNIVARIATE Procedure

Variable: resid (residual from regression versus age)

Moments

N	415	Sum of weights	415
Mean	0	Sum of observations	0
Standard deviation	2.74501226	Variance	7.53509228
Skewness	1.28441431	Kurtosis	2.835934
Uncorrected SS	3119.5282	Corrected SS	3119.5282
Coefficient of variation		Standard error of mean	0.13474735

Basic Statistical Measures

Location		Variability	
Mean	0.00000	Standard deviation	2.74501
Median	−0.43380	Variance	7.53509
Mode	−1.10334	Range	17.89502
		Interquartile range	3.02800

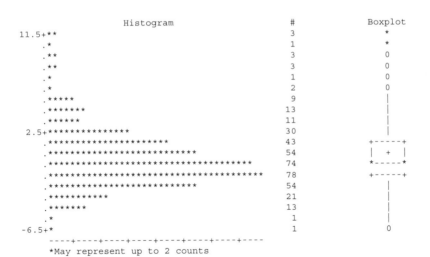

```
              Histogram                              #      Boxplot
 11.5+**                                             3         *
    . *                                              1         *
    . **                                             3         0
    . **                                             3         0
    . *                                              1         0
    . *                                              2         0
    . *****                                          9         |
    . *******                                       13         |
    . ******                                        11         |
  2.5+****************                               30         |
    . *********************                          43      +-----+
    . **************************                     54      |  +  |
    . **************************************         74      *-----*
    . ***************************************        78      +-----+
    . *************************                      54         |
    . **********                                     21         |
    . *******                                        13         |
    . *                                               1         |
 -6.5+*                                               1         0
    ----+----+----+----+----+----+----+----
    *May represent up to 2 counts
```

I.3. Analysis of Days in NICU Versus Birth Weight—Newborn Lung Project

Days in NICU on Birth Weight for Survivors—Newborn Lung Project
Distribution of Number of Days
The UNIVARIATE Procedure

Variable: len (days in NICU)

Moments

N	767	Sum of weights	767
Mean	60.7118644	Sum of observations	46566
Standard deviation	29.2531787	Variance	855.748462
Skewness	0.76237889	Kurtosis	0.35614049
Uncorrected SS	3482612	Corrected SS	655503.322
Coefficient of variation	48.1836276	Standard error of mean	1.05627106

Basic Statistical Measures

Location		Variability	
Mean	60.71186	Standard deviation	29.25318
Median	55.00000	Variance	855.74846
Mode	44.00000	Range	172.00000
		Interquartile range	39.00000

```
                     Histogram                        #      Boxplot
  175+*                                               1         0
    .*                                                2         0
    .*                                                1         0
    .***                                              7         0
    .*                                                2         |
    .*****                                           13         |
    .*********                                       29         |
    .************                                    37         |
    .**************                                  44         |
    .****************                                48         |
    .******************                              55      +-----+
    .********************************                98      |  +  |
    .*********************************************  117      *-----*
    .*********************************************** 126     +-----+
    .********************************                96         |
    .********************                            58         |
    .*********                                       26         |
    5+***                                             7         |
     ----+----+----+----+----+----+----+----+--
     *May represent up to 3 counts
```

Regression of Number of Days in NICU
  The REG Procedure

Model: MODEL1
Dependent Variable: len (days in NICU)

Analysis of Variance

Source	DF	Sum of Squares	Mean Square	F Value	Pr > F
Model	1	280517	280517	572.28	<0.0001
Error	765	374986	490.17803		
Corrected total	766	655503			

Root MSE	22.13996	R-square	0.4279	
Dependent mean	60.71186	Adjusted R-square	0.4272	
Coefficient of variation	36.46728			

Parameter Estimates

Variable	Label	DF	Parameter Estimate	Standard Error
Intercept	Intercept	1	145.15576	3.61932
Birth weight	Birth weight in grams	1	−7.49741	0.31341

Parameter Estimates

Variable	Label	DF	t Value	Pr > $|t|$
Intercept	Intercept	1	40.11	<0.0001
Birth weight	Birth weight in grams	1	−23.92	<0.0001

Days in NICU on Birth Weight for Survivors—Newborn Lung Project
Distribution of Number of Days Conditional on Birth Weight
  The UNIVARIATE Procedure

Variable: resid (residual of number of days versus birth weight)

Moments

N	767	Sum weights	767
Mean	0	Sum observations	0
Standard deviation	22.1255081	Variance	489.53811
Skewness	0.70011397	Kurtosis	1.96459767
Uncorrected SS	374986.193	Corrected SS	374986.193
Coefficient of variation		Standard error of mean	0.7989058

Basic Statistical Measures

Location		Variability	
Mean	0.0000	Standard deviation	22.12551
Median	−1.5933	Variance	489.53811
Mode	−11.9428	Range	186.09306
		Interquartile range	24.74767

```
                      Histogram                         #      Boxplot
    105+*                                               1         *
       .*                                               1         *
       .
       .*                                               4         0
       .**                                              8         0
       .**                                              8         0
       .****                                            15        0
       .********                                        29        |
       .************                                    48        |
     15+*********************                           85     +-----+
       .*****************************************       165    |  +  |
       .****************************************        157    *-----*
       .*******************************                 128    +-----+
       .*****************                               71        |
       .*******                                         28        |
       .****                                            14        |
       .*                                               2         0
       .*                                               2         0
    -75+*                                               1         0
       ----+----+----+----+----+----+----+----+--
       *May represent up to 4 counts
```

CHAPTER TWO

The Maximum Likelihood Approach to Ordinary Regression

In the above, we presented the usual least-squares approach to estimation in ordinary regression. This approach is based on minimizing $\sum (y_i - \hat{\mu}_{y|x})^2$. Minimizing the sum-of-squared distances of the points from the regression line turns out to be a good idea, because the expression is in the numerator of $s_{y|x}^2$ and of the standard errors of regression coefficient estimators. Minimizing the variance of estimators is always a goal, as it means that the estimators are efficient. The least-squares principle is quite general, and estimation can be carried out without any reference to how the points are actually distributed. Note how the assumptions of ordinary regression came into play only gradually. First, no assumption was made in choosing the least-squares principle. Then assumptions on the variance of the points were made, but not on the entire distribution. The normality assumption came into play only in the last step—in constructing the t- and F-tests. This gradual approach has many advantages, as we can decide how many assumptions we wish to make.

2.1 MAXIMUM LIKELIHOOD ESTIMATION

Maximum likelihood takes the completely opposite path. We start with an assumption on the entire distribution of the data. For simple regression, this amounts to assuming both that y is normally distributed around the regression line (i.e., conditionally on x) and that all sample points are independent. Mathematically, the normality assumption is written $y_i|x_i \sim N(\beta_0 + \beta_1 x_i, \sigma_{y|x}^2)$ or $\epsilon_i \sim N(0, \sigma_{y|x}^2)$. The fact that we also assume independence can be written $\epsilon_i \overset{i.i.d.}{\sim} N(0, \sigma_{y|x}^2)$, where the *i.i.d.* stands for "independently, identically distributed."

The likelihood of a sample is often thought of as the joint probability of the particular observations expressed with the parameters of the probability as unknowns. For example, in constructing the likelihood of a sample consisting of

Quantitative Methods in Population Health, by Mari Palta
ISBN 0-471-45505-9   Copyright © 2003 John Wiley & Sons, Inc.

binary observations, where the probability of success π is to be estimated, we multiply together π's for the successes and $(1 - \pi)$'s for the failures. Normally distributed data points, however, are by definition assumed to be continuous. In that case, we are used to seeing probabilities of intervals, rather than probabilities of individual data points—for example, $P(y > 140)$ is of interest if y is systolic blood pressure measured in mmHg. Such probabilities can be obtained from the table of the standardized normal distribution (once the mean and standard deviation of y are known). It makes little sense, however, to speak of a particular observation (say a blood pressure of 115.11111 or 115.1111111111) having a probability. The probability becomes smaller and smaller to a vanishing point as more and more decimals are added. Instead, the limiting probability of an infinitely narrow interval around a point y is based on calculus concepts and is referred to as the density. The density is the function that generates the probabilities of y falling in given intervals by mathematical integration. For discrete y (such as binary or counts) the density is simply equal to the probability of observing y.

The particular integral that generates the probability up to a given point—that is, $F(y) = P(Y \le y)$—is called the distribution function. It is common to denote a density by a lowercase letter and to denote the distribution by the corresponding uppercase letter. For the normal distribution, the density is

$$f(y) = \phi(y) = \frac{1}{\sigma\sqrt{2\pi}} \exp\left(-\frac{(y - \mu)^2}{2\sigma^2}\right)$$

The normal distribution function is often denoted by Φ but cannot be written as a neat formula, only as an integral of ϕ. Luckily, this is the integral that has been evaluated numerically and tabulated in normal distribution tables for the case $\mu = 0$ and $\sigma = 1$. For example, the integral from $-\infty$ to 1.96 equals 0.975. Substituting the parameters we are interested in for describing μ, which are now those of $\mu_{y|x}$ from a regression line, we obtain

$$f(y_i) = \frac{1}{\sigma_{y|x}\sqrt{2\pi}} \exp\left(-\frac{(y_i - \beta_0 - \beta_1 x_i)^2}{2\sigma_{y|x}^2}\right)$$

Maximum likelihood estimators are defined as those that maximize the joint density of the sample. If we were dealing with discrete data, it would also be the joint probability of the sample. Because we assumed that all points are independent, the density of the sample is just the product of the individual densities of the observations

$$L = \prod_{i=1}^{n} \frac{1}{\sigma_{y|x}\sqrt{2\pi}} \exp\left(-\frac{(y_i - \hat\beta_0 - \hat\beta_1 x_i)^2}{2\sigma_{y|x}^2}\right)$$

$$= \left(\frac{1}{\sigma_{y|x}\sqrt{2\pi}}\right)^{n} \exp\left(-\frac{\sum_{i=1}^{n}(y_i - \hat\beta_0 - \hat\beta_1 x_i)^2}{2\sigma_{y|x}^2}\right)$$

where we have applied the rule that when multiplying exponentials one takes the sum of the exponents. Note that the β's have "^" on them to indicate that they are the unknowns to be estimated. Generally, $\sigma_{y|x}$ is unknown too, but let's first consider the situation of known $\sigma_{y|x}$.

For example, if we had a sample with just three people aged 42, 50, and 55, and they had respective systolic blood pressures of 110, 145 and 135, and we knew that the standard error of blood pressure measurements in the population is 12 (say), the likelihood would be

$$
L = \left[\frac{1}{12\sqrt{2\pi}} \exp\left(-\frac{(110 - \hat{\beta}_0 - \hat{\beta}_1 42)^2}{2(12)^2} \right) \right]
$$
$$
\times \left[\frac{1}{12\sqrt{2\pi}} \exp\left(-\frac{(145 - \hat{\beta}_0 - \hat{\beta}_1 50)^2}{2(12)^2} \right) \right]
$$
$$
\times \left[\frac{1}{12\sqrt{2\pi}} \exp\left(-\frac{(135 - \hat{\beta}_0 - \hat{\beta}_1 55)^2}{2(12)^2} \right) \right]
$$
$$
= \left(\frac{1}{12\sqrt{2\pi}} \right)^3 \exp\left(-\frac{\begin{array}{c}(110 - \hat{\beta}_0 - \hat{\beta}_1 42)^2 + (145 - \hat{\beta}_0 - \hat{\beta}_1 50)^2 \\ + (135 - \hat{\beta}_0 - \hat{\beta}_1 55)^2\end{array}}{2(12)^2} \right)
$$

When embarking on the maximization of the likelihood, one always takes the logarithm because it is easier to maximize a sum than a product, and maximizing the log of the likelihood also maximizes the likelihood itself. In our case

$$
\log(L) = -n \log(\sigma_{y|x}\sqrt{2\pi}) - \frac{\sum_{i=1}^{n}(y_i - \hat{\beta}_0 - \hat{\beta}_1 x_i)^2}{2\sigma_{y|x}^2}
$$

It is pretty clear that, regardless of the value of $\sigma_{y|x}$ or how it is obtained (known or estimated), this expression is at its largest when $\sum_{i=1}^{n}(y_i - \hat{\beta}_0 - \hat{\beta}_1 x_i)^2$ is at its smallest. It turns out that way because we assumed all observations to have the same variance $\sigma_{y|x}^2$. We have reproduced the unweighted least-squares equation for estimating β_0 and β_1.

What we have just shown is that, in the case of ordinary regression, under the normality and equal variance assumptions, maximum likelihood and the least-squares approach yield the same estimators of the regression coefficients.

Turning to the estimator of $\sigma_{y|x}$, the situation is not quite so simple. When we proceed to maximize

$$
\log(L) = -n \log(\hat{\sigma}_{y|x}\sqrt{2\pi}) - \frac{\sum_{i=1}^{n}(y_i - \hat{\beta}_0 - \hat{\beta}_1 x_i)^2}{2\hat{\sigma}_{y|x}^2} \tag{2.1}
$$

with respect to $\hat{\sigma}_{y|x}$ we find that

$$\hat{\sigma}_{y|x}^2 = \sum_{i=1}^{n}(y_i - \hat{\beta}_0 - \hat{\beta}_1 x_i)^2/n$$

while our usual estimator is

$$s_{y|x}^2 = \sum_{i=1}^{n}(y_i - \hat{\beta}_0 - \hat{\beta}_1 x_i)^2/(n-2)$$

In the latter estimator, we divide by the sample size, minus the number of parameters in the regression equation for the mean. Both estimators are legitimate and have their proponents. Clearly, when n is very large, they are almost the same anyway. At the moment, most of the statistical community favors the second approach. To obtain this estimator, while remaining in the maximum likelihood framework, they developed a slightly modified maximum likelihood approach called "restricted maximum likelihood" or REML. (The usual maximum likelihood is usually abbreviated ML.) Those who wish to see the mathematical foundation are referred to McCullagh and Searle [5] or Diggle et al. [6] for more details. The basic idea is to base the likelihood, not on the original observations, but on the residuals. The number of independent residuals equals the degrees of freedom in the variance, so $n - 2$ (for example) becomes the sample size for estimating $\sigma_{y|x}^2$.

Both ML and REML can be fit in SAS by the procedure PROC MIXED. OUTPUT PACKET II contains an analysis of the blood pressure data from visit 1 in the Wisconsin Sleep Cohort Study. PROC MIXED will be used extensively in this text.

2.2 EXAMPLE

The first example of OUTPUT PACKET II contains the output from PROC REG for the relationship between systolic blood pressure and age. The commands used were simply

PROC REG; MODEL SBP=AGE;

The second example contains the results from PROC MIXED. As this procedure has very extensive capabilities that we will rely on later, it takes a little longer to run. The commands used for producing the second page were

PROC MIXED METHOD=ML; MODEL SBP=AGE/S;

These commands tell SAS to use the maximum likelihood approach. The /S option (S stands for solution) tells the procedure to print the regression coefficients. Strange as it may sound, this is not automatic in this procedure, as sometimes investigators may want only the significance tests for the model. Looking at the output we see that, as expected, the coefficients are identical to those from PROC REG.

The residual variance estimator $\hat{\sigma}^2_{y|x}$, however, is minutely smaller. While PROC REG estimated $s^2_{y|x} = 205.64520$, ML yields "Residual" $= 205.34$. The difference is very small because $n = 1365$ is large. You may note that PROC MIXED is designed to be able to handle multiple observations per subjects, and that has led to strange labels on parts of the output. As we may understand better later, the commands above (because they don't need a SUBJECT specification) lead SAS to think there is only one subject with multiple observations.

Other features of the output are statistics derived from $\log(L)$, which we will use later. Some are familiar. For example, -5570.9 is the value of $\log(L)$. The "-2 Log likelihood", you may recall, is to be used for comparing nested models by χ^2 tests.

The third example of the output was produced by

PROC MIXED METHOD=REML; MODEL SBP=AGE/S;

We did not actually need to say METHOD=REML as that is the default, We see that this output provides estimates that are all identical to those of PROC REG. Likelihood statistics are now based on the restricted likelihood, and can be treated and used the same way as ordinary likelihood quantities (see Section 5.2).

2.3 PROPERTIES OF MAXIMUM LIKELIHOOD ESTIMATORS

Maximum likelihood estimators have many desirable properties that statisticians look for when judging how good an estimator is. The advantage is, of course, also that these properties hold for all estimators obtained by maximum likelihood, so they don't need to be re-proven for each situation. You will often see these properties referred to in statistical papers and texts. The two involved most often are consistency and efficiency. More information on the properties of maximum likelihood estimators can be found in any text on mathematical statistics—for example, Rice [7].

1. Consistency   This is the most important property. It means that the estimator tends to come closer to the truth when the sample size is increased. Think of it as any bias in the estimation of the parameter, as well as the standard error of the estimator going to 0 as the sample size becomes large.

2. Efficiency   As discussed above, efficiency means that the best possible use is made of the data. Maximum likelihood estimators are "asymptotically efficient," which means that they are precise as possible in large samples. We will return to the standard errors for maximum likelihood estimators in Chapter 5.

3. Invariance   This property means that reparameterization does not produce different maximum likelihood estimators of the same quantities. This is logical and desirable. For example, if $\hat{\beta}_1$ is the maximum likelihood estimator of a regression slope β_1, then $1/\hat{\beta}_1$ is the maximum likelihood estimator of $1/\beta_1$. Formally, if $\hat{\theta}$ is a maximum likelihood estimator of θ, then $g(\hat{\theta})$ is a maximum likelihood estimator of $g(\theta)$. You may have seen this principle illustrated in logistic regression of a 2×2 table. There, we obtain the same estimator of the probabilities p_i, whether we obtain the ML directly or parameterize it according to a logistic model with x equal 0 or 1 to indicate the two columns in the table as $p_i = \frac{\exp(\beta_0 + \beta_1 x i)}{1 + \exp(\beta_0 + \beta_1 x i)}$.

4. Normality   In large samples, maximum likelihood estimators have a normal sampling distribution, with a variance that can be computed from the likelihood (see Chapter 5). Hence, we will have standard errors for the estimators. Since the estimators are normally distributed and, in addition, the errors in the standard errors themselves vanish in large samples, we can always form large sample Z or χ^2 tests for maximum likelihood estimators.

5. Comment   Because of the above properties, maximum likelihood estimators tend to be viewed as kind of a "gold standard." However, sometimes they cannot be obtained because a reasonable distribution cannot be specified, or because it is computationally too hard to maximize $\log(L)$. In addition, because the consistency and efficiency apply to large sample sizes, other estimators can be better in small samples. You may note, for example, that the properties listed do not include "unbiasedness." In fact, maximum likelihood estimators can be biased in small samples (as is indeed the ML estimator of $\sigma^2_{y|x}$).

2.4 HOW TO OBTAIN A RESIDUAL PLOT WITH PROC MIXED

PROC MIXED deals with residual plots slightly differently than PROC REG. The statements needed to produce a residual plot from the regression of SBP on Age are

PROC MIXED; MODEL SBP=AGE/S OUTPRED=oo;
PROC PLOT; PLOT Resid*Pred;

These statements simply create data set "oo", which contains (among other things) the desired quantities.

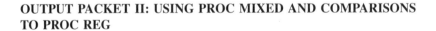

OUTPUT PACKET II: USING PROC MIXED AND COMPARISONS TO PROC REG

Analysis of SBP on Age—Wisconsin Sleep Cohort Study MIXED Versus REG
Using PROC REG
   The REG Procedure

Model: MODEL1
Dependent Variable: SBP

Analysis of Variance

Source	DF	Sum of Squares	Mean Square	F Value	Pr > F
Model	1	11604	11604	56.43	<0.0001
Error	1363	280294	205.64520		
Corrected total	1364	291898			

Root MSE	14.34033	R-square	0.0398	
Dependent mean	125.09145	Adjusted	0.0390	
Coefficient variation	11.46388	R-square		

Parameter Estimates

Variable	DF	Parameter Estimate	Standard Error	t Value	Pr > $|t|$
Intercept	1	107.98092	2.31066	46.73	<0.0001
Age	1	0.36605	0.04873	7.51	<0.0001

Using PROC MIXED with ML
  The Mixed Procedure

Model Information

Data set	WORK.A
Dependent variable	SBP
Covariance structure	Diagonal
Estimation method	ML
Residual variance method	Profile
Fixed effects SE method	Model-based
Degrees-of-freedom method	Residual

Dimensions

Covariance parameters	1
Columns in X	2
Columns in Z	0
Subjects	1
Maximum observations per subject	1378
Observations used	1365
Observations not used	13
Total observations	1378

Covariance Parameter Estimates

Cov Parm	Estimate
Residual	205.34

Fit Statistics

−2 Log Likelihood	11141.9
AIC (smaller is better)	11147.9
AICC (smaller is better)	11147.9
BIC (smaller is better)	11163.6

Solution for Fixed Effects

Effect	Estimate	Standard Error	DF	t Value	Pr > |t|
Intercept	107.98	2.3090	1363	46.77	<0.0001
Age	0.3660	0.04869	1363	7.52	<0.0001

Type 3 Tests of Fixed Effects

Effect	Num DF	Den DF	F Value	Pr > F
Age	1	1363	56.51	<0.0001

Using PROC MIXED with REML
  The Mixed Procedure

Model Information

Data set	WORK.A
Dependent variable	SBP
Covariance structure	Diagonal
Estimation method	REML
Residual variance method	Profile
Fixed effects SE method	Model-based
Degrees-of-freedom method	Residual

Dimensions

Covariance parameters	1
Columns in X	2
Columns in Z	0
Subjects	1
Max observation per subject	1370
Observations used	1365
Observations not used	5
Total observations	1370

Covariance Parameter Estimates

Cov Parm	Estimate
Residual	205.34

Fit Statistics

-2 Log likelihood	11141.9
AIC (smaller is better)	11147.9
AICC (smaller is better)	11147.9
BIC (smaller is better)	11163.6

Solution for Fixed Effects

Effect	Estimate	Standard Error	DF	t Value	Pr > $|t|$
Intercept	107.98	2.3107	1363	46.73	<0.0001
Age	0.3660	0.04873	1363	7.51	<0.0001

Type 3 Tests of Fixed Effects

Effect	Num DF	Den DF	F Value	Pr > F
Age	1	1363	56.43	<0.0001

CHAPTER THREE

Reformulating Ordinary Regression Analysis in Matrix Notation

We have seen that expressing the estimators connected with equation (1.1) algebraically is a pretty easy task. However, as we turn to the situation of multiple regression, including additional predictors on the right-hand side of equation (1.1), it rapidly becomes difficult and then impossible to write the estimators. As an example, with two predictors x_1 and x_2 the formula for $\hat{\beta}_1$ is (only found in textbooks, such as Snedecor and Cochran [8, p. 342])

$$
\hat{\beta}_1 = \frac{\sum_i (x_{1i} - \bar{x}_1)(y_i - \bar{y}) \sum_i (x_{2i} - \bar{x}_2)^2}{\sum_i (x_{1i} - \bar{x}_1)^2 \sum_i (x_{2i} - \bar{x}_1)(x_{2i} - \bar{x}_2)^2}
$$
$$
- \frac{\sum_i (x_{2i} - \bar{x}_2)(y_i - \bar{x}_2)(y_i - \bar{y}) \sum_i (x_{1i} - \bar{x}_1)(x_{2i} - \bar{x}_2)}{\sum_i (x_{1i} - \bar{x}_1)^2 \sum_i (x_{2i} - \bar{x}_1)(x_{2i} - \bar{x}_2)^2}
$$

One practically never finds these types of expressions written out for any situation beyond that of two predictors. Instead, mathematical notation using matrices has been developed that allows estimators to be expressed in simple ways by formulas that explain the structure of the equations, and that can be evaluated by computers. This notation is so universally used in textbooks, methodological papers, and computer manuals that it becomes impossible to learn and utilize recently developed quantitative tools without understanding it. The last page of this chapter summarizes the matrix algebra needed. Readers unfamiliar with any of the matrix operations listed on this page should refer to the Appendix (at the end of this book) for detailed information on matrix algebra.

Quantitative Methods in Population Health, by Mari Palta
ISBN 0-471-45505-9   Copyright © 2003 John Wiley & Sons, Inc.

3.1 WRITING THE ORDINARY REGRESSION EQUATION IN MATRIX NOTATION

Equation (1.1) stated the equation for ordinary regression as

$$y_i = \beta_0 + \beta_1 x_i + \epsilon_i$$

Note how there is actually a separate equation for each subject $i = 1, 2, \ldots, n$, because they have potentially different x_i and almost certainly different ϵ_i. In other words,

$$y_1 = \beta_0 + \beta_1 x_1 + \epsilon_1$$
$$y_2 = \beta_0 + \beta_1 x_2 + \epsilon_2$$
$$\vdots$$
$$y_n = \beta_0 + \beta_1 x_n + \epsilon_n$$

In matrix notation, the outcomes y_i are stacked into a matrix

$$Y = \begin{pmatrix} y_1 \\ y_2 \\ \vdots \\ y_n \end{pmatrix} \quad \text{which equals} \quad \begin{pmatrix} \beta_0 + \beta_1 x_1 + \epsilon_1 \\ \beta_0 + \beta_1 x_2 + \epsilon_2 \\ \vdots \\ \beta_0 + \beta_1 x_n + \epsilon_n \end{pmatrix}$$

However, using the rules of matrix algebra, the right-hand side can be rewritten

$$\begin{pmatrix} \beta_0 + \beta_1 x_1 + \epsilon_1 \\ \beta_0 + \beta_1 x_2 + \epsilon_2 \\ \vdots \\ \beta_0 + \beta_1 x_n + \epsilon_n \end{pmatrix} = \begin{pmatrix} \beta_0 + \beta_1 x_1 \\ \beta_0 + \beta_1 x_2 \\ \vdots \\ \beta_0 + \beta_1 x_n \end{pmatrix} + \begin{pmatrix} \epsilon_1 \\ \epsilon_2 \\ \vdots \\ \epsilon_n \end{pmatrix}$$

where

$$\begin{pmatrix} \beta_0 + \beta_1 x_1 \\ \beta_0 + \beta_1 x_2 \\ \vdots \\ \beta_0 + \beta_1 x_n \end{pmatrix} = \begin{pmatrix} 1 & x_1 \\ 1 & x_2 \\ \vdots & \vdots \\ 1 & x_n \end{pmatrix} \begin{pmatrix} \beta_0 \\ \beta_1 \end{pmatrix}$$

Denoting $\begin{pmatrix} 1 & x_1 \\ 1 & x_2 \\ \vdots & \vdots \\ 1 & x_n \end{pmatrix}$ by X, $\begin{pmatrix} \beta_0 \\ \beta_1 \end{pmatrix}$ by $\boldsymbol{\beta}$, and $\begin{pmatrix} \epsilon_1 \\ \epsilon_2 \\ \vdots \\ \epsilon_n \end{pmatrix}$ by $\boldsymbol{\epsilon}$

the regression equation can now be written in matrix form as

$$Y = X\beta + \epsilon \tag{3.1}$$

It is important to note that X has a row for each of the n subjects, as do Y and ϵ. The number of columns in X is determined by the number of covariates. Interestingly, one can view the intercept as a covariate that is the same (=1) for all subjects. If there were predictors $x_{1i}, x_{2i}, \ldots, x_{mi}$, the matrix X would be

$$\begin{pmatrix} 1 & x_{11} & x_{21} & \cdots & x_{m1} \\ 1 & x_{12} & x_{22} & \cdots & x_{m2} \\ \vdots & \vdots & \vdots & \ddots & \vdots \\ 1 & x_{1n} & x_{2n} & \cdots & x_{mn} \end{pmatrix}$$

but equation (3.1) would look the same. It is clear that equation (3.1) seamlessly generalizes into multiple regression.

3.1.1   Example

The matrix Y containing systolic blood pressures for the first visit to the sleep laboratory for the first five subjects in the Wisconsin Sleep Cohort is

$$Y = \begin{pmatrix} 119.333 \\ 138.333 \\ 119.333 \\ 111.667 \\ 148.333 \end{pmatrix}$$

where the decimals arise from averaging three measurements. When regressing SBP only on age the matrix X for the same five subjects is

$$X = \begin{pmatrix} 1 & 47.1677 \\ 1 & 52.0137 \\ 1 & 53.5359 \\ 1 & 30.1383 \\ 1 & 42.8282 \end{pmatrix}$$

while if both age and BMI are included, we obtain

$$X = \begin{pmatrix} 1 & 47.1677 & 20.1956 \\ 1 & 52.0137 & 24.0509 \\ 1 & 53.5359 & 28.0190 \\ 1 & 30.1383 & 26.2507 \\ 1 & 42.8282 & 27.6095 \end{pmatrix}$$

3.2   OBTAINING THE LEAST-SQUARES ESTIMATOR $\hat{\beta}$ IN MATRIX NOTATION

We examine the least-squares equations (1.2)

$$\frac{\partial LS}{\partial \hat{\beta}_0} = -2 \sum (y_i - \hat{\beta}_0 - \hat{\beta}_1 x_i) = 0 \quad \text{or} \quad \sum (y_i - \hat{\beta}_0 - \hat{\beta}_1 x_i) = 0 \qquad (3.2)$$

$$\frac{\partial LS}{\partial \hat{\beta}_1} = -2 \sum x_i (y_i - \hat{\beta}_0 - \hat{\beta}_1 x_i) = 0 \quad \text{or} \quad \sum x_i (y_i - \hat{\beta}_0 - \hat{\beta}_1 x_i) = 0$$

$$(3.3)$$

Matrix property 15 from the list tells us that (3.2) can be written

$$\begin{pmatrix} 1 & 1 & \cdots & 1 \end{pmatrix} \begin{pmatrix} (y_1 - \hat{\beta}_0 - \hat{\beta}_1 x_1) \\ (y_2 - \hat{\beta}_0 - \hat{\beta}_1 x_2) \\ \vdots \\ (y_n - \hat{\beta}_0 - \hat{\beta}_1 x_n) \end{pmatrix} = \mathbf{0}$$

and equation (3.3) can be written

$$\begin{pmatrix} x_1 & x_2 & \cdots & x_n \end{pmatrix} \begin{pmatrix} (y_1 - \hat{\beta}_0 - \hat{\beta}_1 x_1) \\ (y_2 - \hat{\beta}_0 - \hat{\beta}_1 x_2) \\ \vdots \\ (y_n - \hat{\beta}_0 - \hat{\beta}_1 x_n) \end{pmatrix} = \mathbf{0}$$

But these equalities can be stacked into a larger matrix as

$$\begin{pmatrix} 1 & 1 & \cdots & 1 \\ x_1 & x_2 & \cdots & x_n \end{pmatrix} \begin{pmatrix} (y_1 - \hat{\beta}_0 - \hat{\beta}_1 x_1) \\ (y_2 - \hat{\beta}_0 - \hat{\beta}_1 x_2) \\ \vdots \\ (y_n - \hat{\beta}_0 - \hat{\beta}_1 x_n) \end{pmatrix} = \mathbf{0} \qquad (3.4)$$

Recognizing matrixes and operations introduced above, we see that (3.4) can be written

$$X'(Y - X\hat{\beta}) = \mathbf{0} \qquad (3.5)$$

Thinking through how equations (1.2) arose, we realize that (3.5) would stay the same even if there were additional predictors. Additional predictors would just add additional equations like (3.3), and hence additional rows of $x's$ to X'.

Solving equation (3.5) for $\hat{\beta}$ by matrix operation is not difficult and involves the following steps:

$X'(Y - X\hat{\boldsymbol{\beta}}) = \mathbf{0}$ we can multiply into parentheses

$X'Y - X'X\hat{\boldsymbol{\beta}} = \mathbf{0}$ we can move terms to the other side of the equation

$X'Y = X'X\hat{\boldsymbol{\beta}}$ we can multiply both sides by the same quantity

$(X'X)^{-1}X'Y = (X'X)^{-1}X'X\hat{\boldsymbol{\beta}}$ $(X'X)^{-1}X'X = I$ by definition

$$\hat{\boldsymbol{\beta}} = (X'X)^{-1}X'Y \tag{3.6}$$

The last line in (3.6) presents the ordinary least-squares estimator in matrix notation.

Hidden in the derivation that leads to (3.6) is the assumption that $X'X$ is an invertible matrix. We will take care to make this true in all our analyses. In practice it involves (1) making sure that predictors in X are not linear combinations of other predictors in X and (2) using at most $(k - 1)$ indicator variables to describe k groups. The second point reflects the tradition followed in most observational studies. Analyses of designed experiments sometimes follow other traditions of coding and/or generalizations of (3.6) that allow for $X'X$ not being directly invertible.

We may note that based on only the assumption that $E(Y|X) = X\boldsymbol{\beta}$, we can show that the ordinary least-squares estimator is unbiased (its mean or expected value equals the parameter):

$$\mathbf{E}(\hat{\boldsymbol{\beta}}) = \mathbf{E}[(X'X)^{-1}X'Y|X] = (X'X)^{-1}X'\mathbf{E}(Y|X)$$
$$= (X'X)^{-1}X'X\boldsymbol{\beta} = \boldsymbol{\beta}$$

Since we also know that under the equal variance assumption the ordinary least-squares estimator minimizes $\sigma^2_{y|x}$, and since the estimator is a linear expression in y_i, it is sometimes referred to as the "best linear unbiased estimator" or "BLUE" of $\boldsymbol{\beta}$. More information can be found in McCullagh and Searle [5].

3.2.1   Example: Matrices in Regression Analysis

The following output shows analysis of only the first five subjects in the Wisconsin Sleep Cohort Study and illustrates the matrix computations involved in obtaining regression estimators. The commands ran to show the detail are

PROC PRINT; VAR ID AGE SBP;
PROC REG ALL; MODEL SBP=AGE;

Producing output

Obs	id	age	sbp
1	S1	47.1677	119.333
2	S2	52.0137	138.333

```
            3        S3      53.5359      119.333
            4        S4      30.1383      111.667
            5        S5      42.8282      148.333
```

Model Crossproducts X'X X'Y Y'Y

Variable	Label	Intercept	age
Intercept	Intercept	5	225.68377824
age	uncentered age in years	225.68377824	10538.880935
sbp	systolic blood pressure	636.99999999	28930.815423

Model Crossproducts X'X X'Y Y'Y

Variable	Label	sbp
Intercept	Intercept	636.99999999
age	uncentered age in years	28930.815423
sbp	systolic blood pressure	82089.222219

X'X Inverse, Parameter Estimates, and SSE

Variable	Label	Intercept	age
Intercept	Intercept	5.9837951594	-0.128139364
age	uncentered age in years	-0.128139364	0.0028389139
sbp	systolic blood pressure	104.50122963	0.5073198115

X'X Inverse, Parameter Estimates, and SSE

Variable	Label	sbp
Intercept	Intercept	104.50122963
age	uncentered age in years	0.5073198115
sbp	systolic blood pressure	844.76311845%

However, not all the output produced is shown. (The ALL option produces a lot!) Extracting relevant parts of the information shown, we see the matrices

$$X'X = \begin{pmatrix} 5 & 225.68 \\ 225.68 & 10538.88 \end{pmatrix} \quad \text{and} \quad X'Y = \begin{pmatrix} 636.999 \\ 28930.82 \end{pmatrix}$$

This follows because $X'X$ is printed in the upper 2×2 segment of the "Model Crossproducts," $X'Y$ is printed as the last row (two entries), and $Y'Y$ is the very last entry. $Y'Y$ is not needed for producing $\hat{\beta}$, but is used in obtaining the "Total sum of squares" for the ANOVA table.

Further down, we also see

$$(X'X)^{-1} = \begin{pmatrix} 5.984 & -0.1281 \\ -0.1281 & 0.00284 \end{pmatrix}$$

3.3 LIST OF MATRIX OPERATIONS TO KNOW

1. Matrix dimension $n \times m$ refers to $n = $ #rows, $m = $ #columns. If $m = n$, the matrix is a square matrix.

2. Matrix notation: $A = \begin{pmatrix} a_{11} & \cdots & a_{1\,m} \\ \vdots & \ddots & \vdots \\ a_{n1} & \cdots & a_{nm} \end{pmatrix}$

3. Addition of matrices—straightforward—add corresponding elements. Matrices must be of same dimension.

4. Multiplication of a matrix by a constant—multiply each element by the constant.

5. Multiplication of two matrices—row 1 of the first matrix multiplies corresponding elements of column 1 of the second matrix, then these products are summed up to form product element (1, 1) of the new matrix, row 1 with column 2 forms product element (1, 2), and so on. When multiplying A by B to form AB, # columns in A has to equal # rows in B.

6. Identity matrix I has 1's on the diagonal and 0's elsewhere. It is a square matrix of any dimension. When multiplying A by I, one gets back A. In fact $AI = A$ and $IA = A$, as long as the matrices can be multiplied.

7. Transpose of A denoted by A'. The transpose is obtained by flipping rows and columns. Note that AA' is a square matrix, as is $A'A$. However, the two do not usually equal each other. In fact, if A is $n \times m$ then AA' is $n \times n$, but $A'A$ is $m \times m$.

8. Symmetric matrix—A is symmetric if $A = A'$. Symmetric matrices are important because they will often be encountered in statistics. Both AA' and $A'A$ are symmetric matrices.

9. The transpose of a product. It can be demonstrated that $(AB)' = B'A'$. We will need this when showing how the standard error of the estimators of the regression parameters are obtained.

10. Cofactor of a matrix element a_{ij}—the determinant of the smaller matrix obtained when row i and column j are deleted, multiplied by $(-1)^{i+j}$.

11. Determinant: The determinant of any $n \times n$ matrix is $\sum_{i=1}^{n} a_{ij}(-1)^{i+1} A_{i1}$, where A_{i1} is the determinant of the matrix obtained when the first column and the ith row are deleted, and $(-1)^{i+1} A_{i1}$ is the cofactor of element a_{i1}. Note that the determinant of a 2×2 matrix $\begin{vmatrix} a & b \\ c & d \end{vmatrix} = ad - bc$ (which by the cofactor formula is derived as $(-1)^2 ad + (-1)^3 cb$). In examples, we will only use the determinant of a 2×2 matrix.

12. Inverse A^{-1}. Defined by $AA^{-1} = A^{-1}A = I$. A matrix is invertible if it is square and has nonzero determinant. A noninvertible square matrix is sometimes referred to as singular (and an invertible one as nonsingular). A^{-1}

is obtained by $\frac{1}{determinant}(cofactormatrix)'$. It is handy to know that

$$\begin{pmatrix} a & b \\ c & d \end{pmatrix}^{-1} = \frac{1}{ad - bc}\begin{pmatrix} d & -b \\ -c & a \end{pmatrix}$$

13. Diagonal matrices have especially simple properties. Obtaining the inverse involves inverting each of the diagonal elements (i.e., $1/a_{11}$, etc.). When a diagonal matrix has the same entry along its entire diagonal, multiplying another matrix by it has the same effect as multiplying by that constant. For example,

$$\begin{pmatrix} a & 0 & 0 \\ 0 & a & 0 \\ 0 & 0 & a \end{pmatrix} B = aB$$

14. When there is a string of matrices multiplied by each other, a constant multiplier anywhere in the string can be moved up front. For example,

$$A\begin{pmatrix} k & k \\ k & k \end{pmatrix} B = kA\begin{pmatrix} 1 & 1 \\ 1 & 1 \end{pmatrix} B \quad \text{and} \quad A\begin{pmatrix} k & 0 \\ 0 & k \end{pmatrix} B = kAB$$

15. Based on the rules of matrix multiplication, sums arise from multiplying a row of ones into a column, that is,

$$\begin{pmatrix} 1 & 1 & \cdots & 1 \end{pmatrix}\begin{pmatrix} a_1 \\ a_2 \\ \vdots \\ a_n \end{pmatrix} = \sum_{i=1}^{n} a_i$$

Sums of cross products arise from any multiplication of a row with a column, that is,

$$\begin{pmatrix} b_1 & b_2 & \cdots & b_n \end{pmatrix}\begin{pmatrix} a_1 \\ a_2 \\ \vdots \\ a_n \end{pmatrix} = \sum_{i=1}^{n} b_i a_i$$

CHAPTER FOUR

Variance Matrices and Linear Transformations

Chapter 3 showed how writing variables and parameters in matrix form results in simple-looking equations for regression estimators. Another important application of matrix algebra, as well as of more advanced matrix theory, is in working with variance matrices. Variance matrices are a generalization of the simple variance in that they allow expressing the variances of several variables simultaneously. We will need variance matrices to express the variances (and hence standard errors) of estimators and to be able to write formulas that extend ordinary regression to situations where the usual assumptions do not hold.

This is a multipurpose chapter centered around variance matrices. First of all, it defines variance matrices and provides further practice of matrix operations. We will define a linear transformation and obtain its variance. This sets the framework for future developments. In the process we will look at the variance of a mean and a difference, which are useful in other contexts.

4.1 VARIANCE AND CORRELATION MATRICES

We will make extensive use of the concept of a variance matrix, usually denoted by V. For a single measurement, the variance matrix simply consists of the constant σ^2 (a 1×1 matrix). However, when we have several outcomes, possibly with different variances, it is convenient (for reasons we will soon see) to present the variances along the diagonal of a matrix, for example,

$$V = \mathbf{Var}(Y) = \mathbf{Var}\begin{pmatrix} y_1 \\ y_2 \\ y_3 \end{pmatrix} = \begin{pmatrix} \sigma_1^2 & \cdot & \cdot \\ \cdot & \sigma_2^2 & \\ \cdot & \cdot & \sigma_3^2 \end{pmatrix}$$

Quantitative Methods in Population Health, by Mari Palta
ISBN 0-471-45505-9   Copyright © 2003 John Wiley & Sons, Inc.

The equal variance assumption in Chapter 1 translates to

$$\text{Var}(Y|X) = \text{Var}\begin{pmatrix} \epsilon_1 \\ \epsilon_2 \\ \epsilon_3 \end{pmatrix} = \begin{pmatrix} \sigma^2_{y|x} & \cdot & \cdot \\ \cdot & \sigma^2_{y|x} & \cdot \\ \cdot & \cdot & \sigma^2_{y|x} \end{pmatrix}$$

We have not yet filled in the elements off the diagonal. In a variance matrix, these consist of covariances. While the variance of y_i (where $i = 1, 2, \ldots$ as referring to each outcome) is defined as $\sigma_i^2 = \sigma_{y_i}^2 = E[(y_i - \mu_{y_i})^2]$ (i.e., the mean of all squared deviations) and is usually estimated from n measurements of y_i by

$$s_{y_i}^2 = \sum_j (y_{ij} - \bar{y}_i)^2 / (n - 1)$$

the covariance refers to two y's together and is defined as $\sigma_{y_i y_{i'}} = E[(y_i - \mu_{y_i})(y_{i'} - \sigma_{y_i y_{i'}})] = E[(y_i - \mu_{y_i})(y_{i'} - \mu_{y_{i'}})]$. When $i = i'$, the covariance is the variance. Hence, while the variance refers to a single measurement, the covariance refers to how two measurements behave together or "covary." The covariance can be estimated by

$$s_{ii'} = s_{y_i y_{i'}} = \sum_j (y_{ij} - \bar{y}_i)(y_{i'j} - \bar{y}_{i'}) / (n - 1)$$

An alternative estimator is divided by $n - 2$ (or n minus "degrees of freedom") and forms the basis for an "adjusted" correlation, such as seen on regression analysis output. From remembering the formula for estimating the usual Pearson correlation between y_i and $y_{i'}$

$$r = \frac{\sum_j (y_{ij} - \bar{y}_i)(y_{i'j} - \bar{y}_{i'})}{\sqrt{\sum_j (y_{ij} - \bar{y}_i)^2 \sum_j (y_{i'j} - \bar{y}_{i'})^2}}$$

we see that the covariance estimator is just $r \times (s_{y_i} s_{y_{i'}})$. The same relationship holds for the parameters, that is, $\sigma_{y_i y_{i'}} = \rho \sigma_{y_i} \sigma_{y_{i'}}$. We present the covariance this way because the correlation is a better known entity than the covariance. The fact of the matter is, however, that the correlation arises from the covariance by the definition

$$\rho = \text{Cov}(y_i, y_{i'}) / (\sigma_{y_i} \sigma_{y_{i'}})$$

Now we can fill in the variance matrix as

$$V = \text{Var}(Y) = \text{Var}\begin{pmatrix} y_1 \\ y_2 \\ y_3 \end{pmatrix} = \begin{pmatrix} \sigma_1^2 & \sigma_{12} & \sigma_{13} \\ \sigma_{21} & \sigma_2^2 & \sigma_{23} \\ \sigma_{31} & \sigma_{32} & \sigma_3^2 \end{pmatrix}$$

The row and column indicators correspond to the respective covariance, so that σ_{12} is the covariance between y_1 and y_2, and so on. By the definition of the covariance, $\sigma_{ij} = \sigma_{ji}$. The variance matrix is, therefore, a symmetric matrix, meaning that $V = V'$. Since independent observations are uncorrelated, and $\rho = 0$ implies that the covariance is 0, the independence assumption in Chapter 1 for simple regression analysis results in

$$\text{Var}(Y|X) = \text{Var}\begin{pmatrix} \epsilon_1 \\ \epsilon_2 \\ \epsilon_3 \end{pmatrix} = \begin{pmatrix} \sigma_{y|x}^2 & 0 & 0 \\ 0 & \sigma_{y|x}^2 & 0 \\ 0 & 0 & \sigma_{y|x}^2 \end{pmatrix} = \sigma_{y|x}^2 I$$

where I is the identity matrix.

4.1.1 Example

When measuring blood pressure, it is common to obtain more than one measurement on each individual to improve precision. For two sequential systolic blood pressure measurements (SBP$_1$ and SBP$_2$) on a person, each with standard deviation 10 mmHg, correlated at 0.80, the variance matrix is

$$\text{Var}(Y) = \text{Var}\begin{pmatrix} \text{SBP}_1 \\ \text{SBP}_2 \end{pmatrix} = \begin{pmatrix} 100 & 80 \\ 80 & 100 \end{pmatrix} = 100\begin{pmatrix} 1 & 0.80 \\ 0.80 & 1 \end{pmatrix}$$

The first matrix is the variance matrix and the second is the correlation matrix.

4.2 HOW TO OBTAIN THE VARIANCE OF A LINEAR TRANSFORMATION

A linear transformation refers to a combination of variables, where variables are multiplied by constants and then added or subtracted from each other. The sum of two variables is one simple example, and a variable transformed to a different scale (e.g., $^\circ$F to $^\circ$C by $^\circ$C = ($^\circ$F − 32) × $\frac{5}{9}$) is another. It is useful to know how to obtain the variance of a linear transformation of variables—not only for the purposes here, but in general. Often, one needs to obtain the variance or standard error of a difference of variables, or a combination of regression coefficients, such as may occur if there is an interaction effect. In the latter case (see example at the end of this chapter) we need the standard error of expressions $\hat{\beta}_{x_1} + \hat{\beta}_{x_1 \times x_2} x_2$, meaning the "effect" of variable x_1 at a given level of another interacting variable x_2.

4.2.1 Two Variables

The basic formula for a linear combination of two variables is $t_1 y_1 + t_2 y_2$. For a sum $t_1 = t_2 = 1$, while for a difference $t_1 = 1, t_2 = -1$.

If the two variables are correlated at ρ, the formula for the variance of this linear combination is

$$\text{Var}(t_1 y_1 + t_2 y_2) = t_1^2 \text{Var}(y_1) + t_2^2 \text{Var}(y_2) + 2t_1 t_2 \rho \sqrt{\text{Var}(y_1) \text{Var}(y_2)} \qquad (4.1)$$

or equivalently

$$\text{Var}(t_1 y_1 + t_2 y_2) = t_1^2 \text{Var}(y_1) + t_2^2 \text{Var}(y_2) + 2t_1 t_2 \text{Cov}(y_1, y_2)$$

We do not derive these formulas here, but they follow from the basic definitions of variance and covariance given above. Note that when y_1 and y_2 are independent replicates of the same random variable, and $t_1 = t_2 = 0.5$, so that $t_1 y_1 + t_2 y_2$ is just the usual mean of two independent measurements,

$$\text{Var}(t_1 y_1 + t_2 y_2) = 0.25 \text{Var}(y_1) + 0.25 \text{Var}(y_2) + 0$$

$$= 2(0.25) \text{Var}(y_1) + 0 = \frac{\text{Var}(y_1)}{2}$$

Reasonably enough, the formula simplifies to the usual one for means of independent variables when $\rho = 0$.

For variables y_1, y_2 with equal variance σ^2, more generally we have

$$\text{Var}(y_1 + y_2) = 2\sigma^2(1 + \rho) \quad \text{or} \quad \text{Var}\left(\frac{y_1 + y_2}{2}\right) = \frac{\sigma^2(1 + \rho)}{2}$$

using the formula $\text{Var}(t_1 y) = t_1^2 \text{Var}(y)$. Furthermore,

$$\text{Var}(y_1 - y_2) = 2\sigma^2(1 - \rho)$$

4.2.1.1 Example

Often, when planning data collection for a study, we may wonder how much benefit there will be in obtaining repeat measurements of variables and then use the mean of the repeats. In another setting, we may be planning a study where change in variables is a primary outcome, and wonder how the variability of the difference compares to that of the measurements themselves.

For the blood pressure example above, the variance across persons of the mean blood pressure is

$$\text{Var}\left(\frac{\text{SBP}_1 + \text{SBP}_2}{2}\right) = \frac{10^2(1 + 0.8)}{2} = 90$$

so that the standard deviation of the mean is $\sqrt{90} = 9.5$. Another way to look at this is that we have reduced the variability between people by 10%. Because the two measurements are highly correlated, the standard deviation of the mean is only slightly lower than the standard deviation of a single measurement. Logically, if

$\rho = 1$, so that we have two perfectly correlated measurements, there is no gain at all in using the mean. The lower the correlation, the greater the gain. Of course, a low correlation would imply a great deal of measurement error or moment-to-moment variation in the measurement. We see that it is very worthwhile to take several measurements when there is a lot of measurement error.

For the difference between the two measurements, we obtain

$$\text{Var}(\text{SBP}_1 - \text{SBP}_2) = 2(10)^2(1 - 0.8) = 40$$

Here we see that if ρ were 1, we would have no variability at all. This makes sense, because $\rho = 1$ implies that the two variables are in a fixed relationship to each other. It would in fact not be very interesting to analyze the difference in that situation. With $\rho = 0$, the variability would be twice as high as that of the individual measurements. The relatively high correlation $\rho = 0.8$ works to reduce the variability in the difference considerably.

Note the usefulness of the formula for the difference in projecting the standard error for a paired t-test. The variance of the difference is the basis for the paired test, as the standard error used is the variance across subjects of the differences divided by $\sqrt{n}$. Given some knowledge of the variance of the measurement across unpaired subjects, and the correlation within pairs, one can estimate the standard error for use in sample size and power projections. The last part of the discussion implies that a lot is gained by a paired versus an unpaired t-test, when there is a strong correlation between members of the pair, because that's when $(1 - \rho)$ is small.

4.2.2 Many Variables

With linear combinations involving any number of variables, expression (4.1) generalizes so that

$$\text{Var}\left(\sum t_i y_i\right) = \sum t_i^2 \text{Var}(y_i) + \sum_{i \neq i'} t_i t_{i'} \rho_{ii'} \sqrt{\text{Var}(y_i)\,\text{Var}(y_{i'})} \qquad (4.2)$$

The second part of this formula involves the correlation between each pair of variables. The way the expression is written, each pair of observations is counted twice. There are other ways to write (4.2); for example,

$$\text{Var}\left(\sum t_i y_i\right) = \sum t_i^2 \text{Var}(y_i) + 2\sum_{i < i'} t_i t_{i'} \rho_{ii'} \sqrt{\text{Var}(y_i)\,\text{Var}(y_{i'})}$$

It turns out that a linear combination can be expressed more concisely in matrix form.

$$\sum t_j y_j = \begin{pmatrix} t_1 & t_2 & \cdots & \end{pmatrix} \begin{pmatrix} y_1 \\ y_2 \\ \vdots \end{pmatrix} = T'Y$$

This matrix operation is referred to as a *linear transformation* of Y. It is not necessary that the matrix T have only one column. In cases where there are more columns, we still refer to the multiplication of T' and Y as a linear transformation, but actually several different linear combinations of the elements of Y are being produced (see example below).

Using slightly more algebra, one can show that (4.2) can be expressed as

$$\text{Var}(T'Y) = T' \text{Var}(Y)T \tag{4.3}$$

This is an important formula that will come in handy in future chapters.

4.2.2.1 *Example*

Returning to the above blood pressure example, the mean blood pressure can be written

$$\frac{\text{SBP}_1 + \text{SBP}_2}{2} = \begin{pmatrix} \frac{1}{2} & \frac{1}{2} \end{pmatrix} \begin{pmatrix} \text{SBP}_1 \\ \text{SBP}_2 \end{pmatrix} = T'_{\text{mean}} \begin{pmatrix} \text{SBP}_1 \\ \text{SBP}_2 \end{pmatrix}$$

so that

$$T_{\text{mean}} = \begin{pmatrix} \frac{1}{2} \\ \frac{1}{2} \end{pmatrix}$$

and by the matrix formula

$$\text{Var}\left(\frac{\text{SBP}_1 + \text{SBP}_2}{2} \right) = \begin{pmatrix} \frac{1}{2} & \frac{1}{2} \end{pmatrix} \begin{pmatrix} 100 & 80 \\ 80 & 100 \end{pmatrix} \begin{pmatrix} \frac{1}{2} \\ \frac{1}{2} \end{pmatrix}$$

$$= \begin{pmatrix} \frac{1}{2}100 + \frac{1}{2}80 & \frac{1}{2}80 + \frac{1}{2}100 \end{pmatrix} \begin{pmatrix} \frac{1}{2} \\ \frac{1}{2} \end{pmatrix}$$

$$= \begin{pmatrix} 90 & 90 \end{pmatrix} \begin{pmatrix} \frac{1}{2} \\ \frac{1}{2} \end{pmatrix} = 90\frac{1}{2} + 90\frac{1}{2} = 90$$

as before. For the difference, a similar computation can be carried out with

$$T_{\text{diff}} = \begin{pmatrix} +1 \\ -1 \end{pmatrix}$$

However, formula (4.3) can give us the variance matrix for the mean and difference jointly. Let $Y = \begin{pmatrix} \text{SBP}_1 \\ \text{SBP}_2 \end{pmatrix}$ as before, and combine T_{mean} and T_{diff} into an overall T so that

$$T = \begin{pmatrix} \frac{1}{2} & +1 \\ \frac{1}{2} & -1 \end{pmatrix}$$

Now

$$T'Y = \begin{pmatrix} \frac{SBP_1 + SBP_2}{2} \\ SBP_1 - SBP_2 \end{pmatrix}$$

producing both the mean and the difference by one linear transformation, and

$$\text{Var}(T'Y) = T'\,\text{Var}(Y)T = \begin{pmatrix} \frac{1}{2} & \frac{1}{2} \\ +1 & -1 \end{pmatrix}\begin{pmatrix} 100 & 80 \\ 80 & 100 \end{pmatrix}\begin{pmatrix} \frac{1}{2} & +1 \\ \frac{1}{2} & -1 \end{pmatrix}$$

$$= \begin{pmatrix} 90 & 90 \\ 20 & -20 \end{pmatrix}\begin{pmatrix} \frac{1}{2} & +1 \\ \frac{1}{2} & -1 \end{pmatrix} = \begin{pmatrix} 90 & 0 \\ 0 & 40 \end{pmatrix}$$

We see that the variances we obtained by the more mundane (nonmatrix) approach appear on the diagonal. However, in deriving the entire variance matrix for the mean and difference, we have provided the additional result that the mean and difference are uncorrelated. This is reflected in the off-diagonal elements in the covariance matrix being 0. We will see later that one way to deal with correlated data is to relate risk factor changes to differences in outcome within individuals, clusters, or matched sets. Another way is to do ordinary regression on cluster means. More sophisticated analyses, such as we will do with PROC MIXED in effect, combine the two approaches in ways that we will illustrate in Chapter 9.

4.2.2.2 Example: How to Obtain the Standard Error of Regression Coefficients of Predictors When There Is Interaction

When there is an interaction effect in a model, the main effects of variables and their standard errors have to be interpreted with caution. Assume that we have a model

$$y_i = \beta_0 + \beta_1 x_{1i} + \beta_2 x_{2i} + \beta_3 x_{1i} \times x_{2i} + \epsilon_i$$

This implies that the regression coefficient of variable x_i depends on the value of variable x_2 through the relationship

$$\beta_{x_1|x_2} = \beta_1 + \beta_3 x_2$$

Hence, β_1 represents the coefficient of x_1 when $x_2 = 0$, and unless care is taken in scaling x_2 to a reasonable 0 point, β_1 has no meaning. We ran the following commands for the regression of systolic blood pressure at visit 1 in the Wisconsin (one person was not weighed at visit 1, making all analyses with BMI have one observation less.)

PROC REG; MODEL SBP=BMI AGE AGE_BMI/COVB;

The output is

```
                obtaining the se of beta(bmi) at age 50
obtaining the standard error from the variance matrix of
coefficients
```

```
                     The REG Procedure
           Dependent Variable: SBP systolic blood pressure
```

```
                    Parameter Estimates
```

			Parameter	Standard
Variable	Label	DF	Estimate	Error
Intercept	Intercept	1	65.65235	10.70434
age	uncentered age in years	1	0.88162	0.23313
bmi	uncentered bmi kg/m2	1	1.47030	0.35480
age_bmi	uncentered intercation	1	-0.01826	0.00771

```
                    Parameter Estimates
```

Variable	Label	DF	t Value	Pr > |t|
Intercept	Intercept	1	6.13	<.0001
age	uncentered age in years	1	3.78	0.0002
bmi	uncentered bmi kg/m2	1	4.14	<.0001
age_bmi	uncentered intercation	1	-2.37	0.0180

```
                  Covariance of Estimates
```

Variable	Label	Intercept	age
Intercept	Intercept	114.58288366	-2.462545415
age	uncentered age in years	-2.462545415	0.0543507542
bmi	uncentered bmi kg/m2	-3.715985671	0.0798520374
age_bmi	uncentered intercation	0.0798316556	-0.001761434

```
                  Covariance of Estimates
```

Variable	Label	bmi	age_bmi
Intercept	Intercept	-3.715985671	0.0798316556
age	uncentered age in years	0.0798520374	-0.001761434
bmi	uncentered bmi kg/m2	0.1258847378	-0.002700182
age_bmi	uncentered intercation	-0.002700182	0.0000594663

```
                obtaining the se of beta(bmi) at age 50
       obtaining the standard error by centering the interaction
```

```
                     The REG Procedure
           Dependent Variable: SBP systolic blood pressure
```

```
                        Parameter Estimates


                                                      Parameter
      Variable    Label                         DF     Estimate

      Intercept   Intercept                      1     65.65235
      age         uncentered age in years        1      0.88162
      bmi         uncentered bmi kg/m2           1      0.55731
      agec_bmi    interaction with age centered  1     -0.01826
                  at 50


                        Parameter Estimates


                                                   Standard
    Variable   Label                       DF       Error    t Value

    Intercept  Intercept                    1      10.70434     6.13
    age        uncentered age in years      1       0.23313     3.78
    bmi        uncentered bmi kg/m2         1       0.06732     8.28
    agec_bmi   interaction with age centered 1      0.00771    -2.37
               at 50


                        Parameter Estimates


      Variable    Label                         DF  Pr > |t|

      Intercept   Intercept                      1    <.0001
      age         uncentered age in years        1    0.0002
      bmi         uncentered bmi kg/m2           1    <.0001
      agec_bmi    interaction with age centered  1    0.0180
                  at 50
```

Here AGE_BMI is the interaction AGE*BMI (age in years is not centered, neither is BMI). The option COVB prints the variance matrix of the regression coefficients, which we will use in a minute. For now, notice that the interaction is statistically significant and that the value $\hat{\beta}_{bmi} = 1.47$ is the coefficient of BMI extrapolated to age 0. Clearly, this is meaningless. To obtain the coefficient of BMI at a more reasonable age, say 50 (which is close to the mean age of the sample), we calculate $1.47 - 0.0183 \times 50 = 0.555$. Note that this is a linear transformation

$$\hat{\beta}_1 + \hat{\beta}_3 x_2 = \begin{pmatrix} 1 & x_2 \end{pmatrix} \begin{pmatrix} \hat{\beta}_1 \\ \hat{\beta}_3 \end{pmatrix} = \begin{pmatrix} 1 & 50 \end{pmatrix} \begin{pmatrix} \hat{\beta}_1 \\ \hat{\beta}_3 \end{pmatrix}$$

so that $T = \begin{pmatrix} 1 \\ 50 \end{pmatrix}$. Then we can obtain the standard error of the coefficient of BMI at age 50 via the variance formula for a linear transformation. The above output provides the variance matrix of the BMI and interaction coefficients. Note that the diagonal elements of this matrix are just the standard errors squared. The off-diagonal elements are the covariances. Regression coefficient estimators tend to be correlated because they were fit together. We see that

$$\text{Var}\begin{pmatrix}\hat{\beta}_1 \\ \hat{\beta}_3\end{pmatrix} = \begin{pmatrix} 0.126 & -0.00270 \\ -0.00270 & 0.0000595 \end{pmatrix}$$

so

$$\text{Var}(\hat{\beta}_1 + \hat{\beta}_3 x_2) = \begin{pmatrix} 1 & 50 \end{pmatrix} \begin{pmatrix} 0.126 & -0.00270 \\ -0.00270 & 0.0000595 \end{pmatrix} \begin{pmatrix} 1 \\ 50 \end{pmatrix}$$

$$= \begin{pmatrix} 0.126 - 50 \times 0.00270 & -0.00270 + 50 \times 0.0000595 \end{pmatrix} \begin{pmatrix} 1 \\ 50 \end{pmatrix}$$

$$= 0.126 - 50 \times 0.00270 - 50 \times 0.00270 + 2500 \times 0.0000595$$

$$= 0.00475$$

Then the standard error of the coefficient is $\sqrt{0.0047} = 0.0689$. Obviously, the same procedure can be used to obtain the coefficient for BMI and its standard error at any age, as long as the regression estimators and their variance matrix are provided.

A slightly more accurate and painless method is to center the interaction at the value of AGE at which we want to obtain the regression coefficient of BMI. This was done in the second approach above. Now

$$\hat{\beta}_{\text{BMI}|\text{age}=x_2} = \hat{\beta}_1' + \hat{\beta}_3(x_2 - 50)$$

so that the coefficient of BMI at age 50 is $\hat{\beta}_1' = 0.557$ with standard error 0.0673. We note that the first method is more flexible and does not require access to the original data. However, it is laborious and prone to round-off error unless many decimals are carried along.

4.2.2.3 Another Example: How the Variance of the Difference Affects a Paired t-Test

The next output example shows some results from the Wisconsin Diabetes Registry. GHb levels are being compared between the first (duration DUR $= 0$) and second (DUR $= 1$) years of diabetes for individuals who have provided data for both years. We compute the variance of the difference in GHb between the two years by formula (4.3) and directly from the data. In the process we also compare the results from performing unpaired and paired t-tests.

Because the data for different years were originally in different records, a merged data set was created for performing the paired t-test. Note the command for the paired t-test, which does not use a CLASS statement. The commands run were (except that some additional programming is not shown that was needed to delete from the unpaired t-test individuals with missing data in either year):

```
DATA A;
......
LABEL DUR='year of diabetes';
PROC TTEST; CLASS DUR; VAR GHB;
DATA A1; SET A;
IF DUR=1; GHB0=GHB;
KEEP ID GHB0;
PROC SORT; BY ID;
DATA A2; SET A; IF DUR=2;
GHB1=GHB; KEEP ID GHB1; DATA PAIR; MERGE A1 A2; BY ID;
IF GHB0=.  OR GHB1=.  THEN DELETE;
PROC CORR; VAR GHB0 GHB1;
PROC TTEST; PAIRED GHB0*GHB1;
```

Another way to achieve the merging is:

```
DATA A;
.....
PROC SORT; BY ID DUR;
DATA PAIR (KEEP=GHB0 GHB1);
ARRAY G{2} GHB0-GHB1;
DO I=1 TO 2;
SET A; BY ID DUR;
G{I}=GHB;
IF LAST. ID THEN RETURN;
RUN;
PROC CORR; VAR GHB0 GHB1;
PROC TTEST; PAIRED GHB0*GHB1;
```

which makes use of the SAS array feature and also the ability to pinpoint the last (or first) observation for a person. The output follows.

```
Wisconsin Diabetes Registry, comparing GHb between first two
years
```
unpaired t-test

The TTEST Procedure

Statistics

Variable	dur	N	Lower CL Mean	Mean	Upper CL Mean	Lower CL Std Dev
M_GHB	1	446	9.1101	9.3245	9.539	2.1624
M_GHB	2	446	10.252	10.49	10.729	2.4039
M_GHB	Diff (1-2)		-1.486	-1.166	-0.846	2.3283

Variable dur			Std Dev	Upper CL Std Dev	Std Err	Minimum	Maximum
M_GHB		1	2.3043	2.4664	0.1091	4.75	22.98
M_GHB		2	2.5617	2.7418	0.1213	5.5125	23.2
M_GHB	Diff (1-2)		2.4364	2.5551	0.1632		

		T-Tests			
Variable	Method	Variances	DF	t Value	Pr<|t|
M_GHB	Pooled	Equal	890	-7.15	<.0001

correlation for constructing variance matrix

The CORR Procedure

Pearson Correlation Coefficients, N = 446
Prob > |r| under H0: Rho=0

	ghb0	ghb1
ghb0	1.00000	0.48060 <.0001
ghb1	0.48060	1.00000 <.0001

paired t-test

The TTEST Procedure

Difference	N	Lower CL Mean	Mean	Upper CL Mean	Std Dev	Std Err
ghb0 - ghb1	446	-1.397	-1.166	-0.934	2.4896	0.1179

	T-Tests		
Difference	DF	t Value	Pr > |t|
ghb0 - ghb1	445	-9.89	<.0001

The first part of output consists of an unpaired *t*-test. (This is, of course, not the test that should be done, given that the data were actually paired.) We see that the mean GHb level in the first year was 9.32 with a standard deviation of 9.30. In the second year, the level was 10.49 with a standard deviation of 2.56. The standard error for the difference (not taking correlation into account) is 0.1632. We see that the GHb's from the two years correlate at $r = 0.48060$. This correlation will dictate how much is gained by the matched analysis.

We now know that the variance matrix of these two measurements is

$$V = \begin{pmatrix} 2.3043^2 & (0.4806)(2.3043)(2.5617) \\ (0.4806)(2.3043)(2.5617) & 2.5617^2 \end{pmatrix}$$

To form the difference between the measurements, we choose the matrix

$$T = \begin{pmatrix} 1 \\ -1 \end{pmatrix}$$

and obtain the variance of the difference by formula (4.3) as

$$\begin{pmatrix} 1 & -1 \end{pmatrix} \begin{pmatrix} 2.3043^2 & (0.4806)(2.3043)(2.5617) \\ (0.4806)(2.3043)(2.5617) & 2.5617^2 \end{pmatrix} \begin{pmatrix} 1 \\ -1 \end{pmatrix}$$

$$= \begin{pmatrix} 2.3043^2 - (0.4806)(2.3043)(2.5617) \\ (0.4806)(2.3043)(2.5617) - 2.5617^2 \end{pmatrix}' \begin{pmatrix} 1 \\ -1 \end{pmatrix}$$

$$= \begin{pmatrix} 2.4729 & -3.7254 \end{pmatrix} \begin{pmatrix} 1 \\ -1 \end{pmatrix} = 6.1983$$

The paired t-test at the end provides descriptive statistics for the difference between the two measurements obtained directly from the data. The sample variance of the difference is $2.4896^2 = 6.1981$. The standard error for the paired test is 0.118, a substantial reduction from 0.163 of the unpaired test. We note that the paired t-test value for the difference ($H_0:\mu_{\text{diff}} = 0$) is $t(445) = -9.89$, and the unpaired t-test value (for unequal variance) is (approximately) $t(880) = -7.15$. Because of the large sample size, they are both highly significant. If, however, the sample size had been much smaller (about 20), the unpaired t-test would have been nonsignificant at two-sided $\alpha = 0.05$.

At the design stage of a study, a decision may need to be made whether a matched design is worthwhile. If one has estimates of σ^2 and ρ, one can project the sample size or power both ways and assess the benefits of matching. In this projection, one would use the fact that the variance of an unpaired difference is $2\sigma^2/n$, and that of a paired difference is $2\sigma^2(1-\rho)/n$. A paired design is beneficial when ρ is large—in other words, when the matching characteristics are "strong."

CHAPTER FIVE

Variance Matrices of Estimators of Regression Coefficients

Chapter 4 introduced both the variance of regression coefficient estimators and the covariance between these estimators as provided by PROC REG. We saw how variances and covariances can be compactly summarized in a matrix. In this chapter, we will derive this variance matrix from least-squares and maximum likelihood perspectives.

5.1 USUAL STANDARD ERROR OF LEAST-SQUARES ESTIMATOR OF REGRESSION SLOPE IN NONMATRIX FORMULATION

We first look at the estimator of the ordinary least-squares estimator of the slope β_1 in nonmatrix notation. There is assumed to be only one covariate x, so that

$$\hat{\beta}_1 = \frac{\sum_{i=1}^{n}(x_i - \bar{x})(y_i - \bar{y})}{\sum_{i=1}^{n}(x_i - \bar{x})^2} = \frac{\sum_{i=1}^{n}(x_i - \bar{x})y_i}{\sum_{i=1}^{n}(x_i - \bar{x})^2}$$

We can easily show that the $(-\bar{y})$ is not needed as

$$\sum_{i=1}^{n}(x_i - \bar{x})\bar{y} = \bar{y}\sum_{i=1}^{n}(x_i - \bar{x}) = \bar{y}(n\bar{x} - n\bar{x}) = 0$$

Now, to get the $se(\hat{\beta}_1) = \sqrt{\text{Var}(\hat{\beta}_1)}$, we use the nonmatrix formula for the variance of a sum:

Quantitative Methods in Population Health, by Mari Palta
ISBN 0-471-45505-9   Copyright © 2003 John Wiley & Sons, Inc.

$$\text{Var}(\hat{\beta}_1) = \sum_{i=1}^{n} \left(\frac{x_i - \overline{x}}{\sum_{j=1}^{n}(x_j - \overline{x})^2} \right)^2 \text{Var}(y_i|x_i)$$

$$= \sum_{i=1}^{n} \left(\frac{x_i - \overline{x}}{\sum_{j=1}^{n}(x_j - \overline{x})^2} \right)^2 \text{Var}(\epsilon_i) \tag{5.1}$$

Note that the independence assumption has made $\text{Cov}(\epsilon_i, \epsilon_{i'}) = 0$, eliminating that part of expression (4.2). Now comes the point at which a decision has to be made regarding what to assume about the variance $\text{Var}(y_i|x_i) = \text{Var}(\epsilon_i)$. The equal variance assumption leads to

$$\hat{\text{var}}(\hat{\beta}_1) = \sum_{i=1}^{n} \left(\frac{x_i - \overline{x}}{\sum_{j=1}^{n}(x_j - \overline{x})^2} \right)^2 \hat{\text{Var}}(y_i|x_i) = \hat{\sigma}_{y|x}^2 \sum_{i=1}^{n} \left(\frac{x_i - \overline{x}}{\sum_{j=1}^{n}(x_j - \overline{x})^2} \right)^2$$

$$= \hat{\sigma}_{y|x}^2 \frac{\sum_{i=1}^{n}(x_i - \overline{x})^2}{\left[\sum_{i=1}^{n}(x_i - \overline{x})^2 \right]^2} = \hat{\sigma}_{y|x}^2 \frac{1}{\sum_{i=1}^{n}(x_i - \overline{x})^2}$$

the square root of which is the usual standard error of $\hat{\beta}_1$. The estimator $\hat{\sigma}_{y|x}^2$ can be obtained by the various approaches we have discussed (from the MSE, by ML or by REML), with the MSE being the natural approach with least-squares estimation.

5.2 STANDARD ERRORS OF LEAST-SQUARES REGRESSION ESTIMATORS IN MATRIX NOTATION

As an alternative to the above "pedestrian" approach, we can use the matrix formulas from Chapter 4 to derive the variance matrix of the regression coefficients. The variance matrix of the regression estimators includes variances and covariances of all estimated coefficients.

The estimators are in matrix β with one column containing the intercept and all the regression slopes. First note that formula (3.6) for $\hat{\beta}$ is just a linear transformation of Y, $\hat{\beta} = (X'X)^{-1}X'Y = T'Y$, where using the matrix transpose formula $(AB)' = B'A'$ and the fact that $X'X$ and, therefore, its inverse are symmetric, we obtain

$$T = [(X'X)^{-1}X']' = X[(X'X)^{-1}]' = X(X'X)^{-1}$$

By formula (4.2) we obtain

$$\mathrm{Var}(T'Y|X) = T'\mathrm{Var}(Y|X)T = (X'X)^{-1}X'[\mathrm{Var}(Y|X)]X(X'X)^{-1}$$

Again, if we make the equal variance and independence assumptions, we have

$$\mathrm{Var}(Y|X) = \begin{pmatrix} \sigma^2_{y|x} & 0 & \cdots \\ 0 & \sigma^2_{y|x} & \cdots \\ \vdots & \vdots & \ddots \end{pmatrix} = \sigma^2_{y|x}I$$

Then using property 14 from the matrix formula list, along with the property of an identity matrix, we obtain

$$\widehat{\mathrm{Var}}(\hat{\beta}) = (X'X)^{-1}X'[\hat{\sigma}^2_{y|x}I]X(XX')^{-1}$$

$$= \hat{\sigma}^2_{y|x}(X'X)^{-1}X'X(X'X)^{-1}$$

$$= \hat{\sigma}^2_{y|x}(X'X)^{-1} \qquad (5.2)$$

This is the usual expression for the variance matrix of ordinary least-squares estimator of the regression coefficients.

5.2.1 Example

It is instructive to write out $(X'X)^{-1}$ for the situation of simple regression (only one covariate). Then

$$X = \begin{pmatrix} 1 & x_1 \\ 1 & x_2 \\ \vdots & \vdots \\ 1 & x_n \end{pmatrix}$$

and

$$X'X = \begin{pmatrix} 1 & 1 & \cdots & 1 \\ x_1 & x_2 & \cdots & x_n \end{pmatrix} \begin{pmatrix} 1 & x_1 \\ 1 & x_2 \\ \vdots & \vdots \\ 1 & x_n \end{pmatrix} = \begin{pmatrix} n & \sum_1^n x_i \\ \sum_1^n x_i & \sum_1^n x_i^2 \end{pmatrix}$$

It is useful to remember that $X'X$ is a square matrix that always has the same number of rows and columns as there are regression parameters.

Now, by the formula for matrix inversion we obtain

$$(X'X)^{-1} = \frac{1}{n \sum_1^n x_i^2 - \left(\sum_n^1 x_i\right)^2} \begin{pmatrix} \sum_1^n x_i^2 & -\sum_1^n x_i \\ -\sum_1^n x_i & n \end{pmatrix}$$

$$= \begin{pmatrix} \dfrac{\sum_1^n x_i^2/n}{\sum_1^n x_i^2 - \left(\sum_1^n x_i\right)^2/n} & -\dfrac{\sum_1^n x_i}{n \sum_1^n x_i^2 - \left(\sum_1^n x_i\right)^2} \\ -\dfrac{\sum_1^n x_i}{n \sum_1^n x_i^2 - \left(\sum_1^n x_i\right)^2} & \dfrac{1}{\sum_1^n x_i^2 - \left(\sum_1^n x_i\right)^2/n} \end{pmatrix}$$

Examining the (2, 2) element in this matrix, we find that because

$$\sum (x_i - \bar{x})^2 = \sum x_i^2 - \left(\sum x_i\right)^2/n$$

we have

$$\hat{\mathrm{Var}}(\hat{\beta}_1) = \hat{\sigma}_{y|x}^2 \frac{1}{\displaystyle\sum_{i=1}^n (x_i - \bar{x})^2}$$

as before. However, the matrix approach has also provided the variance of the estimator of the intercept, along with the covariance of the slope and intercept estimators.

5.3 THE LARGE SAMPLE VARIANCE MATRIX OF MAXIMUM LIKELIHOOD ESTIMATORS

You may note that the normality assumption was not involved in the derivation of the variance matrix above. It would enter only when we start using the standard errors to form t-tests, F-tests, and confidence intervals. We will now derive the large sample variance matrix of the estimators based on maximum likelihood, when the equal variance assumption holds. To use maximum likelihood, we do need to assume that the observations or regression errors are normally distributed. This section illustrates the general approach to obtaining the standard errors of maximum likelihood estimators.

Recall the log of the likelihood for a regression analysis with one predictor from equation (2.1). (For simplicity we use just one predictor, although all principles apply to the more general case.) Based on the observations y_i, conditionally on x_i, all being normally distributed with variance $\sigma^2 = \sigma^2_{y|x}$, being independent, and having mean of $\beta_0 + \beta_1 x_i$, we have

$$\log(L) = -n \log(\hat{\sigma}_{y|x} \sqrt{2\pi}) - \sum_{i=1}^{n} \frac{(y_i - \hat{\beta}_0 - \hat{\beta}_1 x_i)^2}{2\hat{\sigma}^2_{y|x}}$$

One of the pleasing properties of maximum likelihood estimators is efficiency (in large samples). The ML estimators are known to be to be efficient, because their large sample (sampling) variance has been derived for all situations and can be obtained directly from $\log(L)$. It is extremely convenient that the large sample variance can be obtained by the same method, no matter what is being estimated. For other estimators the variance often needs to be derived for the specific situation; the only problems encountered in large sample maximum likelihood are numeric.

Estimation of the large sample variance of maximum likelihood estimators when there is more than one parameter being estimated involves the inversion of a matrix. This matrix consists of (minus) second derivatives of $\log(L)$. In general, the matrix must include derivatives with respect to all the parameters, but the regression $\log(L)$ above estimates the $\hat{\beta}$'s and the $\hat{\sigma}_{y|x}$ independently. Because of this we can illustrate the principle by deriving the variance matrix only for the $\hat{\beta}$'s. If we did include the regression parameters and the variance together, they would form separate blocks in the matrix, and these blocks will be separately inverted.

First we obtain the second derivatives (remember, there are three for the two parameters):

$$\frac{\partial^2}{\partial \hat{\beta}_0^2} \log(L) = -\frac{n}{\hat{\sigma}^2_{y|x}}$$

$$\frac{\partial^2}{\partial \hat{\beta}_1^2} \log(L) = -\sum \frac{x_i^2}{\hat{\sigma}^2_{y|x}}$$

$$\frac{\partial^2}{\partial \hat{\beta}_0 \partial \hat{\beta}_1} \log(L) = -\sum \frac{x_i}{\hat{\sigma}^2_{y|x}}$$

Next we remove the—signs and place these in a matrix (known as the information matrix $\mathfrak{J}$)

$$\mathfrak{J} = \begin{pmatrix} \frac{n}{\hat{\sigma}^2_{y|x}} & \sum \frac{x_i}{\hat{\sigma}^2_{y|x}} \\ \sum \frac{x_i}{\hat{\sigma}^2_{y|x}} & \sum \frac{x_i^2}{\hat{\sigma}^2_{y|x}} \end{pmatrix} = \frac{1}{\hat{\sigma}^2_{y|x}} \begin{pmatrix} n & \sum x_i \\ \sum x_i & \sum x_i^2 \end{pmatrix}$$

We know the inverse of this matrix is obtained as

$$\mathfrak{I}^{-1} = \hat{\sigma}_{y|x}^2 \frac{1}{n \sum x_i^2 - \left(\sum x_i\right)^2} \begin{pmatrix} \sum x_i^2 & -\sum x_i \\ -\sum x_i & n \end{pmatrix}$$

$$= \hat{\sigma}_{y|x}^2 \begin{pmatrix} \dfrac{\sum x_i^2}{n \sum x_i^2 - \left(\sum x_i\right)^2} & -\dfrac{\sum x_i}{n \sum x_i^2 - \left(\sum x_i\right)^2} \\ -\dfrac{\sum x_i}{n \sum x_i^2 - \left(\sum x_i\right)^2} & \dfrac{n}{n \sum x_i^2 - \left(\sum x_i\right)^2} \end{pmatrix}$$

The (1, 1) element in this matrix is the variance of the intercept, the (2, 2) element is the variance of the slope, and the (1, 2) element (which equals the (2, 1) element) is the covariance of the two. We see that the estimators of the intercept and the mean are correlated from sample to sample.

The (2, 2) element is again recognizable as the usual

$$\text{Var}(\hat{\beta}_1) = \frac{\hat{\sigma}_{y|x}^2}{\sum (x_i - \bar{x})^2}$$

Here, it is common to obtain $\hat{\sigma}_{y|x}^2$ by ML or REML (which happens to coincide with the MSE approach).

5.4 TESTS AND CONFIDENCE INTERVALS

Both least-squares and maximum likelihood estimators are approximately normally distributed in large samples. This follows from applications of the central limit theorem. When the residuals are normally distributed, least-squares estimators are normally distributed also in small samples. Because the two coincide in the current situation, so are the maximum likelihood estimators for ordinary regression. However, when residuals are not normally distributed, the distributions of maximum likelihood estimators in small samples are pretty much unknown.

Because of the approximately normal sampling distribution in large samples, where errors in $s_{y|x}^2$ vanish, the standard error estimates obtained from $\mathfrak{I}^{-1}$ are used for forming inference based on the normal distribution, or squared to form so-called Wald χ^2-tests for the coefficients. Recall that when a statistic with a standard normal distribution is squared, the new variable follows a χ^2-distribution with 1 degree of freedom. The normally distributed residual case is special in that small sample distributions have been derived that take error in $s_{y|x}^2$ into account and allow us to use the t-test for inference, instead of the Wald test. As we noted earlier: In large samples, the t-distribution is very close to the normal, and the F-distribution is close to the χ^2-distribution (divided by its degrees of freedom).

The reader is assumed to be familiar with other tests and procedures associated with maximum likelihood estimation. Most likelihood-based SAS procedures provide the Wald test for individual regression coefficients (or in the special case of PROC MIXED, the t-test for individual coefficients). Comparisons of nested models is often based on likelihood ratio tests. These are formed as differences in $-2\log(L)$ or $-2\log(REML)$ between models that are nested (i.e., one model contains all the parameters in the other, plus some more). The likelihood ratio test has a χ^2-distribution with degrees of freedom equal to the difference in number of parameters. Generally, likelihood ratio tests have been found to be more stable than Wald tests, and some SAS procedures provide likelihood ratio tests and confidence intervals for the coefficients as an option. Again note that for normally distributed residuals, the likelihood ratio test can be replaced by an F-test.

A piece of terminology used by SAS for F and likelihood ratio tests are Type 1 and Type 3 (Type 2 also exists, but is not used much). Type 1 refers to tests arising from sequential model building; that is, the test is performed on a variable with all preceding, but not any of the subsequent, variables in the model. Type 3 tests are performed with all the other variables in the model. Both types can be very useful.

Finally, we will encounter adjustments to the $-2\log(L)$ or $-2\log(REML)$ that impose a penalty for introducing more parameters, just as the adjusted R^2 equals $1 - \frac{n-1}{n-m-1}(1 - \text{regular } R^2)$ for ordinary regression. These criteria will be explained when we encounter them, and they can be used to compare both nested and not nested models.

5.4.1 Example-Comparing PROC REG and PROC MIXED

The output was created for the visit 1 blood pressure data by the statements below

From now onward, we center age and BMI at values 50 and 27, respectively, unless otherwise noted. This improves interpretability of the age and BMI coefficients, as well as of the intercept, which is now the estimated mean blood pressure at age 50 for a person with BMI of 27. The above example also illustrates the capability of PROC MIXED to generate interactions automatically, while they have to be preconstructed for PROC REG. (PROC REG is an aberration, since most other regression-related procedures in SAS can now generate interactions.) PROC MIXED also has the ability to incorporate the alphabetic variable SEX, via the CLASS statement. As is the default in SAS, the indicator variable that is automatically generated is set to 0 for the "last" value of SEX—that is, for SEX='M'. Again, PROC REG does not have this capability, and the indicator variable GENDER has to be preconstructed.

It is easily seen that the variance matrix for the coefficients obtained by the (default) REML option coincides with the one obtained by PROC REG. PROC MIXED does not (as a default) provide Wald χ^2-tests for the coefficients, but takes advantage of known properties of the normal distribution that lead to more exact t- and F-tests in small samples. (Later, when with non-normal distributions, we will use Wald tests). Note the "Type 3" terminology at the end of the PROC MIXED output.

AGEC=AGE-50; BMIC=BMI-27;
AGEC_BMIC=AGEC*BMIC;
GENDER=0;
IF SEX='F' THEN GENDER=1;
PROC REG; MODEL SBP=GENDER AGEC BMIC AGEC_BMIC/COVB;
PROC MIXED; CLASS SEX;
MODEL SBP=SEX AGEC BMIC AGEC*BMIC/S COVB;

some comparisons of PROC MIXED and PROC REG

The REG Procedure
Dependent Variable: SBP systolic blood pressure

Analysis of Variance

Source	DF	Sum of Squares	Mean Square	F Value	Pr > F
Model	4	50562	12641	71.18	<.0001
Error	1359	241336	177.58357		
Corrected Total	1363	291898			

Root MSE	13.32605	R-Square	0.1732	
Dependent Mean	125.09176	Adj R-Sq	0.1708	
Coeff Var	10.65302			

Parameter Estimates

Variable	Label	DF	Parameter Estimate
Intercept	Intercept	1	127.44900
gender		1	-6.57305
agec	age centered at 50	1	0.36912
bmic		1	0.59454
agec_bmic	interaction with age centered at 50, bmi at 27	1	-0.01892

Variable	Label	DF	Standard Error	t Value
Intercept	Intercept	1	0.52502	242.75
gender		1	0.73184	-8.98
agec	age centered at 50	1	0.04946	7.46
bmic		1	0.06556	9.07
agec_bmic	interaction with age centered at 50, bmi at 27	1	0.00750	-2.52

```
Variable   Label                            DF   Pr > |t|

Intercept  Intercept                         1    <.0001
gender                                       1    <.0001
agec       age centered at 50                1    <.0001
bmic                                         1    <.0001
agec_bmic  interaction with age centered     1    0.0117
           at 50, bmi at 27
```

some comparisons of PROC MIXED and PROC REG

Covariance of Estimates

Variable	Intercept	gender	agec
Intercept	0.275650084	-0.217411056	0.008512363
gender	-0.217411056	0.535586414	0.0015878648
agec	0.008512363	0.0015878648	0.0024459371
bmic	-0.011065139	-0.003033067	-0.000807341
agec_bmic	-0.000839358	0.0000535935	-0.000147062

Covariance of Estimates

Variable	bmic	agec_bmic
Intercept	-0.011065139	-0.000839358
gender	-0.003033067	0.0000535935
agec	-0.000807341	-0.000147062
bmic	0.0042985464	0.0002577128
agec_bmic	0.0002577128	0.0000561809

some comparisons of PROC MIXED and PROC REG

The Mixed Procedure

Model Information

```
Data Set                    WORK.A
Dependent Variable          sbp
Covariance Structure        Diagonal
Estimation Method           REML
Residual Variance Method    Profile
Fixed Effects SE Method     Model-Based
Degrees of Freedom Method   Residual
```

```
                         Class Level Information

            Class     Levels     Values

            sex          2        F M

                              Dimensions

                    Covariance Parameters          1
                    Columns in X                   6
                    Columns in Z                   0
                    Subjects                       1
                    Max Obs Per Subject         1378
                    Observations Used           1364
                    Observations Not Used         14
                    Total Observations          1378


                         Covariance Parameter

                              Estimates

                    Cov Parm       Estimate

                    Residual        177.58

                           Fit Statistics

                  -2 Res Log Likelihood          10945.9
                  AIC (smaller is better)        10947.9
                  AICC (smaller is better)       10947.9
                  BIC (smaller is better)        10953.1
```

some comparisons of PROC MIXED and PROC REG
Solution for Fixed Effects

Effect	sex	Estimate	Standard Error	DF	t Value	Pr > |t|
Intercept		127.45	0.5250	1359	242.75	<.0001
sex	F	-6.5731	0.7318	1359	-8.98	<.0001
sex	M	0	.	.	.	.
agec		0.3691	0.04946	1359	7.46	<.0001
bmic		0.5945	0.06556	1359	9.07	<.0001
agec*bmic		-0.01892	0.007495	1359	-2.52	0.0117

Covariance Matrix for Fixed Effects

Row	Effect	sex	Col1	Col2	Col3	Col4	Col5
1	Intercept		0.2757	-0.2174		0.008512	-0.01107

2	sex	F	-0.2174	0.5356		0.001588	-0.00303
3	sex	M					
4	agec		0.008512	0.001588		0.002446	-0.00081
5	bmic		-0.01107	-0.00303		-0.00081	0.004299
6	agec*bmic		-0.00084	0.000054		-0.00015	0.000258

Covariance
Matrix for
Fixed Effects

Row	Col6
1	-0.00084
2	0.000054
3	
4	-0.00015
5	0.000258
6	0.000056

Type 3 Tests of Fixed Effects

Effect	Num DF	Den DF	F Value	Pr > F
sex	1	1359	80.67	<.0001
agec	1	1359	55.70	<.0001
bmic	1	1359	82.23	<.0001
agec*bmic	1	1359	6.37	0.0117

CHAPTER SIX

Dealing with Unequal Variance Around the Regression Line

We have now set the framework for moving forward with extending regression analysis by considering the situation of unequal variance around the regression line. We will first examine what really goes wrong with the usual unweighted (ordinary) least-squares approach in this situation. In Chapter 3, we showed that the ordinary least-squares estimator is unbiased as long as the model is correctly specified. The problem with unequal variance arises not so much from the estimator itself, as from the fact that standard error estimators are not correct. To derive the standard errors in (5.2), we definitely used the equal variance assumption. We will see how to obtain valid estimators of the standard errors when the equal variance assumption does not hold. Also, of course, the usual estimators are no longer efficient. The latter part of this chapter is devoted to methods for constructing more efficient estimators.

6.1 ORDINARY LEAST SQUARES WITH UNEQUAL VARIANCE

When we demonstrated that the ordinary least-squares estimator is unbiased in Chapter 3, we went through two crucial steps:

1. First we realized that since we condition on X, all expressions that contain only X (i.e., not Y or ϵ) can be treated as constants. This led to evaluation of $E(\hat{\beta})$ as $E[(X'X)^{-1}X'Y|X] = E[\text{matrix of constants} \times Y|X] = \text{matrix of constants} \times E[Y|X]$

2. Then we implemented that we have assumed $E[Y|X] = X\beta$—that is, that the model is correct—and obtain $(\text{matrix of constants}) \times X\beta = \beta$, from matrix properties. Note that $\hat{\beta}$ is not a constant. It is an estimator and varies from sample to sample, but its mean is the (constant) parameter β.

Quantitative Methods in Population Health, by Mari Palta
ISBN 0-471-45505-9   Copyright © 2003 John Wiley & Sons, Inc.

One important aspect of steps 1 and 2 is that the equal variance assumption simply does not enter. Hence, we can rest assured that the ordinary least-squares estimator is unbiased even if the equal variance assumption is violated.

To remember the point at which the equal variance assumption enters in the derivation of the variance of regression parameters, we first look at the estimator of the slope β_1 in nonmatrix notation:

$$\hat{\beta}_1 = \frac{\sum_1^n (x_i - \bar{x})(y_i - \bar{y})}{\sum_1^n (x_i - \bar{x})^2} = \frac{\sum_1^n (x_i - \bar{x}) y_i}{\sum_1^n (x_i - \bar{x})^2}$$

which, as before in (5.1), leads to

$$\text{Var}(\hat{\beta}_1) = \sum_1^n \left(\frac{x_i - \bar{x}}{\sum_1^n (x_j - \bar{x})^2} \right)^2 \text{Var}(y_i | x_i)$$

Previously, we made the decision to assume that $\text{Var}(y_i | x_i)$ is equal for all i. Now, if the equal variance assumption does not hold, some other $\hat{\text{Var}}(y_i | x_i)$ needs to be supplied, and the expression does not simplify as much. It is often the case that, while we suspect that $\text{Var}(y_i | x_i)$ is not equal for all i, its correct value or structure is not known. One approach is to separately estimate this quantity for each i by

$$\hat{\text{Var}}(y_i | x_i) = \hat{\epsilon}_i^2 = (y_i - \hat{\beta}_0 - \hat{\beta}_1 x_i)^2$$

Note that this expression is kind of extreme, because it makes no assumptions about how the variance of the residuals changes along the regression line. Each observation has its own variance estimate, so to say. Of course, this leads to a very poor estimator of the variance for individual i, but can be acceptable in large samples when inserted into the expression for $\text{Var}(\beta_1)$. Then

$$\hat{\text{Var}}(\hat{\beta}_1) = \sum_1^n \frac{(x_i - \bar{x})^2 \hat{\epsilon}_i^2}{\left[\sum_1^n (x_i - \bar{x})^2 \right]^2}$$

In the next section we show how to obtain this estimator with PROC MIXED EMPIRICAL.

To obtain a general expression for the sampling variance of all regression coefficients, we use matrix notation. If we cannot make the equal variance assumption, we again take the extreme approach of making no assumptions on the variance itself. But we stick to the independence assumption, so we need to insert for $\hat{\text{Var}}(Y | X)$ a matrix with 0's off the diagonal and $(y_i - \hat{\beta}_0 - \hat{\beta}_1 x_{1i} - \hat{\beta}_2 x_{2i} \cdots)^2$ on the diagonal.

We can write

$$\hat{\text{Var}}(\hat{\boldsymbol{\beta}}) = (X'X)^{-1}X'\hat{\epsilon}\hat{\epsilon}'X(X'X)^{-1} \tag{6.1}$$

where $\hat{\epsilon}$ is a diagonal matrix with $(y_i - \hat{\beta}_0 - \hat{\beta}_1 x_{1i} - \hat{\beta}_2 x_{2i} \cdots)$ on the diagonal, so that

$$\hat{\epsilon}\hat{\epsilon}' = \begin{pmatrix} (y_1 - \hat{\beta}_0 - \hat{\beta}_1 x_{11} - \hat{\beta}_2 x_{21} \cdots)^2 & 0 & \cdots \\ 0 & (y_2 - \hat{\beta}_0 - \hat{\beta}_1 x_{12} - \hat{\beta}_2 x_{22} \cdots)^2 & \cdots \\ \vdots & \vdots & \ddots \end{pmatrix}$$

Formula (6.1) is a special case of the so-called "sandwich estimator." It gets its name from the ϵ's being sandwiched in between the X's. As it makes few assumptions, it is also known as a "robust" variance estimator. It was originally proposed by Huber [9] and by White [10]. Because the usual (PROC REG) standard errors for the least-squares estimator are derived under assumptions that make the estimator the most efficient (i.e., standard errors small), one can expect that the standard errors from (6.1) will tend to be larger. This is generally the case, but standard errors can turn out to be smaller with (6.1) in a given data set, especially if many observations are in the range where residuals are most variable, and if there are many outliers.

Several procedures in SAS can produce the estimator (6.1). However, as we will be using PROC MIXED for the first part of this text, we first show examples of how to implement the standard error estimation with this procedure. The statements for telling PROC MIXED to provide standard errors based on (6.1) are

PROC MIXED NOCLPRINT EMPIRICAL;
CLASS ID; MODEL $y = x \cdots$/S;
REPEATED/SUBJECT=ID;

EMPIRICAL asks that formula (6.1) be used in obtaining the variance matrix of the regression coefficients. However, because PROC MIXED is so general, the other statements are needed to tell it exactly what to do. More specifically, PROC MIXED needs to know what observations can be assumed to be independent, because it can also deal with correlated observations. The REPEATED/SUBJECT=ID; statement tells MIXED that we are assuming independence between observations on different individuals. Because we have only one observation per person right now, this amounts to total independence.

It is safest to include the variable that indicates individual in a CLASS statement. The CLASS ID; statement tells PROC MIXED that the ID is a label and not a measurement. Finally, the NOCLPRINT prevents the ID's of all the subjects from being printed, as would be the default with the CLASS statement.

6.1.1   Examples

For these examples refer to OUTPUT PACKET III. It contains analyses of GHb, as well as of systolic blood pressure. We reanalyze the GHb data only for the age

**Table 6.1   Regression Coefficients (se) Modeling GHb to
Ages up to 15 Years**

	Ordinary Regression	Ordinary Regression with Empirical
Intercept	8.59 (0.447)	8.59 (0.381)
Age (per year)	0.27 (0.0413)	0.27 (0.0414)

range of rise, up to (and including) age 15. The restriction results in a sample size
of $n = 274$. We first fit an ordinary regression by PROC REG. The regression
coefficients are in Table 6.1, and the original output and residual plot are included
in OUTPUT PACKET III. We see the increase in residual variance with increasing
predicted value of GHb.

Then we used PROC MIXED to obtain robust standard errors as above:

**PROC MIXED NOCLPRINT EMPIRICAL; CLASS ID;
MODEL GHB=AGE/S;
REPEATED/SUBJECT=ID;**

As expected, the estimates of the regression coefficients themselves did not
change with the EMPIRICAL option. This is always true, since EMPIRICAL does
not interfere in that part of the analysis. In our analysis, we see that the standard
errors did not change much either and that there was actually a decrease in the
standard error of the intercept with the empirical option. One may conjecture that
this may be caused by many rather outlying GHb residuals that made the initial $s_{y|x}^2$
large. We can view the robust analysis as a confirmation that tests and confidence
intervals from the original analysis are not too far off. However, we will see below
that the efficiency of the analysis can be improved by taking the unequal variance
into account in estimation in a more pervasive manner.

After adding gender, age, bmi, and the age by bmi interaction to the regression of
systolic blood pressure from visit 1 in the Wisconsin Sleep Cohort Study, inequality
of the residual variance seems to be present also in this analysis. OUTPUT PACKET
III shows a residual plot. We ran the commands

**PROC MIXED NOCLPRINT EMPIRICAL; CLASS SEX ID;
MODEL SBP=SEX AGE BMIC AGEC*BMIC/S;
REPEATED/SUBJECT=ID;
PROC REG; MODEL SBP=GENDER AGEC BMIC AGEC_BMIC;
OUTPUT OUT=RRR=RESID P=PRED; PROC PLOT; PLOT RESID*PRED;**

Here, the variables entered are as defined in the last example in Chapter 5.
Results are summarized in Table 6.2.

We see that in this case the empirical option has generally increased the estimates
of the standard errors.

Table 6.2   Regression Coefficients (se) Modeling SBP in Wisconsin Sleep Cohort

	Ordinary Regression		Ordinary Regression with Empirical	
Intercept	127	(0.525)	127	(0.549)
Female	−6.57	(0.732)	−6.57	(0.726)
Age (per year—centered at age 50)	0.369	(0.495)	0.369	(0.0510)
BMI (centered 27)	0.595	(0.0656)	0.595	(0.0720)
Age *BMI (centered)	−0.0189	(0.00750)	−0.0189	(0.00888)

6.2   ANALYSIS TAKING UNEQUAL VARIANCE INTO ACCOUNT

Although the above analysis using unweighted ordinary regression is not wrong, it is not efficient. In the rest of this chapter we will discuss approaches that more directly deal with situations that violate the equal variance assumption of ordinary regression analysis.

6.2.1   The Functional Transformation Approach

A very standard and technically easy approach is to take a mathematical transformation of the outcome variable Y. There is a formula (derived by Taylor expansion) that is handy for choosing a transformation f:

$$\text{Var}[f(y)] \approx [f'(\mu_y)]^2 \, \text{Var}(y)$$

The most common use of this formula is to see that when $sd(y)$ is proportional to μ_y (i.e., $\text{Var}(y) = c\mu_y^2$), taking the log of y leads to approximately equal variance across μ_y. Because $f'(\mu_y)$ is then $1/\mu_y$, we have

$$[f'(\mu_y)]^2 \, \text{Var}(y) = \left(\frac{1}{\mu_y}\right)^2 (c\mu_y^2) = c$$

that is, constant. When $\text{Var}(y)$ is proportional to μ_y, taking the square root of y works to equalize the variance. The residual plot, or calculating the variance in subgroups of predicted value, may give a clue as to how the variance changes with the mean.

The log and square root transformations have the additional effect of pulling in upper tails of the error distribution. This is often helpful in improving normality. However, in situations with a few low values, the log transformation aggravates the problem of outliers on the low end. Obviously, linearity may also be destroyed after transforming y, making additional transformations of x or polynomial terms

Table 6.3   Regression Coefficients (se) Modeling Transformed GHb on Age

	Inverse GHb	Inverse $\hat{\beta}/se(\hat{\beta})$	Original (Empirical) $\hat{\beta}/se(\hat{\beta})$
Intercept	0.111 (0.00331)	33.4	22.5
GHb per %	−0.00190 (0.000306)	−6.22	6.57

necessary. Technically, linearity cannot hold for both the untransformed and transformed models, although it may nearly hold in some regions of the covariates.

6.2.1.1   Example
The residual plot of GHb as predicted by age shows a rather steep increase in residual standard deviation with predicted values, especially when the predicted value is at the upper end. We may conjecture that the standard deviation increases proportionally to the predicted value squared in this case. Then $\text{Var}(y|x)$ increases proportionally to μ_y^4, so $f'(\mu_y)$ needs to be $\pm 1/\mu_y^2$. Consequently, the function f should be chosen as the inverse $1/y$.

Analyses in OUTPUT PACKET IV are based on taking the inverse of GHb and predicting this transformed variable by age. The residual plot in the PACKET implies that after the transformation, the variance of the residuals is more or less constant. Table 6.3 shows the estimated regression coefficients. We calculated values for $\hat{\beta}/se(\hat{\beta})$ for this model as well as for the empirical option above to assess any gain in efficiency from using a model where the equal variance assumption more nearly holds. We see that there was no gain. (Note that the intercepts cannot be compared.) This is because GHb is quite linear in age, while an equation that is linear in age somewhat overestimates 1/GHb at the higher ages. This nonlinearity of the transformed outcome is not statistically significant, but its presence prevented the gain in efficiency which might otherwise have resulted from equalizing the variance.

The interpretation of the coefficients on the inverse scale is that a unit increase in a covariate leads to a change of $\hat{\beta}$ in mean of the inverse of the outcome. This interpretation is not very satisfactory for practical purposes.

6.2.1.2   Interpretation of log on log Regression- and Another Example
In some applications, investigators have preferred, or become used to, transformed variables. Traditionally, regression coefficients from modeling the log of an outcome on the log of a predictor has held special importance in econometrics. There, the resulting regression coefficient is referred to as an *elasticity*, and it is interpreted as the percent increase in the mean outcome with one percent increase in the predictor. The basis for this interpretation comes from Taylor approximation. Since for μ_{y_2}/μ_{y_1} close to 1 we have

$$\log(\mu_{y_2}) - \log(\mu_{y_1}) = \log(\mu_{y_2}/\mu_{y_1}) \approx \mu_{y_2}/\mu_{y_1} - 1$$

and a similar approximation holds for x, it follows that

$$\log(\mu_{y|x_2}) - \log(\mu_{y|x_1}) = \beta_1[\log(x_2) - \log(x_1)]$$

can be approximated

$$\mu_{y_2}/\mu_{y_1} - 1 \approx \beta_1[x_2/x_1 - 1]$$

and the interpretation follows.

As may be expected, the elasticity concept has been particularly applied to costs and prices. Even there, it may be argued that an absolute interpretation of expenses, and so on, may be more desirable. However, the elasticity has the advantage of being independent of currency used, as well as independent of change in the value of currency over time.

6.2.1.3   *Example*

OUTPUT PACKET IV also contains a regression analysis of the quarterly cost in dollars of medical care in the Wisconsin Sleep Cohort [11] as predicted by an individual's gender and BMI. Analysis on the original scale and its residual plot indicates violation of the linearity assumption, extreme skewness in the residuals, and possibly inequality of variance toward the higher end of predicted value. Skewness of this type is especially common when modeling the cost of care in a basically healthy population.

The outcome variable was transformed as $\log(\text{cost} + 10)$, where 10 was added so that individuals with 0 cost during the data collection period could be included. We see marked improvement in the residual plot (except almost unavoidable nonlinearity for the 0 values, which could be dealt with by more advanced methods such as a tobit model or by a two-part model [12]). The interpretation of the regression coefficients is that a 1% increase in BMI leads to approximately 0.53% increase in cost of medical care (+10) and that men's cost of medical care is $\exp(-0.389) = 0.68$ of women's.

6.2.1.4   *Comment*

Examples 6.2.1.1 and 6.2.1.3 illustrate that the functional transformation approach at first appears convenient. However, it can destroy linearity and normality of the data. Also, the desirability of the transformation approach depends on the application. In some situations the regression coefficients in the transformed equation make perfect sense. Other times, the practical usefulness of the equation is much reduced by transformations. For further discussion of these issues see Manning and Mullahy [13].

6.2.2   The Linear Transformation Approach

When we apply transformations such as the log to the left-hand side of the regression equation, we may destroy linearity. In addition, the meaning of the regression coefficients is changed. To preserve the meaning with a transformation, one would need to transform the whole right-hand side of the regression equation. For example, if the true regression equation is

$$y_i = \beta_0 + \beta_1 x_i + \epsilon_i \tag{6.2}$$

the new equation after taking the log of y, with the meaning of the regression coefficients preserved, would be

$$\log(y_i) = \log(\beta_0 + \beta_1 x_i + \epsilon_i)$$

But this is no longer a linear equation. The coefficients and error term are both inside a log, making estimation complicated.

To preserve the structure of equation (6.1), we need to apply a linear transformation. At the end of this section we will see that the appropriate choice of linear transformation combined with unweighted least-squares estimation is equivalent to weighted least-squares estimation. In fact, it is most common to take the latter shortcut in practice. We first present the linear transformation perspective, because it provides the justification for weighted least-squares estimation. The same derivation, in more mathematical form, is found in almost all other books that present the theory of regression analysis (see, e.g., Draper and Smith [14]).

If we know the variance of each y_i, it turns out to be fairly easy to find a linear transformation that equalizes the variance around the regression line. Of course, this is not usually the case, but we make the assumption for illustration of the transformation principle. Assume that $\mathrm{Var}(y_i|x_i) = \mathrm{Var}(\epsilon_i) = \sigma_i^2$. If we have the regression equation

$$y_i = \beta_0 + \beta_1 x_i + \epsilon_i$$

and divide each side by σ_i, we obtain

$$\frac{y_i}{\sigma_i} = \beta_0 \frac{1}{\sigma_i} + \beta_1 \frac{x_i}{\sigma_i} + \frac{\epsilon_i}{\sigma_i}$$

or

$$\underline{\mathrm{new}}\, y_i = \beta_0 \underline{\mathrm{new}}\,\mathrm{variable} + \beta_1 \underline{\mathrm{new}}\, x_i + \underline{\mathrm{new}}\, \epsilon_i$$

where now, because of the way the transformation was chosen, $\underline{\mathrm{new}}\ \epsilon_i$ have the same variance along the regression line, because $\mathrm{Var}(\underline{\mathrm{new}}\epsilon_i) = \mathrm{Var}(\frac{\epsilon_i}{\sigma_i}) = \frac{1}{\sigma_i^2}\sigma_i^2 = 1$, which is constant. (Recall that $\mathrm{Var}(t_1 y) = t_1^2\,\mathrm{Var}(y)$.) We can also write $\sigma_i^2 = c_i \sigma^2$, and transform the original equation by

$$\frac{y_i}{\sqrt{c_i}} = \beta_0 \frac{1}{\sqrt{c_i}} + \beta_1 \frac{x_i}{\sqrt{c_i}} + \frac{\epsilon_i}{\sqrt{c_i}} \tag{6.3}$$

In this regression equation, the new residual has constant variance σ^2.

We will proceed in matrix notation to see what estimator we end up with. Define the matrix

$$P = \begin{pmatrix} \sigma\sqrt{c_1} & 0 & \cdots \\ 0 & \sigma\sqrt{c_2} & \cdots \\ \vdots & \vdots & \ddots \end{pmatrix}$$

which has $\sqrt{\mathrm{Var}(\epsilon_i)}$ on the diagonal. Because taking the inverse of a diagonal matrix amounts to taking the regular inverses of all the elements on the diagonal, we have

$$P^{-1} = \begin{pmatrix} \frac{1}{\sigma\sqrt{c_1}} & 0 & \cdots \\ 0 & \frac{1}{\sigma\sqrt{c_2}} & \cdots \\ \vdots & \vdots & \ddots \end{pmatrix}$$

Then (6.3) can be written in matrix notation as

$$\sigma P^{-1}Y = \sigma P^{-1}X\beta + \underline{\text{new}\epsilon}$$

where $\mathrm{Var}(\text{new } \epsilon) = \sigma^2 I$. We use P^{-1} rather than T to denote the transformation matrix here to better conform with the notation in this context of standard books on regression analysis and the analysis of variance.

Now we can obtain an efficient (BLUE) estimator by the ordinary least-squares equation using new quantities $\underline{\text{new}}X = \sigma P^{-1}X$, and so on, in matrix form

$$\begin{aligned} \hat{\beta} &= [\underline{\text{new}}X'\underline{\text{new}}X]^{-1}[\underline{\text{new}}X'\underline{\text{new}}Y] \\ &= [(\sigma P^{-1}X)'\sigma P^{-1}X]^{-1}[(\sigma P^{-1}X)'\sigma P^{-1}Y] \\ &= [X'\sigma P^{-1}\sigma P^{-1}X]^{-1}[X'\sigma P^{-1}\sigma P^{-1}Y] \\ &= \frac{1}{\sigma^2}[X'P^{-1}P^{-1}X]^{-1}[X'P^{-1}P^{-1}Y]\sigma^2 \\ &= [X'P^{-1}P^{-1}X]^{-1}[X'P^{-1}P^{-1}Y] \end{aligned}$$

We have applied the usual matrix formula for a linear regression estimator, the formula for the transpose of a product so that $(P^{-1}X)' = X'[P^{-1}]'$, and the fact that P^{-1} is symmetric (all diagonal matrices are symmetric). We now see that

$$P^{-1}P^{-1} = \begin{pmatrix} \frac{1}{\mathrm{Var}(\epsilon_1)} & 0 & 0 \\ 0 & \ddots & 0 \\ 0 & 0 & \frac{1}{\mathrm{Var}(\epsilon_n)} \end{pmatrix} = V^{-1}$$

where V is the variance matrix of ϵ, or equivalently $V = \text{Var}(Y|X)$. Then we can write

$$\hat{\beta} = [X'V^{-1}X]^{-1}[X'V^{-1}Y] \tag{6.4}$$

Equation (6.4) is the ordinary least-squares estimator for the transformed equation. Because of the way we derived it, we know that (6.4) gives an efficient estimator of the original β. For practical purposes, it is good to note that it doesn't matter whether we use the actual V^{-1} or $\sigma^2 V^{-1}$ in formula (6.4). By the rules of how constants multiply matrices (Property 14 in the list in Chapter 3) σ^2 cancels in (6.4), and we only need to specify c_i.

More generally, if we are not sure of V^{-1}, we can write

$$\hat{\beta}_W = [X'WX]^{-1}[X'WY] \tag{6.5}$$

where $\hat{\beta}_W$ is a general weighted least-squares estimator. It is important to note that as long as $E(Y|X) = X\beta$, $E(\hat{\beta}_W) = [X'WX]^{-1}[X'WX]\beta = \beta$, so the estimator (6.5) is unbiased even if W is not V^{-1}. It may not be efficient.

The above framework is hard to implement exactly as presented, because we do not usually know c_i (or σ_i^2), so we can't directly know what V^{-1} to use in (6.4). Using the "empirical" formula $s_i^2 = (y_i - \hat{\beta}_0 - \hat{\beta}_1 x_{1i} - \hat{\beta}_2 x_{2i} \cdots)^2$ for each i is out, because the number of estimators would increase with the number of subjects n, so we would not have consistency. Potentially, subjects could be grouped to produce a limited number of s_i^2. We will illustrate another route that is more in line with the functional approach above, and also with the context of generalized linear models (Chapter 12).

As indicated above, the residual variance often changes systematically with $\mu_{y|x}$, and we may glean information on how, from the residual plot of the residuals on the predicted values. The spread of residuals in that plot is an approximate presentation of how the standard deviation changes with the predicted value. We can then choose c_i as a function of $\mu_{y|x}$, $g(\mu_{y|x})$. In reality this means that we first have to estimate the regression line by ordinary regression and then use the predicted values $\hat{\mu}_{y_i|x_i}$ in the weights. For example, if we think that the residual standard deviation is proportional to the predicted value, we can choose c_i as $(\mu_{y_i|x_i})^2$ and weight by the matrix with $(1/\hat{\mu}_{y_i|x_i})^2$ on the diagonal. Most computer programs require specification of these diagonal elements. It should be noted that we have ignored interpretation and estimation of σ^2 here.

6.2.2.1 Example
OUTPUT PACKET V has further analyses of GHb versus age at approximately four years' diabetes duration. Initial analyses above had shown that the standard deviation around the regression line may be increasing approximately proportionally to the square of the predicted value. To illustrate the above transformation, we

Table 6.4 Regression Coefficients (se) Modeling GHb to Ages up to 15 Years by Weighted Regression

	Weighted Regression		Weighted with Empirical		Ordinary with Empirical	
Intercept	8.63	(0.366)	8.63	(0.346)	8.59	(0.381)
Age (per year)	0.268	(0.0371)	0.268	(0.0376)	0.272	(0.0414)

first fit the ordinary regression line and obtain the predicted values. We then choose

$$W = \begin{pmatrix} \frac{1}{\hat{\mu}_{y_1|x_1}^4} & 0 & 0 \\ 0 & \ddots & 0 \\ 0 & 0 & \frac{1}{\hat{\mu}_{y_n|x_n}^4} \end{pmatrix}$$

so that the diagonal is proportional to the inverse of the variance for each observation. In SAS, formula (6.4) can be implemented by both PROC REG and PROC MIXED, by commands such as those below:

PROC REG; MODEL GHB=AGE;
OUTPUT OUT=RR P=PRED R=RESID;
DATA NEW; SET RR;
WGT=1/PRED**4;
PROC REG;
MODEL GHB=AGE;
WEIGHT WGT;

The results are in the second column of Table 6.4:

Furthermore, we implement the transformation to examine the behavior of the new residuals by the commands:

PROC REG; MODEL GHB=AGE; OUTPUT OUT=RR P=PRED;
DATA NEW; SET RR;
NGHB=GHB/PRED**2;
NINT=1/PRED**2;
NAGE=AGE/PRED**2;
PROC REG; MODEL NGHB=NINT NAGE/NOINT;
OUTPUT OUT=XX R=NRESID P=NPRED;
PROC PLOT; PLOT NRESID*NPRED;

Note that while the weights are inverses of the predicted value to the fourth power, the transformation multiplies by the square root of that weight. The /NOINT option is used to avoid the fitting of the intercept. (Regression equation (6.3) does not have an intercept in the usual sense.) We see in OUTPUT PACKET V that the residual plot from the transformed regression displays a more constant residual variance than the corresponding plot from the untransformed regression.

In Table 6.4 there is a slight difference between the coefficients from the unweighted and weighted estimation. For example, the coefficient of age is 0.272 in the original regression and is 0.268 in the weighted regression. This is a minor change. Because the unweighted estimators are unbiased, there should not be a major difference between the weighted and unweighted estimators when the model is correct. In fact, there is a goodness-of-fit test for regression, called the Hausman test, that is essentially based on this principle [15]. This test is quite widely used in econometrics.

We should be aware that we still have not weighted the regression estimators in the best way because the above procedure obtained the predicted values for the weights from the unweighted regression. The predicted values of GHb from the weighted regression are, of course, slightly different. We can compute them and repeat the estimation process to slightly improve efficiency. We could also apply maximum likelihood directly on the normal, unequal variance structure implied. PROC GENMOD, which we address in Chapter 11, can do this with an *iterative* procedure of updating parameter estimates. Unweighted regression can be fit without iteration by either least-squares or maximum likelihood only because the regression parameter estimates can be obtained independently of the variance estimate in that special case.

6.2.3   Standard Errors of Weighted Regression Estimators

We can derive the variance matrix of a weighted regression estimator by again using formula (4.3) for the variance of a linear transformation. Also, because we may be either quite sure of the variance or not so sure, we can derive the standard errors without and with the empirical approach. In this context the estimators that assume that we know V^{-1} are called "model-based." In formula (6.5) the linear transformation of Y uses the matrix

$$T' = [X'WX]^{-1}[X'W]$$

and we have

$$\hat{\boldsymbol{\beta}}_W = T'Y$$

Then applying the linear transformation variance formula

$$\text{Var}(\hat{\boldsymbol{\beta}}_W) = [X'WX]^{-1}[X'W]\,\text{Var}(Y|X)[W'X][X'WX]^{-1} \qquad (6.6)$$

by the same principles as in the unweighted case. For the model-based situation, we assume

$$W = [\text{Var}(Y|X)]^{-1} = V^{-1}$$

so we can insert W^{-1} for $\text{Var}(Y|X)$, obtaining

$$\text{Var}(\hat{\boldsymbol{\beta}}_W) = [X'WX]^{-1}[X'W]\,\text{Var}(Y|X)[W'X][X'WX]^{-1}$$
$$= [X'WX]^{-1}[X'W]W^{-1}[W'X][X'WX]^{-1}$$
$$= [X'WX]^{-1}[X'WX][X'WX]^{-1}$$

which equals

$$\text{Var}(\hat{\boldsymbol{\beta}}_W) = [X'WX]^{-1} \tag{6.7}$$

Note also that in the special case of equal variance we have

$$W = (\sigma^2 I)^{-1} = \frac{1}{\sigma^2}I$$

and (6.7) simplifies to the usual

$$\text{Var}(\hat{\boldsymbol{\beta}}) = \sigma^2 (X'X)^{-1}$$

In the situation when we are not quite sure of the variance $\text{Var}(Y|X)$ or have used only one iteration to obtain it, we can use the empirical approach, parallel to formula (6.1). Inserting $\hat{\boldsymbol{\epsilon}}\hat{\boldsymbol{\epsilon}}'$ for $\text{Var}(Y|X)$, we obtain

$$\hat{\text{Var}}(\hat{\boldsymbol{\beta}}) = (X'WX)^{-1}X'W\hat{\boldsymbol{\epsilon}}\hat{\boldsymbol{\epsilon}}'WX(X'WX)^{-1} \tag{6.8}$$

The prime has been removed from W as in situations of interest in practice; W is always taken as symmetric. PROC MIXED can be requested to use formula (6.8) by the EMPIRICAL OPTION. Using the ALL option PROC REG ALL; includes the same result under the heading "consistent variance matrix" in the massive output produced, but this seems more cumbersome than using PROC MIXED EMPIRICAL.

Note again that the approach in formula (6.8) is appropriate when we either know or suspect that W is not exactly V^{-1}.

6.2.3.1 Example

Table 6.4 contains both model-based and empirical standard error estimates for the weighted regression of GHb on age. We see that again the model-based and empirical coefficients are the same. Comparison of the empirical estimates for weighted and unweighted options indicates a gain in efficiency with weighting.

OUTPUT PACKET III: APPLYING THE EMPIRICAL OPTION TO ADJUST STANDARD ERRORS

III.1. Regressing GHb on Age in Wisconsin Diabetes Registry

Analysis of GHb Versus Age for Those Less than 15 Years Old
The REG Procedure

Model: MODEL1
Dependent Variable: GHb at about 4 years of diabetes

Analysis of Variance

Source	DF	Sum of Squares	Mean Square	F Value	Pr > F
Model	1	205.87840	205.87840	43.22	<0.0001
Error	272	1295.67016	4.76349		
Corrected total	273	1501.54856			

Root MSE	2.18254	*R*-square	0.1371	
Dependent mean	11.40352	Adjusted *R*-square	0.1339	
Coefficient of variation	19.13921			

Parameter Estimates

Variable	Label	DF	Parameter Estimate	Standard Error	t Value
Intercept	Intercept	1	8.59390	0.44725	19.22
Age	Age	1	0.27154	0.04130	6.57

Parameter Estimates

Variable	Label	DF	Pr > |t|
Intercept	Intercept	1	<0.0001
Age	Age	1	<0.0001

Regression Analyses of GHb Versus Age
Original Residual Plot

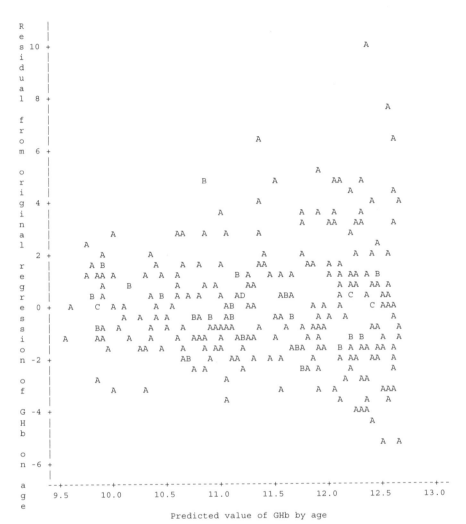

Predicted value of GHb by age

Plot of resid*pred. Legend: A = 1 obs, B = 2 obs, and so on.

Unweighted Regression with Empirical Option
  The Mixed Procedure

Model Information

Data set	WORK.RES
Dependent variable	Ghb
Covariance structure	Variance components
Subject effect	Id
Estimation method	REML
Residual variance method	Parameter
Fixed effects SE method	**Empirical**
Degrees-of-freedom method	Between–within

Dimensions

Covariance parameters	1
Columns in X	2
Columns in Z	0
Subjects	274
Maximum observations per subject	1
Observations used	274
Observations not used	0
Total observations	274

Iteration History[a]

Iteration	Evaluations	−2 Res Log-Likelihood	Criterion
0	1	1210.03720983	
1	1	1210.03720983	0.00000000

[a] Convergence criteria met.

Covariance Parameter Estimates

Covariance Parameter	Subject	Estimate
Residual	id	4.7635

Fit Statistics

−2 Residual log likelihood	1210.0
AIC (smaller is better)	1212.0
AICC (smaller is better)	1212.1
BIC (smaller is better)	1215.7

Null Model Likelihood Ratio Test

DF	Chi-Square	Pr > ChiSq
0	0.00	1.0000

Solution for Fixed Effects

Effect	Estimate	Standard Error	DF	t Value	Pr > $|t|$
Intercept	8.5939	0.3814	272	22.53	<0.0001
Age	0.2715	0.04135	272	6.57	<0.0001

Type 3 Tests of Fixed Effects

Effect	Num DF	Den DF	F Value	Pr > F
Age	1	272	43.12	<0.0001

III.2. Regressing SBP Versus Age, BMI, and Sex—Wisconsin Sleep Cohort

Unequal Variance Example, Wisconsin Sleep Cohort Study
Ordinary Regression and Residual Plot for SBP Versus Age Gender and BMI
The REG Procedure

Model: MODEL1
Dependent Variable: SBP, systolic blood pressure

Analysis of Variance

Source	DF	Sum of Squares	Mean Square	F Value	Pr > F
Model	4	50562	12641	71.18	<.0001
Error	1359	241336	177.58357		
Corrected total	1363	291898			

Root MSE	13.32605	R-square	0.1732	
Dependent mean	125.09176	Adjusted R-square	0.1708	
Coefficient of variation	10.65302			

Parameter Estimates

Variable	Label	DF	Parameter Estimate
Intercept	Intercept	1	127.44900
gender		1	−6.57305
agec	Age centered at 50	1	0.36912
bmic		1	0.59454
agec_bmic	Interaction with age centered at 50, bmi at 27	1	−0.01892

Variable	Label	DF	Standard Error	t Value
Intercept	Intercept	1	0.52502	242.75
gender		1	0.73184	−8.98
agec	Age centered at 50	1	0.04946	7.46
bmic		1	0.06556	9.07
agec_bmic	Interaction with age centered at 50, bmi at 27	1	0.00750	−2.52

Variable	Label	DF	Pr > |t|
Intercept	Intercept	1	<0.0001
gender		1	<0.0001
agec	Age centered at 50	1	<0.0001
bmic		1	<0.0001
agec_bmic	Interaction with age centered at 50, bmi at 27	1	0.0117

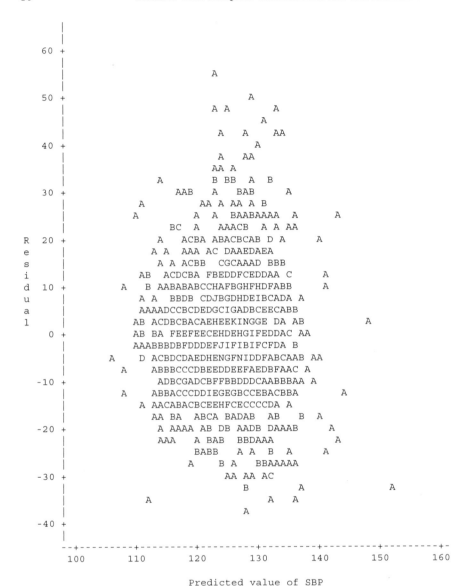

Plot of resid*pred. Legend: A = 1 obs, B = 2 obs, and so on.

Applying the Empirical Option to Regression of SBP Versus Age Gender and BMI
  The Mixed Procedure

Model Information

Data set	WORK.RR
Dependent variable	sbp
Covariance structure	Variance components
Subject effect	id
Estimation method	REML
Residual variance method	Parameter
Fixed effects SE method	Empirical
Degrees-of-freedom method	Between–within

Dimensions

Covariance parameters	1
Columns in X	6
Columns in Z	0
Subjects	1373
Maximum observations per subject	1
Observations used	1370
Observations not used	6
Total observations	1370

Iteration History[a]

Iteration	Evaluations	−2 Res Log-Likelihood	Criterion
0	1	10945.85019390	
1	1	10945.85019389	0.00000000

[a] Convergence criteria met.

Covariance Parameter Estimates

Covariance Parameter	Subject	Estimate
Residual	id	177.58

Fit Statistics

−2 Res log-likelihood	10945.9
AIC (smaller is better)	10947.9
AICC (smaller is better)	10947.9
BIC (smaller is better)	10953.1

Null Model Likelihood Ratio Test

DF	Chi-Square	Pr > ChiSq
0	0.00	1.0000

Solution for Fixed Effects

Effect	Sex	Estimate	Standard Error	DF	t Value	Pr > $|t|$
Intercept		127.45	0.5494	1359	231.96	<0.0001
sex	F	−6.5731	0.7263	1359	−9.05	<0.0001
sex	M	0	.	.	.	.
agec		0.3691	0.05103	1359	7.23	<0.0001
bmic		0.5945	0.07196	1359	8.26	<0.0001
agec*bmic		−0.01892	0.008882	1359	−2.13	0.0334

Type 3 Tests of Fixed Effects

Effect	Num DF	Den DF	F Value	Pr > F
sex	1	1359	81.90	<.0001
agec	1	1359	52.33	<.0001
bmic	1	1359	68.26	<.0001
agec*bmic	1	1359	4.54	0.0334

OUTPUT PACKET IV: ANALYSES WITH TRANSFORMATION OF THE OUTCOME VARIABLE TO EQUALIZE RESIDUAL VARIANCE

IV.1. Analysis of Inverse of GHb Versus Age—Wisconsin Diabetes Registry

Analysis of GHb Versus Age for Those Less than 15 Years Old
Regression of Inverse GHb Versus Age
  The REG Procedure

Model: MODEL1
Dependent Variable: fghb

Analysis of Variance

Source	DF	Sum of Squares	Mean Square	F Value	Pr > F
Model	1	0.01013	0.01013	38.72	<.0001
Error	272	0.07113	0.00026152		
Corrected total	273	0.08126			

Root MSE	0.01617	R-square	0.1246	
Dependent mean	0.09108	Adjusted R-square	0.1214	
Coefficient of variation	17.75486			

Parameter Estimates

Variable	Label	DF	Parameter Estimate	Standard Error	t Value	Pr > |t|
Intercept	Intercept	1	0.11079	0.00331	33.43	<0.0001
Age	Age	1	−0.00190	0.00030604	−6.22	<0.0001

Residual Plot from Regression of Inverse GHb

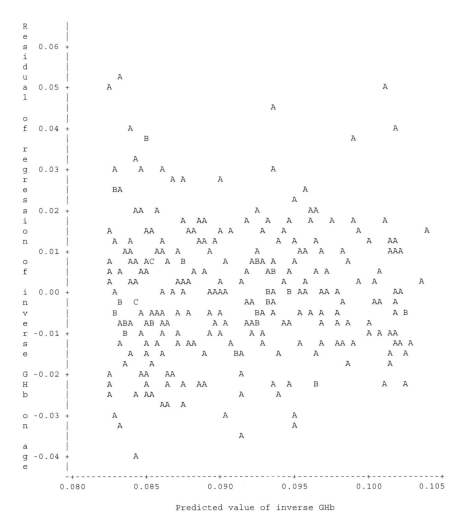

Predicted value of inverse GHb

Plot of fres*fpred. Legend: A = 1 obs, B = 2 obs, and so on.

IV.2. Analysis of Cost Data from Wisconsin Sleep Cohort

Analysis of Medical Cost Data—Wisconsin Sleep Cohort
Regression Analysis of Untransformed Data
The REG Procedure

Model: MODEL1
Dependent Variable: avcost—average cost of medical care per quarter

Analysis of Variance

Source	DF	Sum of Squares	Mean Square	F Value	Pr > F
Model	2	816335	408168	12.03	<.0001
Error	686	23269242	33920		
Corrected total	688	24085578			

Root MSE	184.17431	R-square	0.0339
Dependent mean	150.47676	Adjusted R-square	0.0311
Coefficient of variation	122.39386		

Parameter Estimates

Variable	Label	DF	Parameter Estimate	Standard Error	t Value
Intercept	Intercept	1	117.98755	36.06740	3.27
Gender		1	−62.93287	14.21548	−4.43
BMI	Body Mass Index (kg/m^2)	1	2.37457	1.17892	2.01

Parameter Estimates

Variable	Label	DF	Pr > |t|
Intercept	Intercept	1	0.0011
Gender		1	<0.0001
BMI	Body Mass Index (kg/m^2)	1	0.0444

Residual Plot from Untransformed Analysis

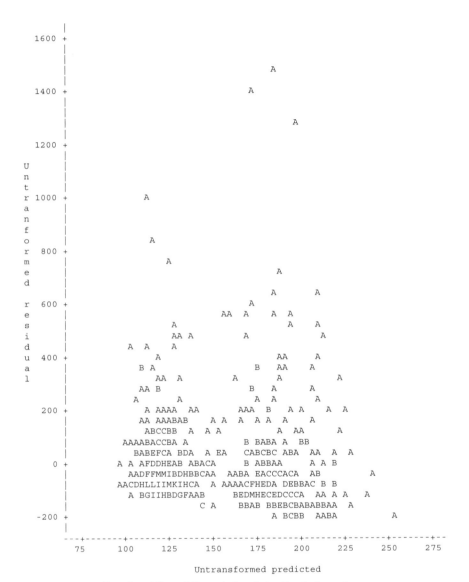

Plot of oresid*ppred. Legend: A = 1 obs, B = 2 obs, and so on.

Histogram of Untransformed Residuals
  The UNIVARIATE Procedure

Variable: oresid (untransformed residual)

Moments

N	689	Sum of weights	689
Mean	0	Sum of observations	0
Standard deviation	183.906425	Variance	33821.5731
Skewness	3.36346689	Kurtosis	17.4059317
Uncorrected SS	23269242.3	Corrected SS	23269242.3
Coefficient of variation	.	Standard error of mean	7.00627679

Basic Statistical Measures

Location		Variability	
Mean	0.0000	Standard deviation	183.90642
Median	−55.7239	Variance	33822
Mode	.	Range	1709
		Interquartile range	136.85957

Tests for Location: Mu0 = 0

Test		Statistic		p Value	
Student's t	t	0	Pr > $|t|$	1.0000
Sign	M	−120.5	Pr > $|M|$	<0.0001
Signed rank	S	−34638.5	Pr > $|S|$	<0.0001

Quantiles (Definition 5)

Quantile	Estimate
100% Max	1493.6630
99%	710.1336
95%	359.8459
90%	198.2884
75% Q3	36.1587
50% Median	−55.7239
25% Q1	−100.7009
10%	−132.7012
5%	−156.5006
1%	−189.8031
0% Min	−215.6743

Extreme Observations

Lowest		Highest	
Value	Observed	Value	Observed
−215.674	543	857.664	339
−211.572	401	1016.734	164
−200.984	207	1294.453	48
−199.359	151	1408.392	683
−198.138	231	1493.663	4

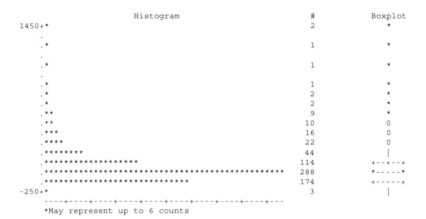

```
                        Histogram                          #         Boxplot
  1450+*                                                    2            *
      .
      .*                                                    1            *
      .
      .*                                                    1            *
      .
      .*                                                    1            *
      .*                                                    2            *
      .*                                                    2            *
      .**                                                   9            *
      .**                                                  10            0
      .***                                                 16            0
      .****                                                22            0
      .********                                            44            |
      .******************                                 114         +--+--+
      .***************************************************288         *-----*
      .****************************                       174         +-----+
  -250+*                                                    3            |
      ----+----+----+----+----+----+----+----+----+---
      *May represent up to 6 counts
```

The UNIVARIATE Procedure

Variable: oresid (untransformed residual)

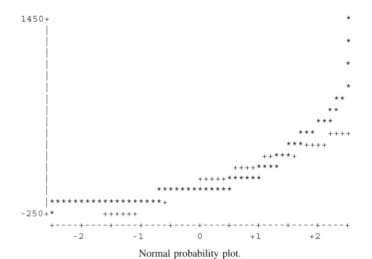

Normal probability plot.

Regression Analysis with Log-Transformed Outcome
  The REG Procedure

Model: MODEL1
Dependent Variable: lcost log cost + 10

Analysis of Variance

Source	DF	Sum of Squares	Mean Square	F Value	Pr > F
Model	2	32.73356	16.36678	16.68	<0.0001
Error	686	673.24538	0.98141		
Corrected total	688	705.97895			

Root MSE	0.99066	R-square	0.0464	
Dependent mean	4.59310	Adjusted R-square	0.0436	
Coefficient of variation	21.56843			

Parameter Estimates

Variable	Label	DF	Parameter Estimate	Standard Error	t Value	Pr > |t|
Intercept	Intercept	1	3.03979	0.64783	4.69	<.0001
Gender		1	−0.38919	0.07645	−5.09	<.0001
lbmi	log bmi	1	0.53116	0.19275	2.76	0.0060

Residual Plot from Transformed Regression Analysis

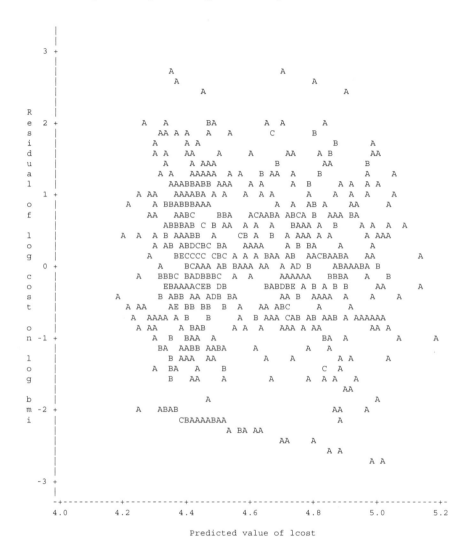

Predicted value of lcost

Plot of resid*pred. Legend: A = 1 obs, B = 2 obs, and so on.

Histogram of Residuals from Transformed Analysis
  The UNIVARIATE Procedure

Variable: resid (residual of log cost on log bmi)

Moments

N	689	Sum of weights	689
Mean	0	Sum of observations	0
Standard deviation	0.98921905	Variance	0.97855434
Skewness	−0.1833497	Kurtosis	0.05761522
Uncorrected SS	673.245384	Corrected SS	673.245384
Coefficient of variation	.	Standard error of mean	0.03768624

Basic Statistical Measures

Location		Variability	
Mean	0.000000	Standard deviation	0.98922
Median	0.025537	Variance	0.97855
Mode	.	Range	5.40296
		Interquartile range	1.27033

Tests for Location: Mu0 = 0

Test		Statistic		p Value	
Student's t	t	0	Pr > $|t|$	1.0000
Sign	M	5.5	Pr > $|M|$	0.7033
Signed rank	S	2126.5	Pr > $|S|$	0.6844

Quantiles (Definition 5)

Quantile	Estimate
100% Max	2.6914562
99%	2.0543739
95%	1.6107023
90%	1.2552759
75% Q3	0.6698180
50% Median	0.0255368
25% Q1	−0.6005144
10%	−1.2781850
5%	−2.0140941
1%	−2.3903305
0% Min	−2.7115048

Extreme Observations

Lowest		Highest	
Value	Observations	Value	Observations
−2.71150	543	2.40959	48
−2.68872	401	2.52120	339
−2.58157	668	2.62856	4
−2.54808	286	2.67868	683
−2.41839	497	2.69146	164

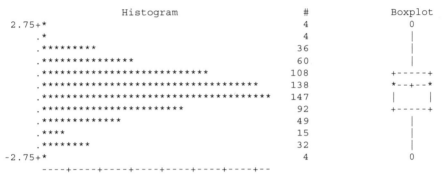

```
              Histogram                    #          Boxplot
 2.75+*                                     4              0
     .*                                     4              |
     .********                             36              |
     .***************                      60              |
     .**************************           108         +-----+
     .************************************ 138         *--+--*
     .*************************************147         |     |
     .**********************                92         +-----+
     .*************                         49              |
     .****                                  15              |
     .********                              32              |
-2.75+*                                      4              0
     ----+----+----+----+----+----+----+--
     *May represent up to 4 counts
```

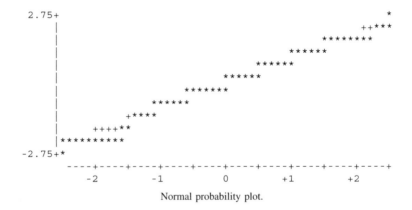

```
 2.75+                                                    *
      |                                               ++***
      |                                            *******
      |                                          ******
      |                                   ******
      |                                 ******
      |                         *******
      |                    ******
      |               +****
      |          ++++**
      |*********
-2.75+*
     ----+----+----+----+----+----+----+----+----+----+
        -2       -1        0       +1        +2
```

Normal probability plot.

OUTPUT PACKET V: WEIGHTED REGRESSION ANALYSES OF GHb DATA ON AGE

Weighted Regression Analyses of GHb—Wisconsin Diabetes Registry
Weighted Regression with Weights Based on Predicted**4
  The REG Procedure

Model: MODEL1
Dependent Variable: ghb GHB at about 4 years of diabetes
Weight: WGT

Analysis of Variance

Source	DF	Sum of Squares	Mean Square	F Value	Pr > F
Model	1	0.01337	0.01337	52.36	<.0001
Error	272	0.06943	0.00025526		
Corrected total	273	0.08280			

Root MSE	0.01598	R-square	0.1614	
Dependent mean	11.12560	Adjusted R-square	0.1583	
Coefficient of variation	0.14360			

Parameter Estimates

Variable	Label	DF	Parameter Estimate	Standard Error	t Value
Intercept	Intercept	1	8.62642	0.36619	23.56
Age	Age	1	0.26826	0.03707	7.24

Parameter Estimates

Variable	Label	DF	Pr > |t|
Intercept	Intercept	1	<0.0001
Age	Age	1	<0.0001

Weighted Regression with Empirical Option
   The Mixed Procedure

Model Information

Data set	WORK.NEW
Dependent variable	ghb
Weight Variable	**WGT**
Covariance structure	Variance components
Subject effect	id
Estimation method	REML
Residual variance method	Parameter
Fixed effects SE method	**Empirical**
Degrees-of-freedom method	Between–within

Dimensions

Covariance parameters	1
Columns in X	2
Columns in Z	0
Subjects	274
Maximum observations per subject	1
Observations used	274
Observations not used	0
Total observations	274

Iteration History[a]

Iteration	Evaluations	−2 Residual Log Likelihood	Criterion
0	1	1180.17787127	
1	1	1180.17787127	0.00000000

[a] Convergence criteria met.

Covariance Parameter Estimates

Covariance Parameter	Subject	Estimate
Residual	id	0.000255

Fit Statistics

−2 Residual log likelihood	1180.2
AIC (smaller is better)	1182.2
AICC (smaller is better)	1182.2
BIC (smaller is better)	1185.8

Null Model Likelihood Ratio Test

DF	Chi-Square	Pr > ChiSq
0	0.00	1.0000

Solution for Fixed Effects

Effect	Estimate	Standard Error	DF	t Value	Pr > $|t|$
Intercept	8.6264	0.3464	272	24.90	<.0001
Age	0.2683	0.03761	272	7.13	<.0001

Type 3 Tests of Fixed Effects

Effect	Num DF	Den DF	F Value	Pr > F
Age	1	272	50.88	<.0001

Linearly Transformed Regression
  The REG Procedure

Model: MODEL1
Dependent Variable: NGHb
Note: No intercept in model. R-square is redefined.

Analysis of Variance

Source	DF	Sum of Squares	Mean Square	F Value	Pr > F
Model	2	2.14599	1.07300	4203.55	<0.0001
Error	272	0.06943	0.00025526		
Uncorrected total	274	2.21542			

Root MSE	0.01598	R-square	0.9687
Dependent mean	0.08822	Adjusted R-square	0.9684
Coefficient of variation	18.10979		

Parameter Estimates

Variable	DF	Parameter Estimate	Standard Error	t Value	Pr > $|t|$
NINT	1	8.62642	0.36619	23.56	<0.0001
NAGE	1	0.26826	0.03707	7.24	<0.0001

Plot of Transformed Residuals

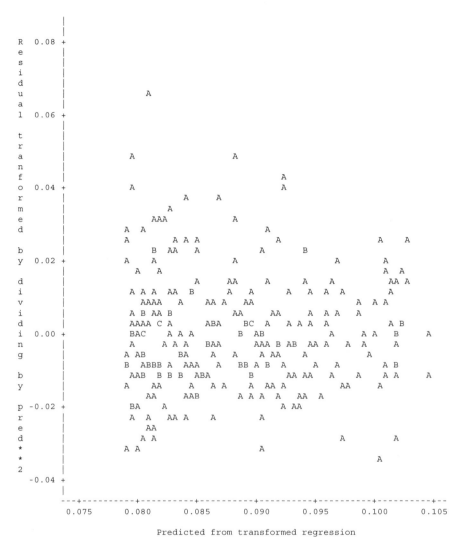

Plot of NRESID*NPRED. Legend: A = 1 obs, B = 2 obs, and so on.

CHAPTER SEVEN

Application of Weighting with Probability Sampling and Nonresponse

In this chapter we digress a bit from the development of regression estimators with general variance structure. While in Chapter 6 we applied weighting to achieve greater efficiency, we now turn to situations where weighting is applied to avoid or reduce bias. These are situations where based on the sample $E(Y|X) \neq X\beta$, but weights are available such that $E(WY|X) = X\beta$. In the situation to be discussed here, weights arise from consideration of how the sample was selected from the population about which inferences are to be made. This chapter is included because of its practical importance for observational studies where either by study design or missing data mechanisms, not every data point in the population has the same probability of ending up in the sample.

In Chapter 6 we discussed weighting in obtaining regression estimators from the viewpoint of improving efficiency of estimators, but the key equation (6.6) can be derived regardless of the choice of weights.

$$\text{Var}(\hat{\beta}_W) = [X'WX]^{-1}[X'W]\text{Var}(Y|X)[W'X][X'WX]^{-1}$$

We saw that this equation can be used to obtain the variance matrix of regression estimators in general situations, by using the "empirical" method for estimating $\text{Var}(Y|X)$. Often the empirical method is used just because, even though we guessed that $\text{Var}(Y|X) = W^{-1}$, we are not sure. So, in order not to overestimate the significance of regression coefficients, we choose the safe route. There are other equally common and important applications of weighted regression estimators and empirical estimation of the variance of regression coefficients in the context of sample surveys and in investigating the effects of selection bias. In these situations, weights W have no relationship to $\text{Var}(Y|X)$.

Quantitative Methods in Population Health, by Mari Palta
ISBN 0-471-45505-9   Copyright © 2003 John Wiley & Sons, Inc.

97

7.1   SAMPLE SURVEYS WITH UNEQUAL PROBABILITY SAMPLING

The conceptually simplest way to perform a survey is to select people with equal probability by what is called "simple random sampling." For example, for a sample of University of Wisconsin employees, we could generate a list of random numbers, count the names sequentially down the phone directory, and select the people whose sequence numbers in the phone book match one of the random numbers. Our analyses up hill now have assumed that the sample arose from such a process. Each observation in the sample can then be thought of as equally "representative" of the underlying population.

However, the method of simple random sampling is sometimes not feasible in practice. Many designs are available for facilitating selection and actual implementation of sampling. National surveys generally employ the procedure of first sampling regions, then smaller units within the region, and finally people within those units. This procedure of selection is called "multistage sampling," and the fact that larger units (than those that are the target of eventual analyses) are selected at some stages is called "cluster sampling." Another feature often used is "oversampling" of certain subcategories. This means that members of subgroups such as rural residents, women, or blacks are invited to participate in proportionately larger numbers. These techniques may be employed because the subgroup can be reached conveniently (for example, there may be less extra cost if we include everyone within a certain community once that community has been selected than if we select yet another city). In a medical record survey of everyone with a given diagnostic code in a hospital record computer file, it may be easier to request all records from hospitals that are contacted anyway. This leads to patients at larger hospitals having greater probability of selection. Most importantly, the technique of oversampling is employed to achieve a sufficiently large sample of subgroups of special interest.

The Wisconsin Sleep Cohort Study employed unequal probability sampling to assemble the sleep cohort from state agencies surveyed [16]. This was done to ensure that there would be sufficiently many subjects with sleep apnea in the sample, an important consideration because the study is to not only determine the prevalence and incidence of sleep disordered breathing, but also map its long- and short-term consequences. Because of this, the initial survey sent to everyone contained questions on snoring and gasping during sleep. A selection algorithm based on these questions was used to identify people who were relatively more likely to have sleep-disordered breathing. The subjects who fell in the high-risk category were all invited to be studied in the sleep laboratory. A random sample of one-third of those in the low-risk category were also invited.

In the situation when all subjects don't have the same probability of being in the sample, estimators of population parameters are not unbiased unless they are weighted. Before considering the more complex case of regression estimation, consider the estimation of a population mean. Also, let's first think of the simple case when there are only two different sampling categories, usually referred to as strata in the population. Assume that there are N_1 people in the first stratum (e.g., habitual snorers and gaspers in the Sleep Cohort Study) and N_2 in the second stratum. Assume that a sample of n_1 people of the first kind are selected and n_2 people of the second kind and that the probabilities of selection are π_1 and π_2, respectively. In the Sleep Cohort Study, $\pi_1 = 1$ and $\pi_2 = 1/3$. If the mean of some variable y in the population is μ_y, it must be that $\mu_y = (N_1\mu_{y_1} + N_2\mu_{y_2})/(N_1 + N_2)$, where μ_{y_1} and μ_{y_2} are the means of the two subgroups. Then the unbiased way to estimate μ_y is as $(N_1\bar{y}_1 + N_2\bar{y}_2)/(N_1 + N_2)$. This is essentially to directly standardize the sample mean to the population composition. Because $\pi_1 = n_1/N_1$ and $\pi_2 = n_2/N_2$, so that $N_1 = n_1/\pi_1$ and $N_2 = n_2/\pi_2$, this can be rewritten

$$\bar{y} = \left(\frac{n_1}{\pi_1}\bar{y}_1 + \frac{n_2}{\pi_2}\bar{y}_2\right) \Big/ \left(\frac{n_1}{\pi_1} + \frac{n_2}{\pi_2}\right) = \left(\frac{n_1}{\pi_1}\frac{\sum_1^{n_1} y_{1i}}{n_1} + \frac{n_2}{\pi_2}\frac{\sum_1^{n_2} y_{2i}}{n_2}\right) \Big/ \left(\frac{n_1}{\pi_1} + \frac{n_2}{\pi_2}\right)$$

$$= \left(\sum_1^{n_1} \frac{y_{1i}}{\pi_1} + \sum_1^{n_2} \frac{y_{2i}}{\pi_2}\right) \Big/ \left(\frac{n_1}{\pi_1} + \frac{n_2}{\pi_2}\right)$$

$$= \left(\sum_1^{n_1} \frac{1}{\pi_1} y_{1i} + \sum_1^{n_2} \frac{1}{\pi_2} y_{2i}\right) \Big/ \left(\sum_1^{n_1} \frac{1}{\pi_1} + \sum_1^{n_2} \frac{1}{\pi_2}\right)$$

which is a weighted average of the sample observations, giving each observation a weight that is the inverse of its sampling probability. In the more general case, if we assume that a random sample $y_1, y_2, \ldots, y_n$ was selected by a mechanism so that the probabilities of being sampled were $\pi_1, \pi_2, \ldots, \pi_n$, the unbiased estimator of the population mean would be

$$\bar{y} = \sum_1^n \frac{y_i}{\pi_i} \Big/ \sum_1^n \frac{1}{\pi_i}$$

The denominator is there to ensure that the weights sum up to one. In the simple random sample case we have $\pi_i = \pi$ and all observations end up receiving equal weight, because

$$\bar{y} = \sum_1^n \frac{y_i}{\pi} \Big/ \sum_1^n \frac{1}{\pi} = \frac{1}{\pi}\sum_1^n y_i \Big/ \left[\frac{1}{\pi}\sum_1^n 1\right] = \sum_1^n y_i/n$$

the ordinary sample mean. Again, "direct standardization" often used in demography and public health is closely related to the weighted formulas provided here, which "standardize the sample to the population composition."

Moving to the regression situation, we first note that while the ordinary mean can be written in matrix notation as

$$
\left(\begin{pmatrix} 1 & 1 & \cdots & 1 \end{pmatrix} \begin{pmatrix} 1 \\ 1 \\ \vdots \\ 1 \end{pmatrix} \right)^{-1} \begin{pmatrix} 1 & 1 & \cdots & 1 \end{pmatrix} \begin{pmatrix} y_1 \\ y_2 \\ \vdots \\ y_n \end{pmatrix} = (X'X)^{-1} X'Y
$$

the weighted mean can be written as

$$
\left(\begin{pmatrix} 1 & 1 & \cdots & 1 \end{pmatrix} \begin{pmatrix} \frac{1}{\pi_1} & 0 & \cdots & 0 \\ 0 & \frac{1}{\pi_2} & \cdots & 0 \\ \vdots & \vdots & \ddots & 0 \\ 0 & 0 & \cdots & \frac{1}{\pi_n} \end{pmatrix} \begin{pmatrix} 1 \\ 1 \\ \vdots \\ 1 \end{pmatrix} \right)^{-1}
$$

$$
\begin{pmatrix} 1 & 1 & \cdots & 1 \end{pmatrix} \begin{pmatrix} \frac{1}{\pi_1} & 0 & \cdots & 0 \\ 0 & \frac{1}{\pi_2} & \cdots & 0 \\ \vdots & \vdots & \ddots & 0 \\ 0 & 0 & \cdots & \frac{1}{\pi_n} \end{pmatrix} \begin{pmatrix} y_1 \\ y_2 \\ \vdots \\ y_n \end{pmatrix}
$$

$$
= \qquad (X'WX)^{-1} X'WY
$$

where W is the matrix with the inverses of the sampling probabilities on the diagonal. The idea generalizes to the regression situation, where X contains not only the column of 1's, but also other columns of covariates x_{ji}. Hence we have the following as an unbiased estimator of regression coefficients in the population for the unequal probability sampling situation:

$$
\hat{\beta}_W = [X'WX]^{-1}[X'WY]
$$

where W is matrix with the inverse sampling probability of each observation on the diagonal. In this case, we are quite sure that W is not the inverse of the variance matrix of the observations. Nor do we wish to make an equal variance assumption, because the sampling strata introduce unknown influences on the variance. (The reasons we chose stratified sampling acknowledges the fact that strata may be different with respect to both mean and variance. Furthermore, the mix of strata represented at different levels of X may differ, again making the variance unequal.) It is therefore customary to use the variance matrix

$$
\mathrm{Var}(\hat{\beta}_W) = (X'WX)^{-1} X'W = (X'WX)^{-1} X'W \hat{\epsilon}\hat{\epsilon}' WX(X'WX)^{-1}
$$

To those familiar with survey sampling, the above discussion will appear to have made a mistake in omitting "finite population" corrections (especially as all snorers were selected for study). The reason such correction was not a concern in, for example, the sleep study (or in many other epidemiologic studies) is that the sampling frame itself was considered a representative sample of an even larger "hyper population" (say "employed middle-aged men and women in the United States") to which the results would be expected to generalize. Further discussion of survey sampling context would lead us far afield from the main emphasis of this course.

SAS version 8 contains several procedures specifically designed for use with complex survey sampling (including PROC SURVEYMEAN; and PROC SURVEYREG;). These will not be covered here, because PROC MIXED serves our present purpose. We have also not covered how to deal with cluster sampling or estimation of weights. Interested readers are referred to the book by Korn and Graubard [17] for more details on how to deal with complex surveys.

7.1.1 Example

The above development implies that we should have taken the sampling into account when fitting regression equations to the blood pressure data from the Sleep Cohort Study. In this situation

$$
W = \begin{pmatrix}
1 & 0 & 0 & \cdots & \cdots \\
0 & 1 & 0 & \cdots & \cdots \\
\cdots & \cdots & \cdots & \cdots & \cdots \\
\cdots & \cdots & 0 & 1/3 & 0 \\
\cdots & \cdots & 0 & 0 & 1/3
\end{pmatrix}
$$

where the number of 1's on the main diagonal equals the number of subjects in the sample from the high-risk group. Because the situation falls under the general case of weighted regression, the following statements were used to obtain the weighted regression estimators and their standard errors. The first PROC MIXED produces an unweighted regression with empirical errors for comparison. To form the weights, the statements make use of the fact that the first letter of the ID in this study indicates the group. The GROUP$ 1 tells SAS to go back and read the letter in the first column of each input record separately. The letter S indicates the oversampled high-risk subjects, all other subjects were sampled with 1/3 probability (In light of the above note, W only needs to indicate the relative size of sampling probabilities as long as we don't care about $\sigma_{y/x}^2$). Outputs are in OUTPUT PACKET VI:

```
DATA A;
INFILE 'filename';
INPUT ID$ VISIT AGE BMI SEX$ SBP GROUP$ 1;
IF VISIT=1;
WGT=3;
IF GROUP='S' THEN WGT=1;
PROC MIXED EMPIRICAL NOCLPRINT;
CLASS ID SEX;
MODEL SBP=AGEC BMIC SEX AGEC*BMIC/S;
PROC MIXED EMPIRICAL NOCLPRINT;
```

Table 7.1   Unweighted and Weighted $\hat{\beta}$ (Empirical se) of Wisconsin Sleep Cohort SBP

	Unweighted		Weighted	
Intercept	127	(0.549)	126	(0.629)
Female	−6.57	(0.726)	−6.25	(0.799)
Age (centered at 50)	0.369	(0.0510)	0.344	(0.0586)
BMI (centered at 27)	0.595	(0.0720)	0.567	(0.0813)
Age *BMI (centered)	−0.0189	(0.00888)	−0.0182	(0.0103)

CLASS ID SEX;
MODEL SBP=AGEC BMIC SEX AGEC*BMIC/S;
WEIGHT WGT;
REPEATED/SUBJECT=ID;

Here again, SEX as an alphabetic variable can be entered in PROC MIXED as long as it is declared a CLASS variable.

We see in OUTPUT PACKET VI and Table 7.1 that the coefficients change slightly with the weighting and that the standard errors become larger. The latter is usually the case, because weighting here is not performed for increasing efficiency, but rather for validity. As the p-value of the interaction coefficient is higher with weighting, it slips to the nonsignificant side of 0.05.

National surveys such as NHANES (conducted by the National Center for Health Statistics) contain variables that provide the weights to be used in analyses (and additional information used to boost standard errors to take clustering into account). There has been some controversy about the importance of weights in analyses that are performed to estimate association. Some of this may have arisen from the fact that the empirical error estimators can be unstable. Even estimators of regression coefficients themselves can be unstable if small sample sizes in subgroups lead to very high weighting of some observations in the sample. (However, techniques for "smoothing" weights exist [18].) Another argument against weighting is that it loses its importance if the variables that form the basis for the weights are included in the model (i.e., adjusted for). Many situations arise, however, where inclusion of the selection variables is undesirable. We would not, for example, want snoring status in the model when examining the relationship between BMI and SBP. This is because high BMI may lead to snoring and both high BMI and snoring may elevate blood pressure. We would be underestimating the total effect of BMI in the population. A variable higher in the causal chain should not be included in the model as a confounder in the epidemiologic investigation of the total effect of a risk factor.

7.2   EXAMINING THE IMPACT OF NONRESPONSE

Up till now, this chapter has dealt with intentionally unequal probabilities of sampling. However, almost every study of human subjects involves unintentionally (as far as the investigators, not necessarily the subjects themselves, are concerned!) unequal probabilities of inclusion in the sample by nonresponse. The difference is only that we may not know all the factors that affect the response, and therefore sampling, probability. Many statisticians recommend that in this situation, one should still determine the sampling probabilities based on *known* factors. In principle this is very similar to statistically analyzing the associations of outcomes with risk factors that have not been assigned by randomization. If, for example, people with less than a high school education are less likely to respond to a survey, one (a) computes the proportion responding out of all subjects in that group and (b) weights the analysis by the inverse of that probability. NHANES provides such weights in addition to the "regular" sampling weights arising from the design. They use the terminology "post-stratification weights" to designate weights that take into account differential nonresponse by factors that were not part of the initial design.

Another set of terminology [19] is popular when there are missing data or nonresponse. You will hear the terms "missing completely at random," designating that nonresponse does not depend on any known or unknown factors, "missing at random," designating that nonresponse depends only on known and measured factors, and "nonignorable missingness," which means that nonresponse depends on unknown or unmeasured factors. The weighting scheme described here assumes that nonresponses are "missing at random."

A complete investigation of all measured factors that may have affected the response is obviously a time-consuming undertaking. Nonetheless, it is a good idea to prepare for such an investigation by collecting as much data as possible on all subjects, including nonresponders. For example, it may be possible to determine the socioeconomic level of the neighborhood even of persons who do not fill out a survey. When nonresponse is found to depend on any of the measured factors, it is useful to perform a sensitivity analysis to ensure that major study conclusions are not changed by reweighting the data by the response probabilities. When important changes occur with weighting, this should be noted in the study report. If differences in results do not change the main study conclusions, the initial unweighted analyses may still be the main results presented.

The above approach is one of several ways to examine the possible biases introduced by missing data and nonresponse. Unfortunately, none of these several appropriate methods are common in the medical or even epidemiologic literature. Instead, one often encounters a "Table 1" with significance testing of differences between respondents and nonrespondents. As you know, the statistical significance of the difference depends on its magnitude and on the absolute numbers of respondents and nonrespondents. The importance of the difference for the actual conclusions, on the other hand, depends on its magnitude and on the proportion of nonresponders. In addition, we hardly care if the differences between nonresponders and responders arose by chance or systematically (which is the only aspect the p-value clarifies). What matters is whether our results would have substantially changed, had we been able to obtain the relevant data on all the nonresponders. Philosophically, the goals when examining biases due to nonresponse are similar those in examining potential confounders, and so are the problems.

One never knows whether all confounders have been adjusted for, or whether all factors influencing response probabilities have been determined and weighted on. Nonetheless, the analysis should take into account everything that is known.

7.2.1 Example (of Reweighting as Well as Some SAS Manipulations)

The Newborn Lung Project consists of several study stages. One stage was the determination of health at age 5 years, which included a functional assessment [20]. Reasonably, one may view all children who were originally admitted to the six neonatal care units and who survived to age 5 as the underlying sample of interest. An effort was made (with the help of the neonatal unit) to identify all deaths up to age 5.

A great number of variables were collected during the neonatal period and could form the basis for reweighting analyses. To keep things somewhat simple, we illustrate the methods using a few variables which predicted participation at age 5. (Nonparticipants here consist mostly of children who could not be located, and a few refusals to participate once located.) The particular variables considered as predictors of participation were available on all neonates.

Table 7.2 shows the usual type "Table 1" seen in papers, although many variables that did not differ between groups would normally be included. For example, oxygen use at 24 hours of age was almost identical in the two groups.

Table 7.2 establishes that children who were larger at birth, who were born at another hospital (and then transported to the NICU), and who were singleton births were less likely to participate. It also shows that these differences were probably not due to chance. The only unexpected finding is that of a birth weight difference. An excess of multiple births among participants reflects the fact that once a parent of multiples is enrolled, one gains several children into the study.

It seems more reasonable to present a table that shows how much the group composition is altered from the original intended by not being able to include the nonresponders in analyses. Table 7.3 is recommended instead of Table 7.2.

Table 7.3 can then be supplemented by examining the sensitivity of the main study analyses to differences in the distributions of these characteristics among the participants from the distribution among all admissions. This is based on reweighting the participant sample to reflect the distribution in the NICU admission group. (Again, note the similarity in spirit to direct standardization.)

Table 7.2 Comparison of Birth Characteristics Between Participants and Nonparticipants in Functional Assessment at Age 5 Years

Birth characteristic	Nonparticipants	Participants	p-Value
n	382	422	
Birth weight (g), mean (sd)	1148 (256)	1105 (254)	0.019
Born at another hospital (%)	17.8	8.8	0.001
Multiple birth (%)	16.0	29.9	0.001

Table 7.3 Comparison of Birth Characteristics Between All Survivors and Participants in Functional Assessment at Age 5 Years

Birth Characteristic	All Survivors	Participants
n	804	422
Birth weight (g), mean (sd)	1125 (256)	1105 (254)
Born at another hospital	13.1	8.8
Multiple birth (%)	23.3	29.9

Some of the study aims were related to the prediction of social function at age 5 from socioeconomic and neonatal clinical characteristics and study year. Social function was a continuous measurement with standardized normative mean of 50 and standard deviation of 10 among "normal" children studied by the developer of the instrument [21]. OUTPUT PACKET VI shows the results of analyses using PROC MIXED. The empirical option was included as a couple of variables has slightly higher standard errors with this option. A summary is provided in Table 7.4. Not shown in the table are the regression coefficients for the indicator variable for NURSE. These were included to adjust for any differences in interview technique that may affect the social function score. Prior to running the regression analysis, an overall socioeconomic score was constructed based on whether the child was living with both parents, parents' occupation, mother's education, and neighborhood income level from census data. Other predictors indicate whether the child had severe respiratory disease at age 30 days and the grade of intraventricular hemorrhage. The effect of birth year was of special interest, because the introduction of surfactant treatment for neonatal lung immaturity during the period study births accrued increased the survival of very premature babies [22]. In the analyses INDYR and SURFYR indicate the years when surfactant was available as an investigational new drug, and generally available, respectively.

We see that, in general, higher socioeconomic level and less neonatal illness is associated with higher social function. Additionally, there appears to have been a

Table 7.4 Unweighted and Weighted Regression Coefficients (empirical se) for Predicting Social Function at Age 5 Years for VLBW Children

	Unweighted	Weighted for participation
Male	−2.15 (1.09)	−2.04 (1.10)
Socioeconomic level	2.75 (0.591)	2.90 (0.584)
Neonatal respiratory disease	−4.41 (1.30)	−4.66 (1.35)
Grade of IVH	−3.23 (0.606)	−3.35 (0.633)
IND period birth	−0.860 (1.49)	−1.28 (1.56)
Surfactant period birth	−4.58 (1.51)	−4.14 (1.56)

decrease in social function associated with the third study year. Girls had slightly higher social function than did boys.

The following statements were now run, where the variable PARTIND=1 if the child was a respondent for 5-year assessment and PARTIND=0 if the child was a nonresponder. Output is in PACKET VI.

```
PROC LOGIST DESCENDING;
MODEL PARTIND=BW BPLACE MULT SURFYR BPLACE*SURFYR;
OUTPUT OUT=PROBS P=PPART;
DATA B; SET PROBS;
FILE 'PROBS. DAT';
PUT ID PPART;
PROC UNIVARIATE PLOT; VAR PPART;
```

Note that PROC LOGIST in version 8 of SAS (in contrast to earlier versions) can handle both interaction effects and categorical variables directly. A new data set called PROBS is created by the OUTPUT that, for each participant, contains the estimated probability of being a participant based on the characteristics included in the model. The probabilities are written to a new file, so that they will be conveniently available for all kinds of further analyses. The UNIVARIATE procedure result illustrates the wide range in predicted participation probabilities from 21% to 83%.

Now, the original data used for analysis were in DATA PART;. This data set was merged with the probabilities in the set PROBS, and a weighted regression analysis was run by PROC MIXED:

```
DATA P;
INFILE 'PROBS. DAT';
INPUT ID$ PPART;
PROC SORT; BY ID;
DATA NEW; MERGE PART P; BY ID;
WGT=1/PPART;
PROC MIXED EMPIRICAL NOCLPRINT;
CLASS SEX NURSE;
MODEL SOC=NURSE SEX SOCIOEC RESPDIS GRADEIVH INDYR SURFYR/S;
WEIGHT WGT;
REPEATED/SUBJECT=ID;
```

Table 7.4 provides a comparison of the key regression coefficients without and with weighting.

We see that the result of reweighting is an increase in the coefficients of almost all variable. The exceptions are that SEX which was borderline significant loses significance further, and that the effect of the third time period is somewhat reduced. These results confirm the importance of the variables, but could lead one to emphasize the time period slightly less. It appears that the changes with weighting came about partly because there were relatively few children born at other hospitals among the participants in the first study year (5.2%) and relatively many among the nonparticipants (17.5%). The imbalance was less in the last study year. By and large, children born at other hospitals did worse. Then, reweighting to reflect more outborn children in the first year tended to imply that this function may have been relatively worse than originally thought. However, the relationships are complex, and the main thing to look at here is the overall effect of reweighting. Although it led to some changes in results, there was no major shift in the main conclusions. This is despite a low participation probability and despite differences in some birth characteristics between participants and nonparticipants.

7.2.2 A Few Comments on Weighting by a Variable Versus Including it in the Regression Model

This section attempts to clarify an issue that seems to arise quite often in studies employing stratified sampling as well as in studies investigating complex causal chains. It can be skipped by individuals who have not yet encountered these problems.

All analyses involve inherent weighting whether explicitly acknowledged or not, as parameter estimates are based on the mixture of characteristics that end up in the sample. The list below differentiates between a few options that may be considered for explicit and implicit weighting in the analysis. To make the comparison more concrete, assume that an analysis is to be undertaken to regress self-reported health ("health") on level of exercise. Also assume that another determinant of "health" is body mass index and that body mass index is lowered by increasing exercise. (For the sake of the argument, we ignore that BMI may influence the likelihood that someone exercises.) In addition we assume that people with lower body mass index are more likely to participate in the study.

Throughout considering the various analytic options, it is necessary to keep in mind exactly what question is to be answered. Most likely it would be either (a) What is the total effect of exercise on "health," regardless of whether the effect occurs directly or through lowering body mass index? or (b) What is the effect of exercise on "health" additional to its effect on body mass index, or in other words: If two people with the same body mass index were compared, how much better would the person feel who exercises more?

The scattergram in Figure 7.1, based on fictitious data, shows the relationship between "health" and exercise in a simple random sample of the population. Empty circles indicate the observations that are not available because of lower response by individuals with high body mass indices. The regression line for health on exercise level is estimated as $\mu_{\text{health}} = -1.68 + 2.10 \times \text{exercise}$ for the complete data set. With data missing as indicated, the line becomes $\mu_{\text{health}} = 0.273 + 1.857 \times \text{exercise}$, so the effect in exercise on health is underestimated.

The following approaches are possible in the analysis:

1. Ignore body weight and just regress "health" on exercise level. This would be fine for answering (a) if there were no selection bias—that is, if response was complete or nonresponse occurred "completely at random." As it is, the sample underrepresents people with higher body mass index. Because

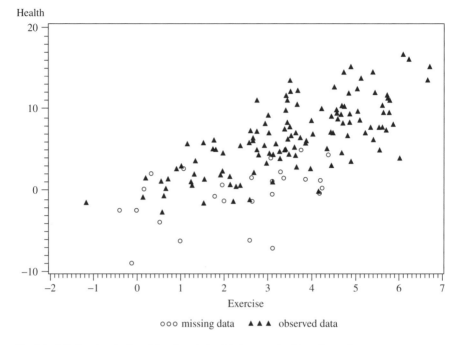

Fig. 7.1   Missing data in describing the relationship between health and exercise.

body mass index is related to exercise and "health," observations on the lower left-hand side of Figure 7.1 are disproportionately missing. The result is underestimation of the total effect of exercise on "health." The inherent weighting in this analysis is to the mix of body mass index in the sample. People at different exercise levels have different mixes of body mass, and the comparison reflects the effect of exercise minus the attenuation imposed by differential exclusion of high body mass among people who exercise less. In effect, people with low exercise levels appear to feel more healthy than they would if there were no nonresponse.

2. Adjust for body mass index in the regression. This is fine for answering question (b). The inherent weighting compares people at the different exercise levels, where the mix of body mass indices is the same at all the levels. The mix to which each exercise level "is standardized" is chosen for maximum statistical efficiency. However, the choice of mix is only important when there are (statistically significant or nonsignificant) interaction effects between body mass index and exercise in their effect on "health." Hence, when there is truly no interaction, reweighting to correct selection bias is not necessary when the variable; underlying selection into the sample is included in the model.

3. Weight the analysis under 1 by inverse sampling probabilities based on body mass index. This will result in comparison of exercise levels, each of which

has the body mass mix, respectively, that they have in the population. The results are relevant to goal (a) above.

4. Weight the analysis under 2 by inverse participation probabilities based on body mass index. This analysis addresses (b) above. It will not differ from 2 except in statistical efficiency (which will be less) and in the resulting influence of potential interaction effects. Instead of representing a mixture of body mass specific exercise effects representing the most efficient mix of the population, it will represent the mix in the underlying population. Thus "external validity" will be greater than for the analysis in 2, at the price of reduced statistical efficiency

The above discussion avoids the even more complex issue that people at lower body mass index may choose to exercise more. Hence body mass index may simultaneously be both a confounder and an intermediate variable. None of the above techniques suffice to deal with this situation. Solutions can be based on the introduction of a new variable that predicts exercise independently of body mass and can be used either as a so-called "instrument" [23] or to produce weights for a weighted analysis similar to above [24]. These techniques are a mainstay of econometric analyses, and they are gaining popularity in AIDS research. It is often difficult to identify appropriate predictive factors in the general epidemiologic setting, but future work in the area will probably help prepare for such analyses.

OUTPUT PACKET VI: SURVEY AND MISSING DATA WEIGHTS

VI.1. Survey Weighted Analyses—Wisconsin Sleep Cohort

Unequal Probability Weighting—Wisconsin Sleep Cohort
Unweighted Regression with Empirical Option
  The Mixed Procedure

Model Information	
Data set	WORK.A
Dependent variable	SBP
Covariance structure	Variance components
Subject effect	id
Estimation method	REML
Residual variance method	Parameter
Fixed effects SE method	**Empirical**
Degrees-of-freedom method	Between–within

Dimensions

Covariance parameters	1
Columns in X	6
Columns in Z	0
Subjects	1370
Maximum observations per subject	1
Observations used	1364
Observations not used	6
Total observations	1370

Iteration History[a]

Iteration	Evaluations	−2 Residual Log Likelihood	Criterion
0	1	10945.85019390	
1	1	10945.85019389	0.00000000

[a]Convergence criteria met.

Covariance Parameter Estimates

Covariance Parameter	Subject	Estimate
Residual	id	177.58

Fit Statistics

−2 Residual log likelihood	10945.9
AIC (smaller is better)	10947.9
AICC (smaller is better)	10947.9
BIC (smaller is better)	10953.1

Null Model Likelihood Ratio Test

DF	Chi-Square	Pr > ChiSq
0	0.00	1.0000

Solution for Fixed Effects

Effect	Sex	Estimate	Standard Error	DF	t Value	Pr > |t|
Intercept		127.45	0.5494	1359	231.96	<0.0001
sex	F	−6.5731	0.7263	1359	−9.05	<0.0001
sex	M	0	.	.	.	.
agec		0.3691	0.05103	1359	7.23	<0.0001
bmic		0.5945	0.07196	1359	8.26	<0.0001
agec*bmic		−0.01892	0.008882	1359	−2.13	0.0334

Type 3 Tests of Fixed Effects

Effect	Num DF	Den DF	F Value	Pr > F
sex	1	1359	81.90	<0.0001
agec	1	1359	52.33	<0.0001
bmic	1	1359	68.26	<0.0001
agec*bmic	1	1359	4.54	0.0334

Weighted Regression with Empirical Option
  The Mixed Procedure

Model Information

Data set	WORK.A
Dependent variable	sbp
Weight variable	**wgt**
Covariance structure	Variance components
Subject effect	id
Estimation method	REML
Residual variance method	Parameter
Fixed effects SE method	**Empirical**
Degrees-of-freedom method	Between–within

Dimensions

Covariance parameters	1
Columns in X	6
Columns in Z	0
Subjects	1370
Maximum observations per subject	1
Observations used	1364
Observations not used	6
Total observations	1370

Iteration History[a]

Iteration	Evaluations	−2 Residual Log Likelihood	Criterion
0	1	11130.31257378	
1	1	11130.31257378	0.00000000

[a]Convergence criteria met.

Covariance Parameter Estimates

Covariance Parameter	Subject	Estimate
Residual	Id	361.91

Fit Statistics

−2 Residual log likelihood	11130.3
AIC (smaller is better)	11132.3
AICC (smaller is better)	11132.3
BIC (smaller is better)	11137.5

Null Model Likelihood Ratio Test

DF	Chi-Square	Pr > ChiSq
0	0.00	1.0000

Solution for Fixed Effects

Effect	Sex	Estimate	Standard Error	DF	t Value	Pr > |t|
Intercept		126.44	0.6292	1359	200.94	<0.0001
sex	F	−6.2500	0.7989	1359	−7.82	<0.0001
sex	M	0	.	.	.	.
agec		0.3441	0.05856	1359	5.88	<0.0001
bmic		0.5668	0.08130	1359	6.97	<0.0001
agec*bmic		−0.01823	0.01031	1359	−1.77	0.0772

Type 3 Tests of Fixed Effects

Effect	Num DF	Den DF	F Value	Pr > F
sex	1	1359	61.21	<0.0001
agec	1	1359	34.52	<0.0001
bmic	1	1359	48.60	<0.0001
agec*bmic	1	1359	3.13	0.0772

VI.2. Weighted Analyses to Adjust for Loss to Follow-up—Newborn Lung Project

Weighting to Adjust for Missing Data in NLP Follow-up
Estimating the Probabilities of Participation
   The LOGISTIC Procedure

Model Information

Data set	WORK.SELECT
Response variable	partind
Number of response levels	2
Number of observations	804
Model	**binary logit**
Optimization technique	Fisher's scoring

Response Profile[a]

Ordered Value	partind	Total Frequency
1	1	422
2	0	382

[a]Probability modeled is partind=1.

The LOGISTIC Procedure

Analysis of Maximum Likelihood Estimates

Parameter	DF	Estimate	Standard Error	Wald Chi-Square	Pr > ChiSq
Intercept	1	1.0847	0.3432	9.9899	0.0016
bw	1	−0.00087	0.000289	9.1383	0.0025
bplace	1	−1.1335	0.2928	14.9886	0.0001
mult	1	0.8224	0.1796	20.9683	<0.0001
surfyr	1	−0.2502	0.1638	2.3349	0.1265
bplace*surfyr	1	0.9398	0.4556	4.2545	0.0391

Description of the Probabilities of Participation
The UNIVARIATE Procedure
Variable: ppart (Estimated Probability)

Moments

N	804	Sum of weights	804
Mean	0.52487562	Sum of observations	422.000002
Standard deviation	0.1200934	Variance	0.01442243

Basic Statistical Measures

Location		Variability	
Mean	0.524876	Standard deviation	0.12009
Median	0.516567	Variance	0.01442
Mode	0.458788	Range	0.62097
		Interquartile range	0.14884

Note: The mode displayed is the smallest of 2 modes with a count of 7.

The UNIVARIATE Procedure
Variable: ppart (Estimated Probability)

Extreme Observations

Lowest		Highest	
Value	Observations	Value	Observations
0.210726	13	0.776052	56
0.212915	493	0.778473	380
0.214384	721	0.791742	249
0.215121	7	0.796033	41
0.215859	729	0.831694	132

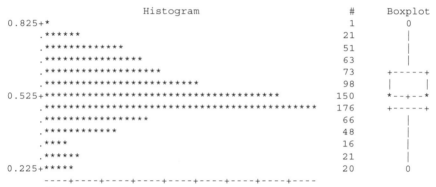

```
                 Histogram                            #     Boxplot
  0.825+*                                              1       0
       .******                                        21       |
       .*************                                 51       |
       .***************                               63       |
       .******************                            73    +-----+
       .************************                      98    |     |
  0.525+*************************************         150   *--+--*
       .***********************************************  176  +-----+
       .*****************                             66       |
       .************                                 48       |
       .****                                         16       |
       .******                                       21       |
  0.225+*****                                        20       0
       ----+----+----+----+----+----+----+----+----
       *May represent up  to 4 counts
```

The Mixed Procedure

Model Information

Data set	WORK.FINAL
Dependent variable	soc
Covariance structure	Variance components
Subject effect	id
Estimation method	REML
Residual variance method	Parameter
Fixed effects SE method	**Empirical**
Degrees of freedom method	Between–within

Dimensions

Covariance parameters	1
Columns in X	19
Columns in Z	0
Subjects	422
Maximum observations per subject	1
Observations used	422
Observations not used	382
Total observations	804

Iteration History[a]

Iteration	Evaluations	−2 Residual Log Likelihood	Criterion
0	1	3079.26827535	
1	1	3079.26827535	0.00000000

[a] Convergence criteria met.

Covariance Parameter Estimates

Covariance Parameter	Subject	Estimate
Residual	id	116.14

Fit Statistics

−2 Residual log likelihood	3079.3
AIC (smaller is better)	3081.3
AICC (smaller is better)	3081.3
BIC (smaller is better)	3085.3

Null Model Likelihood Ratio Test

DF	Chi-Square	Pr > ChiSq
0	0.00	1.0000

Solution for Fixed Effects

Effect		Estimate	Standard Error	DF	t Value	Pr > |t|
Intercept		55.7751	7.3771	404	7.56	<0.0001
nurse	1	−14.7507	7.4541	404	−1.98	0.0484
nurse	2	−2.5405	7.5769	404	−0.34	0.7340
nurse	3	−9.1882	7.3403	404	−1.25	0.2120
nurse	4	−8.6320	7.6529	404	−1.13	0.2591
nurse	5	−6.9527	7.2882	404	−0.95	0.3427
nurse	6	−0.1903	7.8059	404	−0.02	0.9841
nurse	7	−4.3978	7.3942	404	−0.59	0.5555
nurse	8	−11.6370	8.4062	404	−1.38	0.1684
nurse	9	−18.5109	7.4301	404	−2.49	0.0132
nurse	12	−2.9982	7.7448	404	−0.39	0.6967
nurse	13	−22.3962	8.2839	404	−2.70	0.0072
nurse	14	0	.	.	.	.
sex		−2.1474	1.0899	404	−1.97	0.0495
socioec		2.7465	0.5914	404	4.64	<0.0001
respdis		−4.4097	1.3025	404	−3.39	0.0008
gradeivh		−3.2317	0.6055	404	−5.34	<0.0001
indyr		−0.8604	1.4857	404	−0.58	0.5602
surfyr		−4.5842	1.5140	404	−3.03	0.0026

Type 3 Tests of Fixed Effects

Effect	Num DF	Den DF	F Value	Pr > F
nurse	11	404	7.13	<0.0001
sex	1	404	3.88	0.0495
socioec	1	404	21.57	<0.0001
respdis	1	404	11.46	0.0008
gradeivh	1	404	28.48	<0.0001
indyr	1	404	0.34	0.5602
surfyr	1	404	9.17	0.0026

Weighted (for Missingness) Regression with Empirical Option
  The Mixed Procedure

Model Information

Data set	WORK.FINAL
Dependent variable	soc
Weight variable	**wgt**
Covariance structure	Variance components
Subject effect	id
Estimation method	REML
Residual variance method	Parameter
Fixed effects SE method	**Empirical**
Degrees-of-freedom method	Between–within

Dimensions

Covariance parameters	1
Columns in X	19
Columns in Z	0
Subjects	422
Maximum Observations per subject	1
Observations used	422
Observations not used	382
Total observations	804

Iteration History[a]

Iteration	Evaluations	−2 Residual Log Likelihood	Criterion
0	1	3087.25704177	
1	1	3087.25704177	0.00000000

[a]Convergence criteria met.

Covariance Parameter Estimates

Covariance Parameter	Subject	Estimate
Residual	id	218.95

Fit Statistics

−2 Residual log likelihood	3087.3
AIC (smaller is better)	3089.3
AICC (smaller is better)	3089.3
BIC (smaller is better)	3093.3

Null Model Likelihood Ratio Test

DF	Chi-Square	Pr > ChiSq
0	0.00	1.0000

Solution for Fixed Effects

Effect		Estimate	Standard Error	DF	t Value	Pr > $\lvert t \rvert$
Intercept		57.0301	5.9336	404	9.61	<0.0001
nurse	1	−16.0385	6.1600	404	−2.60	0.0097
nurse	2	−3.7356	6.1345	404	−0.61	0.5422
nurse	3	−11.3305	5.8846	404	−1.93	0.0543
nurse	4	−9.7720	6.3061	404	−1.55	0.1219
nurse	5	−8.2304	5.8216	404	−1.41	0.1593
nurse	6	−0.7458	6.4768	404	−0.12	0.9045
nurse	7	−5.2964	5.9019	404	−0.90	0.3687
nurse	8	−12.2269	6.9042	404	−1.77	0.0775
nurse	9	−20.1466	6.0061	404	−3.35	0.0009
nurse	12	−5.1332	6.3858	404	−0.80	0.4242
nurse	13	−24.8656	7.1301	404	−3.49	0.0005
nurse	14	0	.	.	.	.
sex		−2.0350	1.0968	404	−1.86	0.0636
socioec		2.9017	0.5843	404	4.97	<0.0001
respdis		−4.6566	1.3526	404	−3.44	0.0006
gradeivh		−3.3465	0.6338	404	−5.28	<0.0001
indyr		−1.2820	1.5586	404	−0.82	0.4101
surfyr		−4.1405	1.5570	404	−2.66	0.0081

Type 3 Tests of Fixed Effects

Effect	Num DF	Den DF	F Value	Pr > F
nurse	11	404	7.94	<0.0001
sex	1	404	3.44	0.0643
socioec	1	404	24.66	<0.0001
respdis	1	404	11.85	0.0006
gradeivh	1	404	27.88	<0.0001
indyr	1	404	0.68	0.4101
surfyr	1	404	7.07	0.0081

CHAPTER EIGHT

Principles in Dealing
with Correlated Data

Correlated data arise in many situations in health research. On the organismal level, there may be measurements on several tumors, both hands, all teeth, and so on. It is usually expected in such cases that the measurements on a given individual are more similar than those on different individuals. For example, finding decay on one tooth in a person may make decay on another tooth more likely. Other situations often encountered in population studies of health are data arising from clusters of individuals (for example, families) and data collected on a set of individuals longitudinally in time. The first type of correlated data often arises in survey sampling, when sampling units may contain several individuals. When a household has been selected and enrolled based on, for example, random dialing, the effort involved to obtain health data on all its members may be relatively minimal. However, members of a family may be similar in health habits, diet and health status and therefore not well represent the variation in the population. The second type arises in cohort or panel studies. In health studies, we may enroll all patients with a given diagnosis, at the beginning of the disease, and repeatedly remeasure them to document treatment effect or progression of disease. Figure 1.1 (Chapter 1) showed that measurements of GHb taken longitudinally in the Wisconsin Diabetes Registry on the same individual tend to be similar.

Yet another type of correlation between observations arises, even if there are no clusters or repeated measurements on the same individuals, because observations that are close in time may be more similar than those distant from each other in time. Such situations are the concern of so-called time series analyses. Indicators of economic trends and measurements of air quality in a community are examples of data that are often subjected to time series analyses. We will touch on this topic only inasmuch as it intersects with situations of cluster sampled and longitudinal data, which will be the main focus here. Time series analysis has a long history

Quantitative Methods in Population Health, by Mari Palta
ISBN 0-471-45505-9   Copyright © 2003 John Wiley & Sons, Inc.

and rich terminology associated with how it has been adapted to deal with various practical and theoretical problems [25].

The difference in the types of analyses emphasized here and time series analysis enters in how the covariances in the variance matrix $\text{Var}(Y|X)$ are structured. The situations have in common that the measurements are not independent, as assumed in ordinary regression analysis. However, our interest here is in the situation when observations on different individuals or sampling units can still be assumed independent. The independence assumption is violated only for observations on the same individuals or units. In other words, we will deal with situations where the observations are correlated within individual or unit.

We first consider the consequences of analyzing correlated data with ordinary unweighted least-squares, and then proceed to discuss different correlation structures and how they lead to a weighted analysis. In what follows, we will refer to the clusters or units within which observations are correlated as "individuals." This is consistent with our correlated data examples being from longitudinal studies where correlation arises between repeated observations on the same person. The methods discussed apply equally to studies with clusters, such as families.

8.1 ANALYSIS OF CORRELATED DATA BY ORDINARY UNWEIGHTED LEAST-SQUARES ESTIMATION

Exactly as in the case of unequal variance, it can be shown easily that ordinary least-squares estimators are unbiased even when the observations are correlated.

$$\hat{\beta} = (X'X)^{-1}X'Y$$

The part containing the X is a constant, and the mean of Y is $X\beta$. Hence, it follows that

$$E(\hat{\beta}) = E[(X'X)^{-1}X'Y] = [(X'X)^{-1}X'Y]$$
$$= (X'X)^{-1}X'E(Y|X) = (X'X)^{-1}X'X\beta = \beta$$

However, the usual estimators of the standard errors of the regression coefficients do not work. Just as before, we obtain

$$\text{Var}(\hat{\beta}) = \text{Var}[(X'X)^{-1}X'Y] = (X'X)^{-1}X'\text{Var}(Y|X)X(X'X)^{-1} \quad (8.1)$$

but now the residuals are not independent around the regression line, $\text{Var}(Y|X)$ is not a diagonal matrix, and off-diagonal elements need to be estimated in addition to the elements. When data fall into clusters that are independent from each other, it is necessary only to compute these quantities within clusters, while elements corresponding to covariances of residuals in different clusters can be set to 0. We will come back to the estimation of $\text{Var}(Y|X)$ after introducing some new notation.

Before we proceed, it is necessary to introduce notation that allows us to distinguish which observations belong to the same cluster. To this end, we now reserve the previous subscript i for individuals and add a subscript j that differentiates several observations on the same individual. Hence, observations on the first covariate are $x_{1i_1} \cdots x_{1i_{k_i}}$, and so on, where individual i has k_i observations, and the corresponding observations on the outcome are $y_{i1} \cdots y_{ik_i}$. We can include all the covariate values for individual i in a matrix X_i of dimension $k_i \times m$, so that

$$X_i = \begin{pmatrix} 1 & x_{1i_1} & \cdots & x_{mi_1} \\ 1 & x_{1i_2} & \cdots & x_{mi_2} \\ \cdots & \cdots & \cdots & \cdots \\ 1 & x_{1i_{k_i}} & \cdots & x_{mi_{k_i}} \end{pmatrix}$$

Similarly,

$$Y_i = \begin{pmatrix} y_{i1} \\ y_{i2} \\ \vdots \\ y_{ik_i} \end{pmatrix}$$

The overall matrices X and Y can then be written

$$X = \begin{pmatrix} X_1 \\ \vdots \\ X_n \end{pmatrix} \quad \text{and} \quad Y = \begin{pmatrix} Y_1 \\ \vdots \\ Y_n \end{pmatrix}$$

where the n indicates the number of individuals.

To further understand what the special structure with independence between individuals does to the formulas used to produce regression estimators (e.g., in PROC MIXED), we look at a matrix multiplication example.

8.1.1   Example

A matrix that has "submatrices" along the main diagonal and 0's elsewhere is called a "block diagonal" matrix. Such matrices arise naturally with clustered and longitudinal data and are computationally easier to deal with than general matrices that can have nonzero elements anywhere. To see why, we consider an example of matrix multiplication of block diagonal matrices. Note that the expression being evaluated is one that in general form can be written $X'WX$:

$$\begin{pmatrix} 1 & 2 & 10 & 20 \end{pmatrix} \begin{pmatrix} 1 & 2 & 0 & 0 \\ 2 & 3 & 0 & 0 \\ 0 & 0 & 10 & 100 \\ 0 & 0 & 100 & 20 \end{pmatrix} \begin{pmatrix} 1 \\ 2 \\ 10 \\ 20 \end{pmatrix}$$

$$= \begin{pmatrix} 1+4 & 2+6 & 100+2000 & 1000+400 \end{pmatrix} \begin{pmatrix} 1 \\ 2 \\ 10 \\ 20 \end{pmatrix}$$

$$= (1+4) \times 1 + (2+6) \times 2 + (100+2000) \times 10 + (1000+400) \times 20$$

We notice that elements in the upper block only multiply elements from the first two columns of the first matrix and the first two rows of the third matrix, while the lower block multiplies the last two columns and last two rows. In fact, the end result of the multiplication can be written

$$(1 \quad 2)\begin{pmatrix} 1 & 2 \\ 2 & 3 \end{pmatrix}\begin{pmatrix} 1 \\ 2 \end{pmatrix} + (10 \quad 20)\begin{pmatrix} 10 & 100 \\ 100 & 20 \end{pmatrix}\begin{pmatrix} 10 \\ 20 \end{pmatrix}$$

In general, if $X = \begin{pmatrix} X_1 \\ \vdots \\ X_n \end{pmatrix}$ with X_i being of dimension $k_i \times m$, it follows

that $X' = (X'_1, \cdots X'_n)$ and if $W = \begin{pmatrix} W_1 & 0 & 0 \\ 0 & \cdots & 0 \\ 0 & 0 & W_n \end{pmatrix}$ where W_i is $k_i \times k_i$, then

$X'WX = \sum_{i=1}^{n} X'_i W_i X_i$. This greatly reduces the dimension of matrices that need to be inverted to obtain regression estimators and their standard errors.

8.1.2 Deriving the Variance Estimator

Now, consider again the form of an estimator of $\mathrm{Var}(Y|X)$. Since we have not yet introduced any assumptions on the structure of this matrix, we can again take the empirical approach. Variances on the diagonal can be obtained from the residuals as before. With the double subscript notation:

$$\hat{\mathrm{Var}}(\epsilon_{ij}) = \hat{\epsilon}_{ij}^2 = (y_{ij} - \hat{\beta}_0 - \hat{\beta}_1 x_{1ij} - \hat{\beta}_2 x_{2ij} \cdots)^2$$

Off-diagonal covariance elements can be obtained as

$$\hat{\mathrm{Cov}}(\epsilon_{ij}, \epsilon_{ij'}) = \hat{\epsilon}_{ij}\hat{\epsilon}_{ij'}$$
$$= (y_{ij} - \hat{\beta}_0 - \hat{\beta}_1 x_{1ij} - \hat{\beta}_2 x_{2ij} \cdots)(y_{ij'} - \hat{\beta}_0 - \hat{\beta}_1 x_{1ij'} - \hat{\beta}_2 x_{2ij'} \cdots)$$

Note that the cross products are formed only for the same i. Because of the independence assumed between individuals, the entire matrix $\mathrm{Var}(Y|X)$ will have form

$$E = \begin{pmatrix} E_1 & 0 & 0 \\ 0 & \ddots & 0 \\ 0 & 0 & E_n \end{pmatrix}$$

where we use boldface to indicate that the quantities inside the matrix are matrices in themselves. The E_i correspond to clusters or subjects, and the elements inside E_i are estimates of the quantities $\mathrm{Var}(\epsilon_{ij})$ on the diagonal and $\mathrm{Cov}(\epsilon_{ij}, \epsilon_{ij'})$ off the diagonal.

Given the above expressions, we can write

$$E_i = \hat{\epsilon}_i \hat{\epsilon}_i'$$

where the $\hat{\epsilon}_i$ are matrices of form

$$\hat{\epsilon}_i = \begin{pmatrix} \hat{\epsilon}_{i1} \\ \vdots \\ \hat{\epsilon}_{ik} \end{pmatrix} = \begin{pmatrix} y_{i1} - \hat{\beta}_0 - \hat{\beta}_1 x_{1i1} - \hat{\beta}_2 x_{2i1} \cdots \\ \vdots \\ y_{ik} - \hat{\beta}_0 - \hat{\beta}_1 x_{1ik} - \hat{\beta}_2 x_{2ik} \cdots \end{pmatrix}$$

Note that as opposed to the multiplication $X'X$ that "collapses" the two large matrices X' and X into a matrix of dimension $m \times m$, the multiplication $\epsilon_i \epsilon_i'$ expands the matrices with one column and one row, respectively into a $k_i \times k_i$ matrix.

Returning to the issue of "sandwiching" a block diagonal matrix, we can now write middle part of formula (8.1):

$$X' \mathrm{Var}(Y|X) X = \begin{pmatrix} X_1' & \cdots & X_n' \end{pmatrix} \begin{pmatrix} E_1 & 0 & 0 \\ 0 & \ddots & 0 \\ 0 & 0 & E_n \end{pmatrix} \begin{pmatrix} X_1 \\ \vdots \\ X_n \end{pmatrix}$$

Here the X_i are the pieces of X that belong to different subjects. Just as in the example, this multiplication collapses into a sum of "bite-size sandwiches" involving the X_i and the blocks E_i

$$\begin{pmatrix} X_1' & \cdots & X_n' \end{pmatrix} \begin{pmatrix} E_1 & 0 & 0 \\ 0 & \ddots & 0 \\ 0 & 0 & E_n \end{pmatrix} \begin{pmatrix} X_1 \\ \vdots \\ X_n \end{pmatrix} = \sum_{i=1}^{n} X_i' E_i X_i = \sum_{i=1}^{n} X_i' \hat{\epsilon}_i \hat{\epsilon}_i' X_i$$

Thus formula (8.1) becomes

$$\mathrm{Var}(\hat{\beta}) = (X'X)^{-1} \sum_{i=1}^{n} X_i' \hat{\epsilon}_i \hat{\epsilon}_i' X_i (X'X)^{-1}$$

$$= \left(\sum_{i=1}^{n} X_i' X_i \right)^{-1} \sum_{i=1}^{n} X_i' \hat{\epsilon}_i \hat{\epsilon}_i' X_i \left(\sum_{i=1}^{n} X_i' X_i \right)^{-1}$$

Apart from weights, which we will introduce soon, the formula now resembles the one given in the EMPIRICAL option description in the SAS manual for PROC MIXED. In the situations described in previous chapters, when each "cluster" had only one observation, $\epsilon_i \epsilon_i'$ was the special case of a 1×1 matrix. However, the general notation was slightly different in that case.

Table 8.1   Regression Results for All Visits $\hat{\beta}$ (se) and Empirical se

	All Visits		All Visits (Empirical se)
Intercept	126	(0.401)	(0.461)
Female	−6.02	(0.577)	(0.668)
Age (centered at 50)	0.355	(0.0388)	(0.0435)
BMI (centered at 27)	0.677	(0.0457)	(0.0540)
Age *BMI (centered)	−0.0154	(0.00559)	(0.00666)

8.1.3   Example

We now analyze the systolic blood pressure data across all visits. OUTPUT PACKET VII includes analyses by PROC MIXED of all visits with the EMPIRI-CAL option using the commands below. Note that the commands are identical for the first visit and all visits analyses, but the data set is different.

PROC MIXED; CLASS SEX;
MODEL SBP=SEX AGEC BMIC AGEC*BMIC/S;
PROC MIXED NOCLPRINT EMPIRICAL; CLASS ID SEX;
MODEL SBP=SEX AGEC BMIC AGEC*BMIC/S;
REPEATED/SUBJECT=ID;

As before, SUBJECT=ID tells PROC MIXED which observations are independent, so that it knows how to form the "bite-size sandwiches." Comparing the results to Table 6.2 allows us to see how much precision was gained by using all visits, and also how much difference the robust standard error approach made for correlated data. The main results are in summarized in Table 8.1.

We see that while there was a decrease in standard errors when all visits were included, each observation did not add quite as much new information as a new person would have, because it was correlated to other observations on the same individual. The EMPIRICAL option makes quite a difference for both analyses, but the increase in standard error is more consistent across the coefficients for the correlated situation. This is usually the case. We also notice that the regression coefficients are somewhat changed in the longitudinal analysis. We will examine this further in the next chapter.

8.2   SPECIFYING CORRELATION AND VARIANCE MATRICES

Although regression coefficients obtained by ordinary regression are unbiased even when the independence assumption is violated, the estimators are not efficient. In addition, there may be inherent interest in estimating the correlations between observations. The basic solution to how to incorporate correlation into regression analysis is similar to that employed for data where the equal variance assumption does not hold. Again (in theory) a linear transformation is applied to both sides of the regression equation. However, in this case the transformation is more complex, because the new variables must be made to have uncorrelated residuals in addition to equal variance. We address the details of this transformation in the next section. To find the transformation and to perform the weighted analysis that follows, some type of estimable structure needs to be postulated for how the observations are correlated. In this section we demonstrate some options for how this can be done.

First of all it should be noted that the procedure employed by the EMPIRICAL option to supply the $\text{Var}(Y|X)$ piece in the formula for $\text{Var}(\hat{\boldsymbol{\beta}})$ cannot be directly used in estimating the parameters of the distribution of Y given X. It is only a "post hoc" fix-up of the standard errors, considering that the variance structure may have been misspecified. The reason the EMPIRICAL approach cannot be used directly in the estimation is that EMPIRICAL allows each subject to have its own parameters inside the $\text{Var}(Y_i|X_i)$ matrix. For estimators to have desirable properties such as consistency (i.e., the property of coming closer and closer to the parameter as the sample size increases), the number of parameters to be estimated cannot increase together with the sample size. If it did, nothing would be gained even if the sample size was increased indefinitely, because there would be more and more parameters to estimate. For clustered and longitudinal data, the "sample size" usually refers to the number of subjects n. The number of parameters is allowed to increase with the number of observations per subject k, as long as n/k increases with n. Hence, we must choose ways to parameterize the variance matrix that allow pooling information across subjects. Most commonly, the variance matrix is assumed to be the same for all subjects (except for its dimension $k_i \times k_i$, when k varies).

PROC MIXED has a vast array of options for selecting the variance matrix for the observations within a subject. The notation in the manual and outputs for this variance matrix is R_i. So far, we have fit

$$R_i = \sigma_{y|x}^2 I_{k_i \times k_i}$$

where $I_{k_i \times k_i}$ is the $k_1 \times k_i$ identity matrix. This is referred to as the "independence option" and is the default selected by PROC MIXED when no other variance matrix is indicated. Somewhat confusingly, SAS refers to this default option as "variance components." The reason is the option of random effects models that we will address in Chapter 10. In that context an independent error term is one of the several components of variance. Other options can be specified in the REPEATED statement by stating TYPE=xx, where xx stands for one of the variance matrix structures listed in the manual. For example, the statement

REPEATED/SUBJECT=ID TYPE=CS;

fits the so-called "compound symmetry" variance matrix

$$R_i = \sigma_{y|x}^2 \begin{pmatrix} 1 & \rho & \rho & \rho \\ \rho & 1 & \rho & \rho \\ \rho & \rho & 1 & \rho \\ \rho & \rho & \rho & 1 \end{pmatrix}$$

We note that this particular variance matrix assumes that the variance is the same for all observations and that all observations within a subject are equally correlated. This may not be realistic in longitudinal data, where one may expect that observations that are further apart in time have lower correlation with each other. A variance matrix that incorporates this type of pattern is TYPE=AR(1), which is a so-called "autoregressive" structure borrowed from time series analysis. In this case

$$
R_i = \sigma_{y|x}^2 \begin{pmatrix} 1 & \rho^1 & \rho^2 & \rho^3 \\ \rho^1 & 1 & \rho^1 & \rho^2 \\ \rho^2 & \rho^1 & 1 & \rho^1 \\ \rho^3 & \rho^2 & \rho^1 & 1 \end{pmatrix}
$$

so that the exponent of each element equals the absolute difference between the row and column indicators.

Another popular choice is TYPE=UN, the "unstructured" covariance matrix. Here

$$
R_i = \begin{pmatrix} \sigma_1^2 & \sigma_{12} & \sigma_{13} & \sigma_{14} \\ \sigma_{12} & \sigma_2^2 & \sigma_{23} & \sigma_{24} \\ \sigma_{13} & \sigma_{23} & \sigma_3^2 & \sigma_{34} \\ \sigma_{14} & \sigma_{24} & \sigma_{32} & \sigma_4^2 \end{pmatrix}
$$

The only restriction on this variance matrix is that it is assumed to be the same for all subjects. The subscript i is not needed on R if all subjects have the same number of observations. Of all variance matrices the default "independence" variance, the compound symmetry, and the unstructured are the most popular (in decreasing order). In a future chapter we will discuss yet another more complex, but popular, choice that is constructed from random effects.

One may wonder why we are using the TYPE statement to specify the variance matrix for correlated data, but used the WEIGHT statement for unequal variance data. This is because PROC MIXED does not have the ability to let the variance matrix differ between individuals (SUBJECT's). It can only deal with differences in variance between time points within individuals. In fact, the variance is assumed to be the same across all individuals (with some flexibility to specify groups with different matrices). When dealing with unequal variance as in Chapter 6, the differences were between individuals, and the only way to deal with this in PROC MIXED is through the WEIGHT statement.

8.3   THE LEAST-SQUARES EQUATION INCORPORATING CORRELATION

When we dealt with the problem of unequal variance, the solution to the problem of fitting least-squares equations was found in transforming the regression equation so that the assumption of equal variance was made true. Then, in the end, it turned out that this simply meant that analyses were weighted by the inverse of the variance matrix. The same approach is taken to come up with least-squares equations for correlated data. In this case, a linear combination is taken of each cluster of correlated observations, in such a way that the resulting new variables are uncorrelated. We, in fact, did this in Chapter 4. There, we saw that for pairwise correlated observations that have equal variance, their mean was uncorrelated with their difference.

A rather technical approach is employed to find the linear transformation that works to produce new independent residuals. It is based on a theorem from linear algebra [26]:

Theorem 1 (Spectral Theorem) For every symmetric matrix V there exists a matrix T such that $T'VT = D$ is a diagonal matrix and $T'T = TT' = I$.

When V is the variance matrix of Y, it is symmetric. The theorem then tells us that in theory we can always find a transformation $T'Y$ with a variance matrix $T'\text{Var}(Y)T = T'VT$ that has off-diagonal elements 0. Then T' is the kind of transformation we want to apply to Y to be able to fit the least-squares equations. Note that the second part of the theorem implies that the matrix T has T' as its inverse.

8.3.1 Another Application of the Spectral Theorem

While we use the spectral theorem here to motivate a weighted analysis of correlated data, it has many other applications in statistics. We briefly address one of them as well as some additional terminology associated with the theorem.

The theorem above is called the "spectral theorem" because the set of elements on the diagonal of D is known as the "spectrum" of V. The individual elements on this diagonal are known as "eigenvalues" of V. Because $\text{Var}(T'Y) = T'VT$, they are the variances of the linear combinations resulting from $T'Y$. The linear combinations themselves are known as the "principal components" of V. In practice, principal components are thought of as a way to combine variables. In that context, the principal components with the largest eigenvalues are chosen as a way to reduce the number of variables ("reduce dimensionality") [27]. Choosing the linear combinations with the largest eigenvalues captures the most variability in the data, and capturing variability is good in constructing risk factor scores X, or for differentiating between people on a psychological test.

Starting from the estimated variance matrix of several variables from a data set, the principal components can be obtained by SAS by

PROC PRINCOMP; VAR $y_1 \ldots y_k$;

The result is a set of linear combinations of the variables, which are uncorrelated with each other. Investigators usually choose the two or three linear combinations with the largest variances (i.e., corresponding to the largest "eigenvalues") to work with. If the number of original variables k is large, this can simplify model fitting and presentation of results a great deal. However, it makes sense only if the linear combinations appear to be meaningful. Very often the "first" principal component (the one with the largest variance) turns out to be close to the average of all the variables. The variable SOCIOEC in the functional assessment example in Chapter 7 was formed this way from a set of socioeconomic indicators. They were scaled to have mean 0 and variance 1, as is commonly done with principal components. Principal components are not explicitly involved linear regression analysis of correlated data, but both rely on the spectral theorem.

8.4   APPLYING THE SPECTRAL THEOREM TO THE REGRESSION ANALYSIS OF CORRELATED DATA

Given that we have found the matrix T that serves our purpose of "diagonalizing" V, we can apply matrix algebra and the fact that $T'T = I$ to see that

$$V = TDT'$$

and

$$V^{-1} = (TDT')^{-1} = TD^{-1}T'$$

Then the transformation $P^{-1}Y$ with

$$P^{-1} = D^{-\frac{1}{2}}T'$$

will result in least-squares equations

$$
\begin{aligned}
\hat{\beta} &= [(P^{-1}X)'P^{-1}X]^{-1}[(P^{-1}X)'P^{-1}Y] \\
&= [X'(P^{-1})'P^{-1}X]^{-1}[X'(P^{-1})'P^{-1}Y] \\
&= [X'TD^{-\frac{1}{2}}D^{-\frac{1}{2}}T'X]^{-1}[X'TD^{-\frac{1}{2}}D^{-\frac{1}{2}}T'Y] \\
&= [X'V^{-1}X]^{-1}[X'V^{-1}Y]
\end{aligned}
$$

just as before. The difference is that V and its inverse now have nonzero off-diagonal elements arising from the correlation between observations, while when only unequal variance was the problem $P^{-1} = D^{-\frac{1}{2}}$ could be used for the transformation, because only diagonal elements needed to be transformed.

In the situations dealt with by PROC MIXED, we define the blocks on the variance matrix as R_i. As discussed in the section above, they describe how the residuals ϵ_{ij} for individual i vary and covary. Because observations are assumed to be independent between clusters or individuals, matrix V^{-1} in the equation for $\hat{\beta}$ has submatrices along the main diagonal and 0's elsewhere. This means that, for example,

$$V = \begin{pmatrix} \sigma^2 & \rho\sigma^2 & 0 & 0 & \cdots \\ \rho\sigma^2 & \sigma^2 & 0 & 0 & \cdots \\ 0 & 0 & \sigma^2 & \rho\sigma^2 & \cdots \\ 0 & 0 & \rho\sigma^2 & \sigma^2 & \cdots \\ \cdots & \cdots & \cdots & \cdots & \cdots \end{pmatrix}$$

Because of the block diagonal structure, it can be shown that the expression for the estimator can then be written as the weighted least-squares estimator

$$\hat{\beta} = \sum (X_i' R_i^{-1} X_i)^{-1} \sum X_i' R_i^{-1} Y_i \tag{8.2}$$

For the above V, $R_i = \begin{pmatrix} \sigma^2 & \rho\sigma^2 \\ \rho\sigma^2 & \sigma^2 \end{pmatrix}$, a structure that assumes that the two observations for each individual have the same variance σ^2, and the same correlation ρ, for all individuals.

If the variance is correctly specified, it can be shown as was done for formula (6.7) that

$$\text{Var } \hat{\beta} = \left(\sum_{i=1}^{n} X_i' W_i X_i \right)^{-1} \tag{8.3}$$

The robust or "empirical" standard error can also be derived as before and is given by

$$\hat{\text{Var}}(\hat{\beta}) = \left(\sum_{i=1}^{n} X_i' W_i X_i \right)^{-1} \sum_{i=1}^{n} X_i' W_i \hat{\epsilon}_i \hat{\epsilon}_i' W_i X_i \left(\sum_{i=1}^{n} X_i' W_i X_i \right)^{-1} \tag{8.4}$$

8.5 ANALYSIS OF CORRELATED DATA BY MAXIMUM LIKELIHOOD

Again, a similar analysis of correlated data can be presented from the maximum likelihood perspective. In Chapter 2 we briefly discussed regression analysis in a maximum likelihood context. We saw there that for simple regression analysis with the usual assumptions of linearity, independence of errors, equal variance, and normality, the likelihood is

$$L = \prod_{i=1}^{n} \frac{1}{\hat{\sigma}\sqrt{2\pi}} \exp\left(-\frac{(y_i - \hat{\beta}_0 - \hat{\beta}_1 x_i)^2}{2\hat{\sigma}^2} \right)$$

$$= \left(\frac{1}{\hat{\sigma}\sqrt{2\pi}} \right)^n \exp\left(-\frac{\sum_{i=1}^{n}(y_i - \hat{\beta}_0 - \hat{\beta}_1 x_i)^2}{2\hat{\sigma}^2} \right) \tag{8.5}$$

Because $\sum_{i=1}^{n}(y_i - \hat{\beta}_0 - \hat{\beta}_1 x_i)^2$ appears in a negative exponent, the likelihood is maximized when the least-squares expression is minimized. Then ML and the least-squares approach yield exactly the same estimators for the regression coefficients. In this particular case, the estimation of $\hat{\sigma}^2$ can take place completely separately. Recall that maximum likelihood and least-squares do not yield exactly the same estimator of $\hat{\sigma}^2$, but restricted maximum likelihood coincides with the least squares estimator.

We will now see how (8.2) changes when the assumptions of equal variance and independence are abandoned. In the process we will point out how the results related to the least-squares-based development above.

8.5.1 Non equal Variance

If we insert a different variance for each factor of L, we obtain

$$L = \prod_{i=1}^{n} \frac{1}{\hat{\sigma}_i \sqrt{2\pi}} \exp\left(-\frac{(y_i - \hat{\beta}_0 - \hat{\beta}_1 x_i)^2}{2\hat{\sigma}_i^2}\right)$$

$$= \left[\prod_{i=1}^{n} \frac{1}{\hat{\sigma}_i \sqrt{2\pi}}\right] \exp\left(-\frac{1}{2}\sum_{i=1}^{n} \frac{(y_i - \hat{\beta}_0 - \hat{\beta}_1 x_i)^2}{\hat{\sigma}_i^2}\right) \tag{8.6}$$

We see that a weighted least-squares expression comes into the exponent. Several problems arise in minimizing this least-squares expression. The way (8.7) is stated, there are as many $\hat{\sigma}_i^2$ as there are observations. We suggested two ways of dealing with this problem. One was that, perhaps, the relationship between σ_i^2 and $\mu_{y|x}$ is known, so that σ_i^2 can be described by a fixed number of parameters (i.e., the number of parameters no longer increases with n). The other was to assume that there are actually only k different σ_i^2.

It is difficult to directly maximize (8.6) for $\hat{\beta}$'s and $\hat{\sigma}_i^2$ simultaneously, even using derivatives, because the estimators of regression coefficients depend on $\hat{\sigma}_i^2$. For some situations, it has been shown that shown that iteratively pretending that σ_i^2 is known, then estimating the β's, and adjusting $\hat{\sigma}_i^2$ will result in convergence toward the estimators that truly maximize (8.6). This means that if the process of iteration is repeated a lot of times, we can get arbitrarily close to the maximum likelihood estimators [28]. The method is referred to as "iteratively reweighted least squares." In other situations such as when the variance depends directly on the mean, the iteratively reweighted least-squares estimator is still consistent, but only an approximation to the maximum likelihood estimator from (8.6). They will be close in large samples, because weighted least-squares and maximum likelihood estimators are both consistent. Many other numerical techniques exist for obtaining maximum likelihood estimators in the general case.

8.5.2 Correlated Errors

Equation (8.6) is generalized to clusters of correlated data by considering each cluster an observation from the multivariate normal distribution. All the observations in a cluster in effect constitute one "multivariate" observation, and the factors in the likelihood no longer represent single observation, but instead individuals. This makes sense, because individuals are still assumed independent. The multivariate normal distribution is defined by starting with a set of k independently standard normally distributed variables $y_{i1} \cdots y_{ik}$ and placing them in a matrix

$$Y = \begin{pmatrix} y_{i1} \\ y_{i2} \\ \vdots \\ y_{ik} \end{pmatrix}$$

Recall that a univariate normal variable with mean μ and variance σ^2 can be obtained from a standard normal variable Z, by the transformation $Y = \sigma Z + \mu$. For the multivariate situation we apply the more general, but similar, transformation

$$Y = AY + \mu$$

where A is a $k \times k$ matrix of constants and μ is a column of constants. A set of variables Y that can be obtained this way is said to follow a multivariate normal distribution. The constants in μ allow a different mean for each y_{ij}. The multiplication by A changes the variance of each y_{ij} and introduces correlation. We see that the means of the elements of Y are given by μ and that the variance matrix of Y is $V = AA'$. The process just described is the flip side of the development of least-squares estimation above, where we started with a variance matrix and showed that it can be written in form AA'.

The multivariate density describing the joint behavior of the elements of Y can be written

$$f_Y(Y) = \frac{1}{(2\pi)^{\frac{k}{2}} \sqrt{det\,V}} \exp\left[-\frac{1}{2}(Y - \mu)' V^{-1}(Y - \mu) \right]$$

(Proving this is beyond the scope here. It involves the application of so-called "Jacobian" matrices; for example, Ref. 29.) One way to see how the above formula works is to apply it to the case when V^{-1} is diagonal, so there is no correlation. The above formula then results in multiplication of the independent individual normal densities. The likelihood for correlated data is constructed from products of multivariate densities, each containing the observations $Y_i = \begin{pmatrix} y_{i1} \\ \vdots \\ y_{ij} \\ \vdots \\ y_{ik} \end{pmatrix}$ for that cluster and allowing each of these observations to have their own covariate values

$$\mu = \hat{\mu}_i = \begin{pmatrix} \hat{\beta}_0 + \hat{\beta}_1 x_{1i1} + \cdots \\ \vdots \\ \hat{\beta}_0 + \hat{\beta}_1 x_{1ik} + \cdots \end{pmatrix}$$

Again the result is that $\sum_{i=1}^{n}(Y_i - \hat{\mu}_i)'V_i^{-1}(Y_i - \hat{\mu}_i)$ needs to be minimized, which is done by iteratively reweighted least squares. As before, we have a choice of using either ML or REML for estimating the elements inside V. Because the regression coefficient estimators now depend on the variance estimators (which was not the case with the equal variance assumption), ML and REML estimators of the coefficients will differ slightly.

8.5.3 Example

OUTPUT PACKET VII contains outputs from the blood pressure data analysis using the compound symmetry and unstructured options for the within subject variance. This is achieved through the following statements. For the unstructured option, the order of the observations matters, so we sort by ID and VISIT before running PROC MIXED.

PROC SORT; BY ID VISIT;
PROC MIXED NOCLPRINT (EMPIRICAL); CLASS ID SEX;
MODEL SBP=SEX AGEC BMIC AGEC*BMIC/S;
REPEATED/SUBJECT=ID RCORR TYPE=CS;
PROC MIXED NOCLPRINT (EMPIRICAL); CLASS ID SEX;
MODEL SBP=SEX AGEC BMIC AGE*BMIC/S;
REPEATED/SUBJECT=ID TYPE=UN;

The first run for each variance matrix option is without the EMPIRICAL option, and the RCORR option leads to the correlation matrix being printed. The section with "COVARIANCE PARAMETER ESTIMATES" contains the estimator for the matrix R_i for a subject with 3 observations in this case. For subjects with fewer observations, $\hat{R}_i$ is the appropriate upper left block. We also see that the compound symmetry option estimated the (average) within subject correlation to be 0.35. For the unstructured option we have

$$\hat{R}_i = \begin{pmatrix} 179.4 & 84.9 & 17.0 \\ 84.9 & 212.4 & 76.4 \\ 17.0 & 76.4 & 226.7 \end{pmatrix}$$

The correlation matrix is

$$\begin{pmatrix} 1 & 0.44 & 0.08 \\ 0.44 & 1 & 0.35 \\ 0.08 & 0.35 & 1 \end{pmatrix}$$

Table 8.2 $\hat{\beta}$ **(Model-Based se), (Empirical se) Based on Different Correlation Structures**

	Compound Symmetry		Unstructured	
Intercept	126	(0.460), (0.462)	126	(0.458), (0.465)
Female	−5.90	(0.663), (0.664)	−6.08	(0.659), (0.658)
Age (centered at 50)	0.269	(0.0426), (0.0436)	0.282	(0.0425), (0.0427)
BMI (centered at 27)	0.627	(0.0510), (0.0544)	0.630	(0.0515), (0.0539)
Age *BMI (centered)	−0.0152	(0.00597), (0.00679)	−0.0136	(0.00600), (0.00672)

We observe that the variance becomes larger with follow-up time. This is consistent with the higher variance we observed cross-sectionally at higher predicted blood pressure values. It could be due to variable effects of aging (as we will actually examine in Chapter 10) or weight gain across people, or due to the variance (blood pressure lability) biologically depending on the absolute mean blood pressure. We also observe that the correlation is much lower between visits 1 and 3 than between 1 and 2, or between 2 and 3. There are, of course, fewer observations at visit 3, so the correlation estimates with SBP at this visit may be more unstable than that between visits 1 and 2. We may note that the correlation structures we are considering are nested, so we can perform likelihood ratio tests. We see that $-2 \log (REML)$ is 19491.5 for the independence structure with just one variance parameter (the residual variance), 19353.3 for compound symmetry with two variance parameters, and 19300.5 for unstructured variance with six variance parameters. The "Null Model Likelihood Ratio test" on the output tests both of the latter options versus independence. A test for unstructured versus compound symmetry can be constructed as $19353.3 - 19300.5 = 52.8$, which can be compared with a χ^2-distribution with four degrees of freedom. For example, the 95th percentile of this distribution is 9.49. Hence the difference between the unstructured and compound symmetry models is highly statistically significant.

Table 8.2 shows estimated regression coefficients with model based and empirical standard errors with compound symmetry and unstructured variance structures. The same results for the independence structure were in Table 8.1. We see that the unstructured option, although seemingly much more correct, leads to only slight decrease in the standard errors. Hence, there is little efficiency gained. This is not unusual and has led many investigators to routinely choose independence or other simple options for their analysis. The empirical option yields larger standard errors in each case. There is also a change in the estimates of regression coefficients with different covariance structures. This may indicate some lack of model fit. We will further examine it in Chapter 9.

Non-nested models can be compared via the AIC, AICC, and BIC criteria listed on the output. These criteria are based on the $-2 \log (REML)$, but involve a penalty for the number of parameters fitted. The AIC equals $-2 \log (REML)$ plus 2 times the number of variance parameters (i.e., $-2 \log (REML) + 2d$), while the BIC equals $-2 \log (REML) + d \log(n)$. The penalty makes sense because efficiency is

Table 8.3 $\hat{\beta}$ **(Model-Based se), (Empirical se) Based on Autoregressive AR(1) Variance Structure**

	Autoregressive	
Intercept	126	(0.461), (0.463)
Female	−5.96	(0.665), (0.661)
Age (centered at 50)	0.278	(0.0429), (0.0431)
BMI (centered at 27)	0.637	(0.0513), (0.0539)
Age *BMI (centered)	−0.0138	(0.00602), (0.0671)

lost when too many parameters are fitted, yet $-2\log(REML)$ will decrease with adding parameters to a model. BIC has become popular, especially in the social sciences, and there is some evidence that it performs better than AIC [30]. Certainly BIC, as compared to AIC, will favor models that have simpler structure. For independence and the models in Table 8.2 we have BIC 19498.7, 19367.7, and 19343.8, respectively, so the unstructured option appears best of the three. Yet another variance structure is the autoregressive AR(1) mentioned above. It has two variance parameters, just as compound symmetry, so the two are not nested. (Independence is nested into all structures, and all structures specified by REPEATED are nested in the unstructured.) AR(1) yields a BIC of 19331.6. Hence, the autoregressive model appears even better based on the BIC. The $-2\log REML$ for the autoregressive model is 19317.1, still statistically significantly worse than the unstructured. The results from fitting the autoregressive model are in Table 8.3.

We see that the results are quite similar to those for the unstructured option in Table 8.2. As the above discussion indicates, the choice of the best model is not always clear-cut and depends on the purposes of the analysis. If understanding the correlation structure is of inherent interest, more emphasis may be put on the likelihood ratio tests and the BIC. If, as is often the case, the regression coefficients themselves are of primary interest, a simple structure such as independence or compound symmetry will often suffice and not lead to notable lack of efficiency. It has become common in recent years to include consideration of the empirical standard errors rather than to rely on the model-based option with correlated data.

Finally, OUTPUT PACKET VII shows the unstructured analysis using ML rather than REML. It is included to show that because the estimators taking correlation and unequal variance into account depend on the variance estimators, ML and REML estimators differ slightly.

OUTPUT PACKET VII: ANALYSIS OF LONGITUDINAL DATA IN WISCONSIN SLEEP COHORT

VII.1. Unweighted Least-Squares Approach

Analysis of SBP—All Visits Wisconsin Sleep Cohort
Independence Correlation Structure—Model-Based Standard Error
  The Mixed Procedure

Model Information

Data set	WORK.A
Dependent variable	SBP
Covariance structure	**Variance components**
Subject effect	id
Estimation method	REML
Residual variance method	Parameter
Fixed effects SE method	**Model-based**
Degrees-of-freedom method	Between–within

Dimensions

Covariance parameters	**1**
Columns in X	6
Columns in Z	0
Subjects	1370
Maximum Observations per subject	3
Observations used	2404
Observations not used	33
Total observations	2437

Iteration History[a]

Iteration	Evaluations	−2 Residual Log Likelihood	Criterion
0	1	19491.46408153	
1	1	19491.46408154	0.00000000

[a]Convergence criteria met.

Covariance Parameter Estimates

Covariance Parameter	Subject	Estimate
Residual	Id	193.39

Fit Statistics

−2 Residual Log Likelihood	19491.5
AIC (smaller is better)	19493.5
AICC (smaller is better)	19493.5
BIC (smaller is better)	**19498.7**

Null Model Likelihood Ratio Test

DF	Chi-Square	Pr > ChiSq
0	0.00	1.0000

Solution for Fixed Effects

Effect	Sex	Estimate	Standard Error	DF	t Value	Pr > $|t|$
Intercept		125.58	0.4006	1368	313.50	<.0001
sex	F	−6.0230	0.5770	1368	−10.44	<.0001
sex	M	0	.	.	.	.
agec		0.3550	0.03875	1031	9.16	<.0001
bmic		0.6765	0.04571	1031	14.80	<.0001
agec*bmic		−0.01539	0.005587	1031	−2.76	0.0060

Type 3 Tests of Fixed Effects

Effect	Num DF	Den DF	F Value	Pr > F
sex	1	1368	108.98	<.0001
agec	1	1031	83.95	<.0001
bmic	1	1031	219.08	<.0001
agec*bmic	1	1031	7.59	0.0060

Independence Correlation Structure—Empirical Standard Error

Model Information

Data set	WORK.A
Dependent variable	SBP
Covariance structure	**Variance components**
Subject effect	id
Estimation method	REML
Residual variance method	Parameter
Fixed effects SE method	**Empirical**
Degrees-of-freedom method	Between−within

Solution for Fixed Effects

Effect	Sex	Estimate	Standard Error	DF	t Value	Pr > |t|
Intercept		125.58	0.4612	1368	272.27	<.0001
sex	F	−6.0230	0.6675	1368	−9.02	<.0001
sex	M	0	.	.	.	.
agec		0.3550	0.04352	1031	8.16	<.0001
bmic		0.6765	0.05404	1031	12.52	<.0001
agec*bmic		−0.01539	0.006659	1031	−2.31	0.0210

Type 3 Tests of Fixed Effects

Effect	Num DF	Den DF	F Value	Pr > F
sex	1	1368	81.42	<0.0001
agec	1	1031	66.56	<0.0001
bmic	1	1031	156.70	<0.0001
agec*bmic	1	1031	5.34	0.0210

VII.2. Fitting Compound Symmetry Variance

Analysis of SBP—All Visits Wisconsin Sleep Cohort
Compound Symmetry—model-based Standard Error
   The Mixed Procedure

Model Information

Data set	WORK.A
Dependent variable	SBP
Covariance structure	**Compound symmetry**
Subject effect	id
Estimation method	REML
Residual variance method	Profile
Fixed effects SE method	**Model-based**
Degrees-of-freedom method	Between–within

Dimensions[a]

Covariance parameters	**2**
Columns in X	6
Columns in Z	0
Subjects	1370
Maximum Observations per subject	3
Observations used	2404
Observations not used	33
Total observations	2437

[a]Convergence criteria met.

Estimated *R* Correlation: Matrix for id S0001

Row	Col1	Col2	Col3
1	1.0000	0.3498	0.3498
2	0.3498	1.0000	0.3498
3	0.3498	0.3498	1.0000

Covariance Parameter Estimates

Covariance Parameter	Subject	Estimate
CS	id	68.0259
Residual		126.45

Fit Statistics

−2 Residual log likelihood	19353.3
AIC (smaller is better)	19357.3
AICC (smaller is better)	19357.3
BIC (smaller is better)	**19367.7**

Null Model Likelihood Ratio Test

DF	Chi-Square	Pr > ChiSq
1	138.20	<0.0001

Solution for Fixed Effects

Effect	Sex	Estimate	Standard Error	DF	*t* Value	Pr > |*t*|
Intercept		125.55	0.4598	1368	273.07	<0.0001
sex	F	−5.9026	0.6634	1368	−8.90	<0.0001
sex	M	0	.	.	.	.
agec		0.2694	0.04255	1031	6.33	<0.0001
bmic		0.6267	0.05104	1031	12.28	<0.0001
agec*bmic		−0.01516	0.005972	1031	−2.54	0.0113

Type 3 Tests of Fixed Effects

Effect	Num DF	Den DF	*F* Value	Pr > *F*
sex	1	1368	79.17	<.0001
agec	1	1031	40.08	<.0001
bmic	1	1031	150.74	<.0001
agec*bmic	1	1031	6.44	0.0113

Model Information

Data set	WORK.A
Dependent variable	SBP
Covariance structure	**Compound symmetry**
Subject effect	id
Estimation method	REML
Residual variance method	Profile
Fixed effects SE method	**Empirical**
Degrees-of-freedom method	Between–within

Solution for Fixed Effects

Effect	Sex	Estimate	Standard Error	DF	t Value	Pr > |t|
Intercept		125.55	0.4620	1368	271.75	<0.0001
sex	F	−5.9026	0.6642	1368	−8.89	<0.0001
sex	M	0	.	.	.	.
agec		0.2694	0.04364	1031	6.17	<0.0001
bmic		0.6267	0.05440	1031	11.52	<0.0001
agec*bmic		−0.01516	0.006786	1031	−2.23	0.0257

Type 3 Tests of Fixed Effects

Effect	Num DF	Den DF	F Value	Pr > F
sex	1	1368	78.96	<0.0001
agec	1	1031	38.10	<0.0001
bmic	1	1031	132.73	<0.0001
agec*bmic	1	1031	4.99	0.0257

VII.3. Fitting Unstructured Variance

Analysis of SBP—All Visits Wisconsin Sleep Cohort
Unstructured—Model-Based Standard Error
  The Mixed Procedure

Model Information

Data set	WORK.A
Dependent variable	SBP
Covariance structure	**Unstructured**
Subject effect	id
Estimation method	REML
Residual variance method	None
Fixed effects SE method	**Model-based**
Degrees-of-freedom method	Between–within

Dimensions

Covariance parameters	**6**
Columns in X	6
Columns in Z	0
Subjects	1370
Maximum observations per subject	3
Observations used	2404
Observations not used	33
Total observations	2437

Estimated R Correlation: Matrix for id S0001

Row	Col1	Col2	Col3
1	1.0000	0.4350	0.08442
2	0.4350	1.0000	0.3484
3	0.08442	0.3484	1.0000

Covariance Parameter Estimates

Covariance Parameter	Subject	Estimate
UN(1,1)	Id	179.40
UN(2,1)	Id	84.9037
UN(2,2)	Id	212.40
UN(3,1)	Id	17.0236
UN(3,2)	Id	76.4409
UN(3,3)	Id	226.66

Fit Statistics

-2 Residual log likelihood	19300.5
AIC (smaller is better)	19312.5
AICC (smaller is better)	19312.5
BIC (smaller is better)	**19343.8**

Null Model Likelihood Ratio Test

DF	Chi-Square	Pr > ChiSq
5	190.99	<0.0001

Solution for Fixed Effects

Effect	Sex	Estimate	Standard Error	DF	t Value	Pr > |t|
Intercept		125.76	0.4578	1368	274.74	<0.0001
sex	F	−6.0757	0.6594	1368	−9.21	<0.0001
sex	M	0	.	.	.	.
agec		0.2816	0.04249	1368	6.63	<0.0001
bmic		0.6301	0.05148	1368	12.24	<0.0001
agec*bmic		−0.01364	0.005996	1368	−2.27	0.0231

Type 3 Tests of Fixed Effects

Effect	Num DF	Den DF	F Value	Pr > F
sex	1	1368	84.89	<0.0001
agec	1	1368	43.92	<0.0001
bmic	1	1368	149.79	<0.0001
agec*bmic	1	1368	5.17	0.0231

Model Information

Data set	WORK.A
Dependent variable	SBP
Covariance structure	**Unstructured**
Subject effect	Id
Estimation method	REML
Residual variance method	None
Fixed effects SE method	**Empirical**
Degrees-of-freedom method	Between−within

Solution for Fixed Effects

Effect	Sex	Estimate	Standard Error	DF	t Value	Pr > |t|
Intercept		125.76	0.4645	1368	270.74	<0.0001
sex	F	−6.0757	0.6575	1368	−9.24	<0.0001
sex	M	0	.	.	.	.
agec		0.2816	0.04265	1368	6.60	<0.0001
bmic		0.6301	0.05391	1368	11.69	<0.0001
agec*bmic		−0.01364	0.006723	1368	−2.03	0.0427

Type 3 Tests of Fixed Effects

Effect	Num DF	Den DF	F Value	Pr > F
sex	1	1368	85.40	<.0001
agec	1	1368	43.59	<.0001
bmic	1	1368	136.58	<.0001
agec*bmic	1	1368	4.11	0.0427

VII.4. Fitting AR(1) Variance

Analysis of SBP—All Visits Wisconsin Sleep Cohort
Autoregressive—Model-Based Standard Error
   The Mixed Procedure

Model Information

Data set	WORK.A
Dependent variable	SBP
Covariance structure	**Autoregressive**
Subject effect	id
Estimation method	REML
Residual variance method	Profile
Fixed effects SE method	**Model-based**
Degrees-of-freedom method	Between–within

Dimensions

Covariance parameters	**2**
Columns in X	6
Columns in Z	0
Subjects	1370
Maximum observations per subject	3
Observations used	2404
Observations not used	33
Total observations	2437

Estimated R Correlation: Matrix for id A0001

Row	Col1	Col2	Col3
1	1.0000	0.4032	0.1626
2	0.4032	1.0000	0.4032
3	0.1626	0.4032	1.0000

Covariance Parameter Estimates

Covariance Parameter	Subject	Estimate
AR(1)	id	0.4032
Residual		194.20

Fit Statistics

−2 Residual log likelihood	19317.1
AIC (smaller is better)	19321.1
AICC (smaller is better)	19321.1
BIC (smaller is better)	**19331.6**

Null Model Likelihood Ratio Test

DF	Chi-Square	Pr > ChiSq
1	174.35	<0.0001

Solution for Fixed Effects

Effect	Sex	Estimate	Standard Error	DF	t Value	Pr > |t|
Intercept		125.52	0.4608	1368	272.37	<0.0001
sex	F	−5.9596	0.6654	1368	−8.96	<0.0001
sex	M	0	.	.	.	.
agec		0.2783	0.04286	1031	6.49	<0.0001
bmic		0.6370	0.05128	1031	12.42	<0.0001
agec*bmic		−0.01375	0.006016	1031	−2.29	0.0225

Type 3 Tests of Fixed Effects

Effect	Num DF	Den DF	F Value	Pr > F
Sex	1	1368	80.21	<0.0001
Agec	1	1031	42.15	<0.0001
Bmic	1	1031	154.29	<0.0001
agec*bmic	1	1031	5.23	0.0225

Model Information

Data set	WORK.A
Dependent variable	SBP
Covariance structure	**Autoregressive**
Subject effect	id
Estimation method	REML
Residual variance method	Profile
Fixed effects SE method	**Empirical**
Degrees-of-freedom method	Between–within

Solution for Fixed Effects

Effect	Sex	Estimate	Standard Error	DF	t Value	Pr > |t|
Intercept		125.52	0.4628	1368	271.24	<0.0001
sex	F	−5.9596	0.6613	1368	−9.01	<0.0001
sex	M	0	.	.	.	.
agec		0.2783	0.04308	1031	6.46	<0.0001
bmic		0.6370	0.05393	1031	11.81	<0.0001
agec*bmic		−0.01375	0.006714	1031	−2.05	0.0408

Type 3 Tests of Fixed Effects

Effect	Num DF	Den DF	F Value	Pr > F
sex	1	1368	81.23	<0.0001
agec	1	1031	41.72	<0.0001
bmic	1	1031	139.54	<0.0001
agec*bmic	1	1031	4.20	0.0408

CHAPTER NINE

A Further Study of How the Transformation Works with Correlated Data

The transformations applied to correlated data in constructing least-squares estimators are quite technical and messy. In practice, of course, analyses are performed by the application of weighting, rather than by directly transforming the equation. Nonetheless, we will briefly illustrate the transformation approach for two observations per individual ($k = 2$) to generate insight into the components that go into the estimator. More specifically, we will see that clustered or longitudinal models combine information on how covariates relate to the outcome between and within individuals. This chapter, although somewhat technical and ultimately philosophical, is important for understanding the implications of analyses of correlated data in observational studies.

Consider the situation of two correlated observations per individual discussed in Chapter 4. This means that we assume each individual to have two observations y_{i1} and y_{i2}, multivariately seen as

$$Y_i = \begin{pmatrix} y_{i1} \\ y_{i2} \end{pmatrix}$$

which are related to X_i by the regression equation

$$Y_i = X_i \boldsymbol{\beta} = \begin{pmatrix} \beta_0 + \beta_1 x_{i1} + \epsilon_{i1} \\ \beta_0 + \beta_1 x_{i2} + \epsilon_{i2} \end{pmatrix} \tag{9.1}$$

Quantitative Methods in Population Health, by Mari Palta
ISBN 0-471-45505-9   Copyright © 2003 John Wiley & Sons, Inc.

where ϵ_{ij} have equal variance σ^2. Note that both observations follow the same regression equation. We found in Chapter 4 that the transformation matrix

$$T = T_i = \begin{pmatrix} \frac{1}{2} & +1 \\ \frac{1}{2} & -1 \end{pmatrix}$$

produced the means and differences, and that these were uncorrelated linear combinations. The previous development dealt with unconditional y. However, the same transformation can be applied to both sides of a regression equation, and the mean and difference of $\epsilon_{i1}, \epsilon_{i2}$ will be uncorrelated (as long as the equal variance assumption holds).

To make T_i into the T_i of the spectral theorem in Chapter 8, we have to rescale its columns so that $T_i T_i' = I$. The following matrix works, as can verified by performing the multiplication $T_i T_i'$:

$$T_i = \frac{1}{\sqrt{2}} \begin{pmatrix} 1 & 1 \\ 1 & -1 \end{pmatrix}$$

We have just multiplied the mean and difference by constants, so the two resulting linear combinations are still independent. We showed before that

$$\text{Var}(\overline{y}_i | x_{i1}, x_{i2}) = \text{Var}\left[\frac{y_1 + y_2}{2} \Big| x_{i1}, x_{i2} \right]$$

$$= \text{Var}\left(\frac{\epsilon_{i1} + \epsilon_{i2}}{2} \right) = \frac{\sigma^2(1 + \rho)}{2}$$

$$\text{Var}(\Delta y) = \text{Var}(y_1 - y_2) = \text{Var}(\epsilon_{i1} - \epsilon_{i2}) = 2\sigma^2(1 - \rho)$$

where we have substituted ϵ_{i1} and ϵ_{i2} for y_1 and y_2. Now taking $\frac{1}{\sqrt{2}}(\epsilon_{i1} + \epsilon_{i2})$ and $\frac{1}{\sqrt{2}}(\epsilon_{i1} - \epsilon_{i2})$ as the linear transformation matrix T_i implies

$$\text{Var}\left(\frac{1}{\sqrt{2}}(\epsilon_{i1} + \epsilon_{i2}) \right) = \frac{1}{2}[2\sigma^2(1 + \rho)] = \sigma^2(1 + \rho)$$

$$\text{Var}\left(\frac{1}{\sqrt{2}}(\epsilon_{i1} - \epsilon_{i2}) \right) = \frac{1}{2}[2\sigma^2(1 - \rho)] = \sigma^2(1 - \rho)$$

We have found the matrix T_i of the spectral theorem that makes the variance diagonal

$$T'VT = D = \begin{pmatrix} \sigma^2(1 + \rho) & 0 \\ 0 & \sigma^2(1 - \rho) \end{pmatrix}$$

but we still have to make the variances on the diagonal equal by creating P^{-1} of Chapter 8:

$$P^{-1} = D_i^{-\frac{1}{2}} T_i' = \frac{1}{\sqrt{2}} \begin{pmatrix} \frac{1}{\sqrt{(1+\rho)\sigma^2}} & 0 \\ 0 & \frac{1}{\sqrt{(1-\rho)\sigma^2}} \end{pmatrix} \begin{pmatrix} 1 & 1 \\ 1 & -1 \end{pmatrix}$$

$$= \frac{1}{\sqrt{2}} \begin{pmatrix} \frac{1}{\sqrt{(1+\rho)\sigma^2}} & \frac{1}{\sqrt{(1+\rho)\sigma^2}} \\ \frac{1}{\sqrt{2(1-\rho)\sigma^2}} & -\frac{1}{\sqrt{(1-\rho)\sigma^2}} \end{pmatrix}$$

so that

$$P^{-1} Y_i = \begin{pmatrix} \frac{1}{\sqrt{2(1+\rho)\sigma^2}}(y_{i1} + y_{i2}) \\ \frac{1}{\sqrt{2(1-\rho)\sigma^2}}(y_{i1} - y_{i2}) \end{pmatrix} = \begin{pmatrix} \sqrt{w_1}\, \bar{y}_i \\ \sqrt{w_2} \Delta y_i \end{pmatrix}$$

where now $w_1 = \frac{2}{(1+\rho)\sigma^2}$ and $w_2 = \frac{1}{2(1-\rho)\sigma^2}$. With corresponding expressions for the terms on the right-hand side of (9.1)

$$P^{-1} X_i = \begin{pmatrix} \sqrt{w_1} & \sqrt{w_1}\, \bar{x}_i \\ 0 & \sqrt{w_2}\, \Delta x_i \end{pmatrix}$$

so that

$$\begin{pmatrix} \sqrt{w_1}\, \bar{y}_i \\ \sqrt{w_2} \Delta y_i \end{pmatrix} = \begin{pmatrix} \sqrt{w_1}[\beta_0 + \beta_1 \bar{x}_i] \\ \sqrt{w_2}\beta_1 \Delta x_i \end{pmatrix} + \begin{pmatrix} e_{i1} \\ e_{i2} \end{pmatrix}$$

We have two regressions with independent errors, represented by the two rows. One is based on the mean y's of each individual's observations, and the other is based on the difference of the two observations for each individual. The second one has no intercept, because when forming the differences, the intercept cancels out. The weights w_1 and w_2 serve to make e_{i1} and e_{i2} have the same variance, so that the least-squares equations from the two regression can be combined for estimating β_1. In effect, the resulting estimator $\hat{\beta}_1$ combines between individual information on how y changes with x (through the regression of $\bar{y}_i$ on $\bar{x}_i$) and within individual information on how y changes with x (through directly considering the change Δy_i in y with a change Δx_i in x). *It is important to realize that since both equations have the same slope β_1, these two aspects of the $y - x$ relationship are assumed to be the same.* We will refer to a regression slope based on between individual information as β_B and will refer to a regression slope based on within individual change as β_W.

9.1 WHY WOULD β_W AND β_B DIFFER?

Although the discovery that β_W and β_B may differ goes back at least to 1938 [31], it has received little attention in longitudinal and clustered analyses in biostatistics until recently [32–36]. This is despite the fact that such differences have been reported in many applications [37–39].

The topic has been much more vigorously addressed in econometrics [40–44] and in survey research [45]. This is probably because biostatistics has traditionally emphasized randomly assigned X such that $X_i = X$. As we see above, β_B can affect the analysis only when $\overline{x}_{i.}$ differ between individuals.

Logical considerations imply that if the regression coefficient measures a causal effect of x on y, one would expect that the difference in y observed after a given change in x would be the same as the difference in y between individual having that difference in x. For example, we may assume that if a study shows that people who run a mile a day have 10 mmHg lower blood pressure on average than do sedentary people, then starting to run a mile a day will lower a person's blood pressure on average 10 mmHg. An obvious problem is that within-individual changes in x may not have an immediate impact on y. For example, if a person starts running, blood pressure may not decrease right away. Hence, the first reason we may observe differences in β_W and β_B is that there are "lagged" or "carry-over" effects of x [35]. When investigating factors x that may not affect y immediately, or that are cumulative, longitudinal analyses may be difficult to interpret. On the other hand, β_W can capture short-term effects not reflected in β_B. For example, exercise just before taking the blood pressure may increase it, while regular exercise may decrease blood pressure.

The coefficients β_W and β_B may also differ because confounders do not equally affect both. For example, there may be characteristics (e.g., related to health consciousness) that influence whether a person runs a mile a day and also have an effect on blood pressure separate from that of the exercise itself. These characteristics may differ between individuals, but stay relatively constant within individual. As discussed in Chapter 1, confounding regularly happens also in ordinary regression, but may be hard to detect. Luckily, the circumstance of longitudinal data offers greater potential for discovering the omission, because it may affect between and within individual regressions differently.

In a longitudinal model, omitted covariates can be split into within and between individual components. The below formulas expand (1.2) and (1.3) for the longitudinal data situation. Within-individual correlations and variances are annotated by asterisks while corresponding quantities without asterisks denote between-individual quantities.

$$y_{ij} = \beta_0 + \beta'_1 x_{ij} + \beta_2(w_i + w^*_{ij}) + e_{ij}$$

Where w_{ij} has mean 0, is independent from w_i and represents within individual changes from the overall w_i for individual i. It can be shown [32] that then

$$\beta_W = \beta'_1 + \beta_2 \rho^*_{xw} \frac{\sigma^*_w}{\sigma^*_x}$$

and

$$\beta_B = \beta_1' + \beta_2 \left[(1 - \eta_x) \rho_{xw}^* \frac{\sigma_w^*}{\sigma_x^*} + \eta_x \rho_{xz} \frac{\sigma_w}{\sigma_x} \right]$$

$$\eta_x = \frac{\sigma_x^2}{\sigma_x^2 + \sigma_x^{*2}/k}$$

We see that if $\rho_{xw} \frac{\sigma_w}{\sigma_x} \neq \rho_{xw}^* \frac{\sigma_w^*}{\sigma_x^*}$, β_W and β_B differ, and the omission can be detected by methods we outline below.

An important example concerns aging effects, which are commonly examined in longitudinal analyses. Individuals who differ in age during the time frame of a study were also born in different years. There may be differences associated with birth year in the outcome y. For example, persons born in earlier years may have had a different childhood diet. Thus "age" in the model reflects not only the effects of aging, but also those of birth year and different unmeasured variables w_i correlated with birth year. Such effects are called "cohort effects." More generally, cohort effects may be considered to include not only birth cohort phenomena, but also aberrations such as attracting a different type of person into a multiyear study in different study years.

On the other hand, longitudinal studies must remain alert to time trends in general and drifts in measurement technique of the study. Such effects, which are also a form of confounding or omitted covariates w_{ij}^*, are referred to as "period effects." Other unmeasured covariates may act similar to cohort and period effects and also cause β_W and β_B to differ. Cohort effects change β_B while period effects can change both β_B and β_W (see, e.g., Dwyer et al. [46] for additional examples).

Measurement error in covariates can cause β_W and β_B to differ [47, 48]. In that situation, under the most common models for measurement error, both coefficients are biased, but β_B will tend to be less biased and also stronger. Another, more mathematical reason for differing β_W and β_B, is nonlinearity, or poorly chosen functions for the relationship of x to y. It has been shown that in most situations, if the relationship is not truly linear, the two coefficients will emphasize different parts of the curve and then not be the same [49]. Finally, differential dropout of individuals with different time trends can cause the two coefficients to differ.

The above scenarios of between and within individual differences are discussed in further detail by Shen [50] and Palta and Seplaki [51].

9.2 HOW THE BETWEEN- AND WITHIN-INDIVIDUAL ESTIMATORS ARE COMBINED

We explicitly derived the process involved in combining between and within individual estimators only for the case of two observations per person. The development can be generalized to any number of observations k, when $\text{Var}(Y_i | X_i)$ is assumed

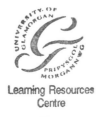

to have compound symmetry structure. It may be noted that when $k = 2$, all correlation structures (that do not vary with individual), except independence, are the same. The compound symmetry estimator, written as an expression combining between and within individual regressions, is known in econometrics as the Balestra–Nerlove estimator [52]. It can be derived by a generalization of the above transformation approach. This estimator is written as

$$\hat{\beta}_1 = \frac{\text{weight}_B \hat{\beta}_B + \sum\limits_{i=1}^{n} \text{weight}_{W_i} \hat{\beta}_{W_i}}{\text{weight}_B + \sum\limits_{i=1}^{n} \text{weight}_{W_i}}$$

$$= \frac{\dfrac{1}{(1 - \rho + k\rho)} \sum\limits_{i=1}^{n} (\bar{x}_i - \bar{x})^2 \hat{\beta}_B + \dfrac{1}{(1 - \rho)k} \sum\limits_{i=1}^{n} \sum\limits_{j=1}^{k} (x_{ij} - \bar{x}_i)^2 \hat{\beta}_{W_i}}{\dfrac{1}{(1 - \rho + k\rho)} \sum\limits_{i=1}^{n} (\bar{x}_i - \bar{x})^2 + \dfrac{1}{(1 - \rho)k} \sum\limits_{i=1}^{n} \sum\limits_{j=1}^{k} (x_{ij} - \bar{x}_i)^2} \tag{9.2}$$

In formula (9.2), $\text{weight}_B = \frac{1}{(1-\rho+k\rho)} \sum_{i=1}^{n} (\bar{x}_i - \bar{x})^2$ is proportional to the inverse of the variance of $\hat{\beta}_B$, and $\text{weight}_{W_i} = \frac{1}{(1-\rho)k} \sum_{j=1}^{k} (x_{ij} - \bar{x}_i)^2$ is proportional to the inverse of the variance of each $\hat{\beta}_{W_i}$. $\hat{\beta}_B$ and all $\hat{\beta}_{W_i}$ are mutually independent estimators of $\hat{\beta}_1$. Hence, to optimally use all the information, they should be combined (as (9.2) does) with inverse variance weights. If analysis is based only on between-individual information $\hat{\beta}_B$ from regression of $\bar{y}_i$ on $\bar{x}_i$ could be used. If only within-individual information is to be used, the overall within-individual estimator can be obtained by

$$\hat{\beta}_W = \frac{\sum\limits_{i=1}^{n} \sum\limits_{j=1}^{k} (x_{ij} - \bar{x}_i)^2 \hat{\beta}_{W_i}}{\sum\limits_{i=1}^{n} \sum\limits_{j=1}^{k} (x_{ij} - \bar{x}_i)^2}$$

Formula (9.2) is another demonstration of the well-known principle that when statistics are assumed to estimate the same parameters they should be combined, weighted by the inverse of their respective variances. The compound symmetry variance structure dictates the form of the variances of the relevant between- and within-individual regression estimators.

Although, for $k > 2$, formula (9.3) holds only to compound symmetry variance structure, the principles it reflects apply to other cases. These principles are:

1. The higher the correlation within cluster, the more weight a combined estimator gives to the within-individual change in y with x. In other words: When

within-individual correlation is high, the regression estimators from PROC MIXED (say) will emphasize the effects of within individual change in x. This at first appears counterintuitive, but remember from Chapter 4 that the variance of a difference is smaller the higher the correlation between the measurements. Within-individual changes are like within-individual differences, and they are given more weight when their variance is smaller.

2. The more $\bar{x}_i$ varies between individuals, the more weight a combined estimator gives to differences in $\bar{y}_i$ between individuals with different $\bar{x}_i$. In other words: If there tend to be larger differences in x between individuals than within (e.g., if a study includes a wide age range, but follows individuals for a relatively short time), the regression estimators from PROC MIXED (say) will represent comparison of individuals at different levels of x. When $x_{ij} = x_j \hat{\beta} = \hat{\beta}_w$.

3. The larger k is, the more weight a combined estimator gives to the within-individual change in y with x. In other words: When each individual has a large number of observations, the regression estimator from PROC MIXED (say) tends to emphasize within individual change.

9.3 HOW TO PROCEED IN PRACTICE

It is a good idea to check the equality of β_W and β_B for all covariates that change within individual before finalizing a model. This can be done either by explicitly forming the estimators $\hat{\beta}_B$ and $\hat{\beta}_W$ given above or by simplifying $\hat{\beta}_W$ to the unweighted average

$$\hat{\beta}_W = \sum_{i=1}^{n} \hat{\beta}_{W_i}/n$$

Even simpler in most situations, especially when there are several covariates, is to fit the model

$$y_{ij} = \beta_0 + \beta_1' x_{ij} + \gamma \bar{x}_i + \epsilon_{ij}$$

or with several x,

$$y_{ij} = \beta_0 + \beta_1' x_{1ij} + \gamma_1 \bar{x}_{1i} + \beta_2' x_{2ij} + \gamma_2 \bar{x}_{2i} + \cdots + \epsilon_{ij} \tag{9.3}$$

From this model we see that

$$\bar{y}_i = \beta_0 + \beta_1' \bar{x}_{1i} + \gamma_1 \bar{x}_{1i} + \cdots + \bar{\epsilon}_i$$

so that $\beta_B = \beta_1' + \gamma_,$. Subtracting the first equation from the second, we obtain

$$y_{ij} - \bar{y}_i = \beta_1'(x_{1ij} - \bar{x}_{1i}) + \cdots + \epsilon_{ij} - \bar{\epsilon}_i$$

So β_1' is actually the regression of within-individual changes in y on within-individual changes in x. By definition, then $\beta_1' = \beta_W$ and $\gamma = \beta_B - \beta_W$. We recommend first fitting model (9.3) and checking whether the β_B and β_W differ substantially by testing the hypothesis $H_0 : \gamma_1 = \gamma_2 = \cdots = 0$ [53]. These checks are quite sensitive for lack of model fit in situations where $\bar{x}_i$ varies considerably between individuals. When it is found that between- and within-individual effects differ significantly and substantively, it becomes necessary to either find the cause and correct for it, or to fit a model with separate within- and between-individual components

$$y_{ij} = \beta_0 + \beta_W(x_{ij} - \bar{x}_i) + \beta_B\bar{x}_i + \epsilon_{ij}$$

Unfortunately, this model can be difficult to interpret when β_B and β_W differ, but it would be equally unfortunate to take the combined longitudinal estimator at face value. As a general rule, investigators tend to put more faith in the causal nature of β_W, but as we discussed above, this assumes a high level of continuous quality control of measurement, no lags or aberrant short-term effects, and also that no events intervened either as a consequence of the study or externally, as we see happening in the example below. Another problem is that efficiency is usually reduced when β_B and β_W cannot be combined. Because of the relatively short duration of most studies in population health, $\hat{\beta}_W$ usually has the larger standard error. We see this to be the case in our example below.

Finally, it should be pointed out that there are other ways to define between- and within-individual effects. For example, Diggle et al. [6] recommend fitting the terms x_{i1} and $(x_{ij} - x_{i1})$. Different choices may be appropriate for different data accrual patterns. We emphasize $(x_{ij} - \bar{x}_{i.})$ and $\bar{x}_i$ due to the connection to compound symmetry estimators and because of the economics tradition.

9.3.1 Example

We analyze the systolic blood pressure on age data in the above light, with outputs shown in OUTPUT PACKET VII. We already observed in Chapter 8 that the combined coefficients for AGE are $\hat{\beta}_{age} = 0.355$ with independence structure and $\hat{\beta}_{age} = 0.269$ with compound symmetry structure. This indicates (based on point 1 above) that the blood pressure may increase less with aging within persons than expected based on comparison of individuals at different ages. To examine this further, we include mean age in the model. The following commands were used:

```
DATA A;
PROC SORT; BY ID;
PROC MEANS NOPRINT; BY ID; VAR AGEC;
OUTPUT OUT=MM MEAN=AGEM;
DATA COMB; MERGE A MM; BY ID;
PROC MIXED NOCLPRINT; CLASS ID SEX;
MODELS SBP= SEX AGEC AGEM BMIC AGEC*BMIC AGEM*BMIC/S;
REPEATED/SUBJECT=ID TYPE=CS;
```

We see that the coefficient of AGEM is significant at $p < 0.001$, indicating a difference in age effect between and within individuals. However, the interaction

Table 9.1 $\hat{\beta}$ **(Empirical se) Fitting an Overall Model by Compound Symmetry, and Fitting Separate Between- and Within-Individual Effects for Age**

	Overall Model		Between and Within Effects	
Intercept	126	(0.462)	126	(0.458)
Female	−5.90	(0.664)	−5.82	(0.659)
Age (centered at 50)	0.269	(0.0436)		
Age between (centered at 50)			0.419	(0.0451)
Age within (centering cancels)			−0.710	(0.104)
BMI (centered at 27)	0.627	(0.0544)	0.678	(0.0551)
Age *BMI (centered)	−0.0152	(0.00679)		
Age between *BMI (centered)			−0.0124	(0.00695)

effects did not differ significantly for between and within age components. The final model was fit to specifically obtain $\hat{\beta}_W$ and $\hat{\beta}_B$ for age. We could have proceeded several ways with the interaction effect. Since the within and between interactions did not differ significantly, and since the between interaction was estimated with more precision we chose to include the latter only. This choice also makes the model easily interpretable.

AGED=AGEC-AGEM;
PROC MIXED NOCLPRINT; CLASS ID SEX;
MODEL SBP=SEX AGED AGEM BMIC AGEM*BMIC/S;
REPEATED/SUBJECT=ID TYPE=CS;

Table 9.1 shows the results of fitting within- and between-individual effects as compared to the results of fitting the overall model.

Here we see that $\hat{\beta}_B = 0.419$ (at BMI of 27). Because the age range of the subjects is large, relative to the age change during the study, and there are only 1–3 observations per subject, the original combined coefficient for AGE is closer to the between-individual age effect. As expected, the within-individual effect has a much larger standard error than does the between-individual effect.

Somewhat surprisingly, we see that $\hat{\beta}_W = -0.710$ is negative. The reason is the increase during the study in the use of hypertensive medication. Using the above terminology, this would be referred to as primarily "period effect," although medication use may well have lowered the coefficient of the between individual age as well. A downward trend in blood pressure and an increase in the use of hypertensive medications has been reported nationally over the last several decades [54]. Due to the difficulties in determining underlying blood pressure in medicated individuals, longitudinal analyses published from the study have concentrated on the binary outcome "hypertensive" versus "nonhypertensive," including medicated individuals in the former category [55]. We pursue this approach in Chapter 15, and we find that doing so removes the difference in within and between individual effects.

OUTPUT PACKET VIII: INVESTIGATING AND FITTING WITHIN- AND BETWEEN-INDIVIDUAL EFFECTS

VIII.1. Testing for the Presence of Different Effects—Wisconsin Sleep Cohort

Investigating Between- and Within-Individual Effects of Age
Testing Significance of Age (Mean)
   The Mixed Procedure

Model Information

Data set	WORK.AB
Dependent variable	SBP
Covariance structure	Compound symmetry
Subject effect	id
Estimation method	REML
Residual variance method	Profile
Fixed effects SE method	Empirical
Degrees-of-freedom method	Between–within

Covariance Parameter Estimates

Covariance Parameter	Subject	Estimate
CS	id	71.6869
Residual		116.65

Fit Statistics

Residual log likelihood	−9627.1
Akaike's information criterion	−9629.1
Schwarz's Bayesian criterion	−9634.3
−2 Residual log likelihood	19254.2

Solution for Fixed Effects

Effect	Sex	Estimate	Standard Error	DF	t Value	Pr > |t|
Intercept		125.56	0.4589	1367	273.64	<0.0001
sex	F	−5.8178	0.6594	1367	−8.82	<0.0001
sex	M	0	.	.	.	.
agec		−0.6339	0.1099	1030	−5.77	<0.0001
agem		**1.0527**	**0.1144**	**1367**	**9.20**	**<0.0001**
bmic		0.6818	0.05517	1030	12.36	<0.0001
agec*bmic		−0.02414	0.01740	1030	−1.39	0.1656
agem*bmic		0.01168	0.01835	1030	0.64	0.5247

VIII.2. Fitting Within- and Between-Individual Effects—Wisconsin Sleep Cohort

Investigating Between- and Within-Individual Effects of Age
Explicitly Fitting Within and Between Effects
   The Mixed Procedure

Model Information

Data set	WORK.AB
Dependent variable	sbp
Covariance structure	Compound symmetry
Subject effect	id
Estimation method	REML
Residual variance method	Profile
Fixed effects SE method	Empirical
Degrees-of-freedom method	Between–within

Covariance Parameter Estimates

Covariance Parameter	Subject	Estimate
CS	id	71.4929
Residual		116.87

Fit Statistics

Residual log likelihood	−9625.0
Akaike's information criterion	−9627.0
Schwarz's Bayesian criterion	−9632.3
−2 Residual log likelihood	19250.1

Solution for Fixed Effects

Effect	Sex	Estimate	Standard Error	DF	t Value	Pr > |t|
Intercept		125.55	0.4588	1367	273.66	<0.0001
sex	F	−5.8223	0.6590	1367	−8.83	<0.0001
sex	M	0	.	.	.	.
agem		**0.4191**	**0.04509**	**1367**	**9.29**	**<0.0001**
aged		**−0.7100**	**0.1044**	**1031**	**−6.80**	**<0.0001**
bmic		0.6775	0.05510	1031	12.30	<0.0001
agem*bmic		−0.01241	0.006953	1031	−1.79	0.0745

CHAPTER TEN

Random Effects

So far we have dealt with correlated data by directly stating the correlation structure within each unit such as an individual. This was done by implementing the REPEATED statement in PROC MIXED. This chapter introduces an alternative approach to modeling correlation, which involves a logical two step process and also introduces additional flexibility. The approach builds on so-called "random effects," which are implemented by PROC MIXED via the RANDOM statement. Models with random effects (also called *mixed* effects models) became popular in biostatistics following the publication of a paper by Laird and Ware in 1982 [56].

10.1 RANDOM INTERCEPT

In the simplest possible random effects model, we assume that correlation within individuals arises from each individual having a different overall level of response. This is captured by individual specific intercepts. It is convenient and most common to write this intercept as a sum of the overall intercept and a random individual component γ_i (which is assumed to have mean 0 at each combination of values of the covariates). Therefore the model can be written

$$y_{ij} = \beta_0 + \gamma_i + \beta_1 x_{ij} + \epsilon_{ij} \tag{10.1}$$

for $j = 1, \ldots, k$ and $i = 1, \ldots, n$
With the equation for the mean y at a given value of x_{ij} [57], we obtain

$$\mu_{y|x} = \beta_0 + \beta_1 x_{ij} \qquad \text{as before}$$

If there were a limited number of individuals of interest (i.e., our n people in the study are the whole population), we could have let the γ_i represent the parameters needed—that is, $(n - 1)$ indicator variables in the MODEL statement. Statistical

Quantitative Methods in Population Health, by Mari Palta
ISBN 0-471-45505-9   Copyright © 2003 John Wiley & Sons, Inc.

properties of the estimators would then be based on increasing the number of observations k_i for each individual. The approach is referred to as modeling by "fixed" effects for individuals. But this is not how data in observational studies usually arise. As implied in previous chapters, we tend to view the n individuals in the study as a sample from a larger population. The reader is referred to McCullagh and Searle [5] for further discussion of the choice of fixed versus random effects. The specific γ_i's in our sample are a random sample from a distribution of individual level intercepts. Our interest becomes modeling the parameters of that distribution. The distribution of γ_i can be modeled as, for example, normal so that there are only two parameters μ_γ and σ_γ^2, rather than the whole set of $\{\gamma_i, i = 1, \ldots, n - 1\}$. In addition to having mean 0, the random γ_i are assumed independent of each other and of ϵ_{ij}.

One way to understand the γ_i is to consider them as unmeasured subject characteristics that influence the response; that is, $\gamma_i = aw_i$ for some unknown covariate w_i. Since we have made the assumption that the mean of γ_i is 0 at each x_{ij} so that γ_i are uncorrelated with x_{ij}, these characteristics are inherently defined not to be confounders. Only unmeasured covariates that are not confounders can be modeled as random effects. This is different from the omitted covariate situation discussed in Chapter 9 that dealt with confounders. If w_i were known, the strength of their influence on the outcome would be measured by the magnitude of a. Now, because the exact values of w_i are not known, we measure their influence by the variance of γ_i. This makes sense, because if we standardize w to have variance 1, then we obtain $\text{Var}(\gamma_i) = a^2$.

Depending on the discipline of application, models such as (10.1) are presented either as "hierarchical," where there are two stages of regression, one for the outcomes conditionally on the individual parameters [58]

$$y_{ij} = \beta_{0i} + \beta_1 x_{ij} + \epsilon_{ij}$$

and another for the individual specific parameters

$$\beta_{0i} = \beta_0 + \gamma_i$$

or as an overall model

$$y_{ij} = \beta_0 + \beta_1 x_{ij} + \gamma_i + \epsilon_{ij} = \beta_0 + \beta_1 x_{ij} + e_{ij}$$

where $e_{ij} = \gamma_i + \epsilon_{ij}$ now defines the error term. With the second way of formulating the model, the variance is said to have several "components." This refers to the variance of the error term e_{ij} having contributions from variability between individuals and from "pure" residual error. The presentation of PROC MIXED in the SAS manual is aligned with the second formulation, but the two representations describe exactly the same model. We also usually assume that all the ϵ_{ij} are independent (although PROC MIXED does have options to specify dependence between ϵ_{ij} with the same i). If, in addition, the variance of ϵ_{ij} is assumed to be constant, we have $\text{Var}(\epsilon_{ij}) = \sigma^2$. We note that for the summed error terms in (10.1),

$$\text{Var}(\gamma_i + \epsilon_{ij}) = \sigma_\gamma^2 + \sigma^2$$

with σ_γ^2 and σ^2 being the two variance components.

With the random intercept model, independence of γ_i from ϵ_{ij} and of $\epsilon_{ij'}$ from each other leads to

$$\begin{aligned}
\text{Cov}(\gamma_i + \epsilon_{ij}, \gamma_i + \epsilon_{ij'}) &= \text{Cov}(\gamma_i, \gamma_i) + \text{Cov}(\gamma_i, \epsilon_{ij'}) \\
&\quad + \text{Cov}(\epsilon_{ij}, \gamma_i) + \text{Cov}(\epsilon_{ij}, \epsilon_{ij'}) \\
&= \sigma_\gamma^2 + 0 + 0 + 0
\end{aligned}$$

so that

$$\text{Var}\begin{pmatrix} e_{i1} \\ e_{i2} \\ \vdots \\ e_{ik_i} \end{pmatrix} = \begin{pmatrix} \sigma_\gamma^2 + \sigma^2 & \sigma_\gamma^2 & \cdots & \sigma_\gamma^2 \\ \sigma_\gamma^2 & \sigma_\gamma^2 + \sigma^2 & \cdots & \sigma_\gamma^2 \\ \vdots & \vdots & \ddots & \vdots \\ \sigma_\gamma^2 & \sigma_\gamma^2 & \cdots & \sigma_\gamma^2 + \sigma^2 \end{pmatrix}$$

which is a compound symmetry matrix because all the diagonal elements are the same, and so are all the covariances. The within-individual correlation is $\sigma_\gamma^2/(\sigma_\gamma^2 + \sigma^2)$. In the SAS manual, compound symmetry matrices are presented this way, with σ_γ^2 being denoted by σ_1^2. Hence, the model with a random intercept is identical to a model with no random intercept, but a compound symmetry variance structure. Nothing very exciting has been gained mathematically, but the random effects perspective helps in interpreting the model.

PROC MIXED uses special notation to describe the variance components of random effects models. The variance matrix of the random effects is denoted by G. In the above case of random intercepts we have

$$G = (\sigma_\gamma^2)$$

a 1×1 matrix. Just as the ordinary covariates (associated with the β's) for a person are summarized in the matrix X_i, covariates for the random effects are summarized in a parallel matrix Z_i and the regression equation (10.1) is written.

$$Y_i = Z_i \gamma_i + X_i \beta + \epsilon_i$$

In the random intercept case, Z_i consists of the intercept column, so that

$$Z_i = \begin{pmatrix} 1 \\ 1 \\ \vdots \\ 1 \end{pmatrix}$$

PROC MIXED retains the notation R_i for the variance matrix of the ϵ_{ij}. With the above assumptions, R_i is a $k_i \times k_i$ matrix

$$
R_i = \begin{pmatrix} \sigma^2 & 0 & \cdots & 0 \\ 0 & \sigma^2 & \cdots & 0 \\ \vdots & \vdots & \ddots & \vdots \\ 0 & 0 & \cdots & \sigma^2 \end{pmatrix}
$$

We see from the variance formula for a linear transformation, along with the independence of $\boldsymbol{\gamma}_i$ and ϵ_{ij}, that the general form for the variance matrix for subject i is

$$
V_i = \mathrm{Var}(Z_i \boldsymbol{\gamma}_i + \epsilon_i) = \mathrm{Var}(Z_i \boldsymbol{\gamma}_i) + \mathrm{Var}(\epsilon_i) = Z_i G Z_i' + R_i
$$

All of the development above depend only on the assumptions of independence between covariates, error terms, and the random effect. To actually fit the model (by REML or ML), PROC MIXED makes the additional assumption that the random effects are normally distributed, so that the multivariate normal likelihood approach can be applied. We have made the assumption for ϵ_{ij} all along, and when γ_i is also assumed normally distributed, it follows that $\gamma_i + \epsilon_{ij}$ is normally distributed, as were all previous error terms modeled by PROC MIXED.

10.1.1   Example

We fit the systolic blood pressure data from the sleep cohort both by compound symmetry by the REPEATED statement and by a random intercept model. Outputs are found in OUTPUT PACKET IX. Because of the finding in Chapter 9 that within and between effects of age differ, we retain these components. The following statements were used with AGEM and AGED defined as in Chapter 9.

```
PROC MIXED NOCLPRINT; CLASS ID SEX;
MODEL SBP=AGEM AGED SEX BMIC AGEM*BMIC/S;
REPEATED/SUBJECT=ID TYPE=CS;
PROC MIXED NOCLPRINT; CLASS ID SEX;
MODEL SBP=AGEM AGED SEX BMIC AGEM*BMIC/S DDFM=BW;
RANDOM INTERCEPT/SUBJECT=ID;
```

The option DDFM=BW is needed for the degrees of freedom to be correct for the random effects model and for the option COVTEST-induced Wald tests of random effects to be performed. The DDFM=BW option and a likelihood ratio test versus a null model happen automatically with the REPEATED statement. With the large sample sizes we tend to have in studies of population health, degrees of freedom usually do not matter very much. OUTPUT PACKET IX shows that the results of the compound symmetry and random intercept models are identical, with a slight change in the labeling of the output. However, the RANDOM statement took longer to run in SAS. Results of these runs were already tabulated

Table 10.1 $\hat{\beta}$ (se) and Variance Components (se) Random Intercept Model

	Fixed Effects		Random Components
Intercept	126	(0.457)	
Female	−5.82	(0.659)	
Age between (centered at 50)	0.419	(0.0455)	
Age within (centering cancels)	−0.710	(0.952)	
BMI (centered at 27)	0.678	(0.0515)	
Age between *BMI (centered)	−0.0124	(0.00635)	
Variance of intercepts			71.4 (6.21)
Variance of residuals			117 (5.06)

for the compound symmetry structure in Table 9.1 with empirical standard errors. Following the current tradition for random effects models, we provide the results from the random intercept model with model-based standard errors in Table 10.1. It should be noted that Wald standard errors have been found unstable for the variance components and that likelihood ratio tests should be performed in borderline cases.

In Chapter 9 we saw that $\overline{x}_{i.}$ was significant when added to the original model, and we showed that this provides evidence that within- and between-individual effects of age differ. In a random effects model we can also consider the test of the coefficient of $\overline{x}_{i.}$ a check on whether γ_i is correlated with x_{ij} — that is, whether γ_i inadvertently contains confounders. From a hierarchical perspective, this amounts to modeling the intercept as

$$\beta_{0i} = \beta_0 + \gamma_F \overline{x}_{i.} + \gamma_i'$$

leading to the overall model

$$y_{ij} = \beta_0 + \gamma_F \overline{x}_i + \beta_1 x_{ij} + \gamma_i' + \epsilon_{ij}$$

and testing the significance of γ_F. Now γ_i' is assumed independent of x_{ij} and ϵ_{ij}, making the model assumptions of independent variance components correct. (It can be shown that the assumption holds, for example, for a missing covariate structure similar to the one in Chapter 9 [32]). Just as in Chapter 9, if $\overline{x}_i$ is included in the model and found significant, it makes sense to subtract $\overline{x}_i$ from x_{ij} to separately model the within- and between-individual effects.

In general, since the covariates can either vary with j ("time-varying," such as age) or be constant for a person (such as gender), one can hierarchically consider the latter included in the model for the intercept as well. Then the model for the observations, conditionally on the parameters, becomes

$$y_{ij} = \beta_{0i} + \beta_{1W}(x_{1ij} - \overline{x}_i) + \epsilon_{ij}$$

while the individual specific parameter model is

$$\beta_{0i} = \beta_0 + \gamma_{1F} \overline{x}_i + \beta_2 x_{2i} + \gamma_i'$$

with γ_{1F} having the interpretation β_{1B}. Here x_{2i} is another covariate, such as gender, that does not change within individual. From the perspective of PROC MIXED we fit the resulting overall model

$$y_{ij} = \beta_0 + \beta_{1W}(x_{1ij} - \bar{x}_{1i.}) + \beta_{1B}\bar{x}_{1i.} + \beta_2 x_{2i} + \gamma_i' + \epsilon_{ij}$$

Again the hierarchical and PROC MIXED models are identical, but the hierarchical perspective helps in interpretation. As in any regression model, when we add important fixed effects, we delegate less information to the variance components, and statistical precision tends to improve.

10.1.2 Example

From the hierarchical perspective, in the model in Table 10.1 for the intercept for an individual is

$$\beta_{0i} = 126 + 0.418 \times (\text{mean age} - 50) - 5.92 \times (\text{female}) + \gamma_i'$$

where the intercept is defined at BMI $= 27$ and $\text{Var}(\gamma_i') = 71.4$. For the observations we have

$$y_{ij} = \beta_{0i} - 0.710 \times (\text{age} - \text{mean age}) + (0.678 + \text{mean age} - 50)$$
$$\times (\text{BMI} - 27) + \epsilon_{ij}$$

where the variance of the residual error is $\text{Var}(\epsilon_{ij}) = 117$.

10.2 RANDOM SLOPES

The next step in random effects modeling is to add random components also to other coefficients—that is, random slopes to coefficients of time varying covariates. This can be thought of as adding interaction terms between measured factors and unknown individual level variables that are not confounders. If for the intercept we have

$$\beta_{0i} = \beta_0 + \gamma_{0i} \qquad \text{where} \quad \gamma_{0i} = a w_i$$

and for the slope

$$\beta_{1i} = \beta_1 + \gamma_{1i} \qquad \text{where} \quad \gamma_{1i} = b w_i$$

the overall model is

$$y_{ij} = \beta_{0i} + \beta_{1i} x_{ij} + \epsilon_{ij} = \beta_0 + a w_i + \beta_1 x_{ij} + b w_i x_{ij} + \epsilon_{ij}$$

This is clearly a model with an interaction effect between the unmeasured covariate w_i and the measured covariate x_{ij}. Just as when including interaction effects between measured covariates in a model, one needs to be careful to

1. Include the corresponding main effects (in this case x_{ij} and a random intercept).
2. Interpret the main effects according to how centering was done. In this case, the unmeasured factor is already centered at 0, so interpretation of the effect of x_{ij} is clear. However, interpretation of the variance and covariance of the random intercept depends on where x_{ij} is centered. In a model with random slopes, it is especially inappropriate to let the 0 point of x_{ij} lie outside its observed range (e.g., let age be centered at 0 years in a study of elderly adults). The overall model statistics are not affected by the choice of centering, but interpretation of the variance components is.

In PROC MIXED notation, adding random slopes involves adding columns to Z_i. Because random slopes are akin to interaction effects, it has become a convention to include in Z_i only columns that are also in X_i. (This applies in the case we are discussing here, where the added columns correspond to slopes. PROC MIXED has other applications, where added columns represent multiple levels of clusters, which may proceed differently than outlined here.) If there are m covariates and p random slopes, we obtain

$$Y_i = Z_i \gamma_i + X_i \beta + \epsilon_i$$

where

$$X_i = \begin{pmatrix} 1 & x_{1i1} & \cdots & x_{pi1} & \cdots & x_{mi1} \\ 1 & x_{1i2} & \cdots & x_{pi2} & \cdots & x_{mi1} \\ \vdots & \vdots & \ddots & \vdots & \ddots & \vdots \\ 1 & x_{1ik_i} & \cdots & x_{pik_i} & \cdots & x_{mik_i} \end{pmatrix}$$

$$Z_i = \begin{pmatrix} 1 & x_{1i1} & \cdots & x_{pi1} \\ 1 & x_{1i2} & \cdots & x_{pi2} \\ \vdots & \vdots & \ddots & \vdots \\ 1 & x_{1ik_i} & \cdots & x_{pik_i} \end{pmatrix}$$

$$\gamma_i = \begin{pmatrix} \gamma_{0i} \\ \gamma_{1i} \\ \vdots \\ \gamma_{pi} \end{pmatrix}$$

$$\beta = \begin{pmatrix} \beta_0 \\ \beta_1 \\ \vdots \\ \beta_p \\ \vdots \\ \beta_m \end{pmatrix}$$

In a variance component model

$$Y_i = X_i \boldsymbol{\beta} + e_i \tag{10.2}$$

the new error term e_i has variance

$$\text{Var}(e_i) = V_i = Z_i G Z_i' + R_i \tag{10.3}$$

Expression (10.3) holds for the error term of Model (10.2) regardless of the number of random effects (which follows from the formula $\text{Var}(Z_i \boldsymbol{\gamma}_i) = Z_i \text{Var}(\boldsymbol{\gamma}_i) Z_i'$ and the assumption that the error terms are independent). To examine the variance structure closer, we complete the matrix multiplications for the case $p = 1$. To avoid too many subscripts, we let

$$G = \begin{pmatrix} \sigma_a^2 & \sigma_{ab} \\ \sigma_{ab} & \sigma_b^2 \end{pmatrix}$$

when there is a random slope γ_{0i} and random intercept γ_{1i}. Looking at the implications of formula (10.3), we then see that

$$
\text{Var}(e_i) = \begin{pmatrix} 1 & x_{i1} \\ 1 & x_{i2} \\ \vdots & \vdots \\ 1 & x_{ik} \end{pmatrix} \text{Var}\begin{pmatrix} \gamma_{0i} \\ \gamma_{1i} \end{pmatrix} \begin{pmatrix} 1 & 1 & \cdots & 1 \\ x_{i1} & x_{i2} & \cdots & x_{ik} \end{pmatrix} + \text{Var}\begin{pmatrix} \epsilon_{i1} \\ \epsilon_{i2} \\ \vdots \\ \epsilon_{ik} \end{pmatrix}
$$

$$
= \begin{pmatrix} \sigma_a^2 + x_{i1}\sigma_{ab} & \sigma_{ab} + x_{i1}\sigma_b^2 \\ \sigma_a^2 + x_{i2}\sigma_{ab} & \sigma_{ab} + x_{i2}\sigma_b^2 \\ \vdots & \vdots \\ \sigma_a^2 + x_{ik}\sigma_{ab} & \sigma_{ab} + x_{ik}\sigma_b^2 \end{pmatrix} \begin{pmatrix} 1 & 1 & \cdots & 1 \\ x_{i1} & x_{i2} & \cdots & x_{ik} \end{pmatrix}
$$

$$
+ \text{Var}\begin{pmatrix} \epsilon_{i1} \\ \epsilon_{i2} \\ \vdots \\ \epsilon_{ik} \end{pmatrix}
$$

$$
= \begin{pmatrix} \sigma_a^2 + 2x_{i1}\sigma_{ab} + x_{i1}^2\sigma_b^2 & \cdots \\ \sigma_a^2 + x_{i1}\sigma_{ab} + x_{i2}\sigma_{ab} + x_{i1}x_{i2}\sigma_b^2 & \cdots \\ \vdots & \vdots \\ \sigma_a^2 + x_{ik}\sigma_{ab} + x_{ik}\sigma_{ab} + x_{i1}x_{ik}\sigma_b^2 & \cdots \end{pmatrix} + \text{Var}\begin{pmatrix} \epsilon_{i1} \\ \epsilon_{i2} \\ \vdots \\ \epsilon_{ik} \end{pmatrix}
$$

It follows that the covariance (and therefore correlation) emerging from the random effects structure with random slopes incorporates dependence of the pairwise correlation on the x's. If there were random effects associated with x_{2ij}, and so on, the expression would expand to include the variance of that random effect as well as its covariance with all the other random effects.

To fit (10.3) with PROC MIXED, we need to specify

1. Which random effects are to be fitted. This is done by listing the corresponding variable names in the random statement.
2. The structure of $G = \text{Var}(\gamma)$—that is, how σ_a^2, σ_b^2, $\sigma_{ab} \cdots$ are to be fitted. This is done by the TYPE option in the random statement. It is most common to fit TYPE=UN, unstructured. There is usually no reason to believe that different random effects have the same variance, and we usually want to allow the effects to be correlated, at least as the first step.
3. The structure of $R_i = \text{Var} \begin{pmatrix} \epsilon_{i1} \\ \epsilon_{i2} \\ \vdots \\ \epsilon_{ik} \end{pmatrix}$. This is done by the REPEATED state-

ment as before. One has to be quite careful, however, to avoid requesting the estimation of parameters that overlap with the random effects part (a situation referred to as "overparameterization" or "nonidentifiability"). We already saw that a compound symmetry model can be fitted either by the REPEATED statement or by the RANDOM statement with a random intercept. Specifying both a random intercept and TYPE=CS with REPEATED will result in error, as the program would then ask for several parameters that are actually the same. Partly because of this danger, it is most common to fit R_i as independence and equal variance, and we hope that the random effects part will adequately capture the correlation structure by itself. Independence is the default when no REPEATED statement is present. Authorities on mixed effects data analysis currently suggest fitting nonindependence structures that reflect diminishing correlation between measurements that are further apart together with random effects. This is beyond the scope here. Also, you will find that PROC MIXED is rather slow with random effects. Sometimes the estimators "do not converge". Specifying "starting values" for the parameters by the PARMS statement sometimes helps. The reader interested in these further issues is recommended to read *Linear Mixed Models in Practice*, by Verbeke and Molenberghs [57].

The question is often asked, How many random effects should be included in the variance structure? Note that what is being estimated are the variance parameters of the random effects. Models with different numbers of random effects can then be viewed as models "nested within each other," and the difference in $-2 \log(L)$ (or $-2 \log(REML)$) can be used to test the significance of random effects. The procedure is the same as when comparing different numbers of regression parameters. If a model has two random effects as above, and the correlation structure of the random effects was specified as unstructured, it has three random effects covariance parameters (σ_a^2, σ_b^2, and σ_{ab}). If that model is compared to a model with just a random intercept, two parameters will be dropped. Then $-2 \log(L_2) - [-2 \log(L_1)]$ has the χ^2-distribution with two degrees of freedom (in general, $df =$ difference in number parameters), and the statistical significance of the added random effects can be tested against this distribution. The COVTEST option in the PROC MIXED statement produces the line "Null Model Likelihood Ratio Test," which is this chi-square of the variance structure versus an independence/equal variance model. In other words, it is a test of whether we needed to bother with PROC MIXED at all (vis-à-vis PROC REG).

10.2.1 Example

We now fit the blood pressure data from the Wisconsin Sleep Cohort with two random effects, one for the intercept and another for the age effect. Since random slopes make sense only for time-varying covariates, the new random component is added for the within-individual age component. We allow this random slope to be both uncorrelated and correlated with the random intercept. Outputs are in OUTPUT PACKET IX. The statements used were

PROC MIXED NOCLPRINT COVTEST;
CLASS ID SEX;
MODEL SBP=SEX AGEM AGED BMIC AGEM*BMIC/S;
RANDOM INTERCEPT AGED/SUBJECT=ID (TYPE=UN GCORR);

The GCORR option computes the correlation between random effects. We also fitted a random intercept model and an AR(1) model for comparison. The latter was chosen because it allows correlation between time points to differ and also because it was found to be the best choice based on BIC in Chapter 8. Looking at the output, we first see that $-2\log(L)$ for the random intercept, random slope and intercept, and correlated intercept and slope models are 19250.1, 19233.7, and 19223.0, respectively, with one-degree-of-freedom difference with each subsequent model ($\chi^2_{0.95}(1) = 3.84$). Their corresponding BIC are 19264.5, 19255.4, and 19251.9. Hence, it appears worthwhile to retain the full random effects covariance structure.

There is a significant correlation of 0.30 between the random intercept and slope, which indicates that individuals with higher blood pressure at their study midpoint (adjusted for gender, BMI, and mean age) also have more increase (or less decrease) in the blood pressure across the study years. It is of interest to know that this correlation refers to true blood pressure, as the covariance is inherently adjusted for short-term fluctuations in the measurement. For a long time there was a debate over the issue whether people who have higher blood pressures also tend to greater increases with age. This is because a simple correlation between initial blood pressure and rise is affected by regression to the mean (more on this below). The issue was finally settled by Blomquist [59] by an analysis similar to the one here. In our study we encounter the interfering effects of medication which make biological interpretation of the correlation difficult.

Note again that the meaning of the intercept effect and its variability changes when x is centered differently. In the present situation, UN(1, 1) is the between-individual variability in a person's blood pressure at the study midpoint, adjusted for all the fixed effects. UN(2, 2) is variability adjusted for all fixed effects. Its size 1.88 is large relative to the mean slope of -0.678. The "Residual" on the output is

Table 10.2 $\hat{\beta}$ **(se) from a model with random slope and from an AR(1) Model**

	Random Slope		AR(1)	
Intercept	126	(0.457)	126	(0.455)
Female	−5.96	(0.657)	−5.89	(0.657)
Age between (centered at 50)	0.410	(0.0452)	0.416	(0.454)
Age within (centering cancels)	−0.678	(0.102)	−0.671	(0.101)
BMI (centered at 27)	0.683	(0.0516)	0.681	(0.0515)
Age between *BMI (centered)	−0.0117	(0.00634)	−0.0126	(0.00635)

Var(ϵ) and is estimated at 93.8 (so sd = 9.69). This variance is interpreted as the variability not due to age, sex, BMI, or random individual specific characteristics. It includes components such as diurnal and day-to-day variability in blood pressure and variability due to measurement error.

While the random effects analysis above gives us a lot of information, the BIC of the autoregressive model is actually the smallest at 19244.3. The variance structure of this analysis offers us only the information that adjacent blood pressures correlate at 0.40, while those two visits apart correlate at 0.17. The residual variance is 188.14, but it should be remembered that this contains all the random variation. In contrast, the random variation in the random effects model has been split into components. Clearly, the random effects analysis is more interesting because it provides insight into the sources of variation. However, if the sole purpose of the analysis is estimation of the fixed effects, Table 10.2 shows that the best random effects model and the autoregressive model yield very similar results. Sometimes, models fitted by the REPEATED approach (such as AR(1) here) are termed "marginal" or "population averaged". Random effects models are then referred to as "cluster specific".

Finally we interpret Table 10.2 from a hierarchical perspective. We now have models that contain random components for the intercept β_{0i} and the age slope β_{1i}, while slope for BMI depends only on a fixed effect, mean age. We can write

$$\hat{\beta}_{BMI} = 0.683 - (\text{mean age} - 50) \times 0.117$$

$$\beta_{0i} = 126 - 5.96 \times \text{female} + 0.410 \times (\text{mean age}) + \gamma_{0i}$$

$$\beta_{age,i} = -0.678 + \gamma_{age,i}$$

$$y_{ij} = \beta_{0i} + \beta_{age,i} \times (\text{age} - \text{mean age}) + \hat{\beta}_{BMI} \times (\text{BMI} - 27) + \epsilon_{ij}$$

where the covariance matrix for the random effects γ_{0i} and $\gamma_{age,i}$ is

$$\begin{pmatrix} 85.5 & 3.84 \\ 3.84 & 1.88 \end{pmatrix}$$

and the variance of ϵ_{ij} is Var(ϵ_{ij}) = 93.8.

10.3 OBTAINING "THE BEST" ESTIMATES OF INDIVIDUAL INTERCEPTS AND SLOPES

We noted at the beginning of Chapter 10 that it is not possible to estimate the random effects for each individual as separate parameters. The situation is similar to when using the empirical standard error: Individual random effects cannot be estimated as model parameters, but after the model is fitted, the parameters can be used to estimate the individual effects. PROC MIXED provides such estimates as we will see in the example below. They are based on a method called "empirical Bayes" [60].

A "naive" approach is to obtain individual random effects estimates by simply fitting separate regression lines to each individual separately. The intercepts would then be estimates of $\beta_0 + \gamma_{0i}$ and the slopes of the appropriate x, estimates of $\beta_1 + \gamma_{1i}$. The first problem one encounters with this approach is that there is no way of allowing for some slopes not having random components. Fitting separate lines, in effect, fits a random slope for every covariate. One will also notice that slopes fit this way tend to be unstable unless the number of observations for each individual i, i.e. k_i is large. Typically there are several individuals with very high or low intercepts or slopes because they had few observations. To remedy this problem, one needs to discount the part of the "extremeness" that is due to error in estimation. You probably recall the concept of "regression to the mean." This phenomenon arises from the fact that observations that are relatively extreme are likely to be that way because they happened to be measured with an error in the direction of the extremeness. In other words, the true value is likely to be closer to the overall mean of the sample distribution than we first think. Then, of course, the individual may be found to be less extreme on subsequent measurements, hence the name of the phenomenon. Regression to the mean is very important, and it may have caused thousands of erroneous scientific conclusions. In fact, it may be a contributor to the famous "placebo effect" in clinical trials and practice [61].

Empirical Bayes estimation is a way to obtain estimates that have been adjusted for regression to the mean. Essentially, because we know that extreme measurements are closer to the mean than we think, especially if they are based on relatively little information (e.g., small k_i), the method uses an appropriately weighted average of the actual measurement, or individual estimate, and the overall mean across the sample as the new estimate. Those familiar with the methods used at the National Center for Health Statistics will recognize the approach, because it is often applied to estimate "small area" mortality rates [62]. The appropriate weights to be used in the averaging process depend on both the underlying distribution and the relative magnitude of the measurement or estimation variance. PROC MIXED is able to choose the weights based on its inherent normality assumption and on the estimates of residual versus random effects variance.

10.3.1 Example

Returning to the sleep cohort blood pressure analysis with random intercept and age slope, we use PROC MIXED commands that store the estimated realizations of the random slope and intercept. These commands utilize the so-called "Output Delivery System"=ODS introduced in SAS version 8. This system has extensive capabilities to modify the printing of SAS output, as well as to save all or parts of it in SAS data files. In the example below, we simply (1) tell SAS that we don't want all the random slopes and intercepts printed (this would be very cumbersome because there are 1374 subjects) and (2) save the part of the output that contains these quantities.

Different parts of the PROC MIXED output is referred to by SAS names, listed in the SAS manual. The output that is relevant here is named SolutionR, where capitalizing the S and the R is essential for SAS to recognize the name. There is a separate record for each random effect, identified by a variable called "EFFECT." This variable takes on values "Intercept" (again, the capitalized I is essential for recognition), and the name of the variable associated with the random effect ("aged" in our case).

OUTPUT PACKET IX contains histograms of the estimated random effects. The commands to produce the graphs were as follows:

```
PROC MIXED NOCLPRINT; CLASS IS SEX;
MODEL SBP=SEX AGEM AGED BMIC AGEM*BMIC/S;
RANDOM INTERCEPT AGED/SUBJECT=ID S;
ODS LISTING EXCLUDE SolutionR;
ODS OUTPUT SolutionR=EFF;
DATA INT; SET EFF;
IF EFFECT='Intercept';
TITLE 'random intercepts';
PROC UNIVARIATE PLOT; VAR ESTIMATE;
DATA SLOPE; SET EFF;
IF EFFECT='aged';
PROC UNIVARIATE PLOT; VAR ESTIMATE;
```

Note that the S is needed in the RANDOM statement to instigate the estimation of the individual effects. We can now view the distribution of these estimated random effects. To obtain actual intercept and slopes, one needs to add the fixed effect intercept 126 and slope -0.678 to each. From the histograms we can judge whether the distribution of the random effects is indeed normal (as assumed) and whether there were any influential observations. We see that there is some skewness and that especially the slopes have some outliers. We may wish to examine these further.

Note 1   We see that while the mean of the random effects is 0 as expected, the estimates do not reflect the correct variance, which we know from PROC MIXED to be 85.5 for the intercepts and 1.88 for the slopes. There are methods for correcting this [63].

Note 2   It has been shown that the regression estimators are still valid, when there is non-normality of the random effects distribution. However, the EMPIRICAL option should be specified to obtain the correct standard errors in such cases [57, page 88].

Note 3   Methods such as those presented above for estimating the random effects are very important in small area estimation. If the random intercepts were mortality rates rather than blood pressure, they would be plotted on a map. Also, they would have been obtained from different distributional assumptions—typically a Poisson distribution for ϵ and a gamma distribution for the random effects [62].

OUTPUT PACKET IX: FITTING RANDOM EFFECTS MODELS

IX.1. Random Intercept Model Compared to Compound Symmetry

Comparing Compound Symmetry and Random Intercept Models
Compound Symmetry Model
  The Mixed Procedure

Model Information

Data set	WORK.AB
Dependent variable	sbp
Covariance structure	**Compound symmetry**
Subject effect	id
Estimation method	REML
Residual variance method	Profile
Fixed effects SE method	**Model-based**
Degrees-of-freedom method	**Between–within**

Dimensions

Covariance parameters	**2**
Columns in X	7
Columns in Z	0
Subjects	1370
Maximum observations per subject	3
Observations used	2404
Observations not used	33
Total observations	2437

Iteration History[a]

Iteration	Evaluations	−2 Residual Log Likelihood	Criterion
0	1	19417.87183223	
1	2	19250.10105675	0.00000087
2	1	19250.09453612	0.00000000

[a]Convergence criteria met.

Covariance Parameter Estimates

Covariance Parameter	Subject	Estimate
CS	**id**	**71.4929**
Residual		**116.87**

Fit Statistics

−2 Residual log likelihood	19250.1
AIC (smaller is better)	19254.1
AICC (smaller is better)	19254.1
BIC (smaller is better)	**19264.5**

Null Model Likelihood Ratio Test

DF	Chi-Square	Pr > ChiSq
1	167.78	<0.0001

Solution for Fixed Effects

Effect	Sex	Estimate	Standard Error	DF	t Value	Pr > |t|
Intercept		125.55	0.4567	1367	274.89	<0.0001
sex	F	−5.8223	0.6587	1367	−8.84	<0.0001
sex	M	0	.	.	.	.
agem		0.4191	0.04548	1367	9.22	<0.0001
aged		−0.7100	0.09518	1031	−7.46	<0.0001
bmic		0.6775	0.05153	1031	13.15	<0.0001
agem*bmic		−0.01241	0.006347	1031	−1.96	0.0508

Type 3 Tests of Fixed Effects

Effect	Num DF	Den DF	F Value	Pr > F
sex	1	1367	78.12	<0.0001
agem	1	1367	84.92	<0.0001
aged	1	1031	55.65	<0.0001
bmic	1	1031	172.87	<0.0001
agem*bmic	1	1031	3.82	0.0508

Random Intercept Model
  The Mixed Procedure

Model Information

Data set	WORK.AB
Dependent variable	sbp
Covariance structure	**Variance components**
Subject effect	id
Estimation method	REML
Residual variance method	Profile
Fixed effects SE method	**Model-based**
Degrees-of-freedom method	**Between–within**

Dimensions

Covariance parameters	**2**
Columns in X	7
Columns in Z per subject	1
Subjects	1370
Maximum observations per subject	3
Observations used	2404
Observations not used	33
Total observations	2437

Iteration History[a]

Iteration	Evaluations	−2 Residual log likelihood	Criterion
0	1	19417.87183223	
1	2	19250.10105675	0.00000087
2	1	19250.09453612	0.00000000

[a]Convergence criteria met.

Covariance Parameter Estimates

Covariance Parameter	Subject	Estimate	Standard Error	Z Value	Pr Z
Intercept	**id**	**71.4929**	**6.2137**	**11.51**	**<0.0001**
Residual		**116.87**	**5.0618**	**23.09**	**<0.0001**

Fit Statistics

−2 Residual log likelihood	19250.1
AIC (smaller is better)	19254.1
AICC (smaller is better)	19254.1
BIC (smaller is better)	**19264.5**

Solution for Fixed Effects

Effect	Sex	Estimate	Standard Error	DF	t Value	Pr > |t|
Intercept		125.55	0.4567	1367	274.89	<0.0001
sex	F	−5.8223	0.6587	1367	−8.84	<0.0001
sex	M	0	.	.	.	.
agem		0.4191	0.04548	1367	9.22	<0.0001
aged		−0.7100	0.09518	1031	−7.46	<0.0001
bmic		0.6775	0.05153	1031	13.15	<0.0001
agem*bmic		−0.01241	0.006347	1031	−1.96	0.0508

Type 3 Tests of Fixed Effects

Effect	Num DF	Den DF	F Value	Pr > F
sex	1	1367	78.12	<0.0001
agem	1	1367	84.92	<0.0001
aged	1	1031	55.65	<0.0001
bmic	1	1031	172.87	<0.0001
agem*bmic	1	1031	3.82	0.0508

IX.2. Fitting Models with Random Slope

Fitting Models with Random Slope
Random Slope for Age with Correlation Between Intercept and Slope
   The Mixed Procedure

Model Information

Data set	WORK.AB
Dependent variable	sbp
Covariance structure	**Unstructured**
Subject effect	id
Estimation method	REML
Residual variance method	Profile
Fixed effects SE method	**Model-based**
Degrees-of-freedom method	**Between–within**

Dimensions[a]

Covariance parameters	**4**
Columns in X	7
Columns in Z per subject	2
Subjects	1370
Maximum observations per subject	3
Observations used	2404
Observations not used	33
Total observations	2437

[a]Convergence criteria met.

Estimated G Correlation Matrix

Row	Effect	id	Col1	Col2
1	Intercept	S0001	1.0000	0.3031
2	Aged	S0001	0.3031	1.0000

Covariance Parameter Estimates

Covariance Parameter	Subject	Estimate	Standard Error	Z Value	Pr Z
UN(1,1)	id	85.5144	6.7758	12.62	<0.0001
UN(2,1)	**id**	**3.8434**	**1.1910**	**3.23**	**0.0013**
UN(2,2)	id	1.8808	0.4692	4.01	<0.0001
Residual		93.7882	6.2991	14.89	<0.0001

Fit Statistics

−2 Residual log likelihood	**19223.0**
AIC (smaller is better)	19231.0
AICC (smaller is better)	19231.0
BIC (smaller is better)	**19251.9**

Null Model Likelihood Ratio Test

DF	Chi-Square	Pr > ChiSq
3	194.92	<0.0001

Solution for Fixed Effects

Effect	Sex	Estimate	Standard Error	DF	t Value	Pr > $\|t\|$
Intercept		125.59	0.4571	1367	274.73	<0.0001
sex	F	−5.9648	0.6567	1367	−9.08	<0.0001
sex	M	0	.	.	.	.
agem		0.4099	0.04515	1367	9.08	<0.0001
aged		−0.6783	0.1016	1031	t-6.68	<0.0001
bmic		0.6833	0.05158	1031	13.25	<0.0001
agem*bmic		−0.01172	0.006342	1031	−1.85	0.0649

Type 3 Tests of Fixed Effects

Effect	Num DF	Den DF	F Value	Pr > F
sex	1	1367	82.49	<0.0001
agem	1	1367	82.44	<0.0001
aged	1	1031	44.57	<0.0001
bmic	1	1031	175.47	<0.0001
agem*bmic	1	1031	3.41	0.0649

Random Slope for Age with no Correlation Between Intercept and Slope

Model Information

Data set	WORK.AB
Dependent variable	sbp
Covariance structure	**Variance components**
Subject effect	id
Estimation method	REML
Residual variance method	Profile
Fixed effects SE method	**Model-based**
Degrees-of-freedom method	**Between−within**

Dimensions[a]

Covariance parameters	**3**
Columns in X	7
Columns in Z per subject	2
Subjects	1370
Maximum observations per subject	3
Observations used	2404
Observations not used	33
Total observations	2437

[a]Convergence criteria met.

Covariance Parameter Estimates

Covariance Parameter	Subject	Estimate	Standard Error	Z Value	Pr Z
Intercept	id	84.0447	6.8030	12.35	<0.0001
aged	id	1.6816	0.4585	3.67	0.0001
Residual		95.8804	6.4227	14.93	<0.0001

Fit Statistics

−2 Residual log likelihood	**19233.7**
AIC (smaller is better)	19239.7
AICC (smaller is better)	19239.7
BIC (smaller is better)	**19255.4**

Solution for Fixed Effects

Effect	Sex	Estimate	Standard Error	DF	t Value	Pr > |t|
Intercept		125.55	0.4576	1367	274.34	<0.0001
sex	F	−5.8065	0.6598	1367	−8.80	<0.0001
sex	M	0	.	.	.	.
agem		0.4151	0.04549	1367	9.12	<0.0001
aged		−0.6778	0.1013	1031	−6.69	<0.0001
bmic		0.6758	0.05165	1031	13.08	<0.0001
agem*bmic		−0.01235	0.006348	1031	−1.95	0.0520

Type 3 Tests of Fixed Effects

Effect	Num DF	Den DF	F Value	Pr > F
sex	1	1367	77.44	<0.0001
agem	1	1367	83.25	<0.0001
aged	1	1031	44.73	<0.0001
bmic	1	1031	171.17	<0.0001
agem*bmic	1	1031	3.78	0.0520

Autoregressive Model
  The Mixed Procedure

Model Information

Data set	WORK.AB
Dependent variable	sbp
Covariance structure	**Autoregressive**
Subject effect	id
Estimation method	REML
Residual variance method	Profile
Fixed effects SE method	**Model-based**
Degrees-of-freedom method	Between–within

Dimensions[a]

Covariance parameters	**2**
Columns in X	7
Columns in Z	0
Subjects	1370
Maximum observation per subject	3
Observations used	2404
Observations not used	33
Total observations	2437

[a]Convergence criteria met.

Estimated R Correlation: Matrix for id S001

Row	Col1	Col2	Col3
1	1.0000	0.4156	0.1727
2	0.4156	1.0000	0.4156
3	0.1727	0.4156	1.0000

Covariance Parameter Estimates

Covariance Parameter	Subject	Estimate	Standard Error	Z Value	Pr Z
AR(1)	id	0.4156	0.02586	16.07	<0.0001
Residual		188.14	5.8275	32.28	<0.0001

Fit Statistics

−2 Residual log likelihood	19229.9
AIC (smaller is better)	19233.9
AICC (smaller is better)	19233.9
BIC (smaller is better)	**19244.3**

Null Model Likelihood Ration Test

DF	Chi-Square	Pr > ChiSq
1	188.00	<0.0001

Solution for Fixed Effects

Effect	Sex	Estimate	Standard Error	DF	t Value	Pr > |t|
Intercept		125.52	0.4553	1367	275.67	<0.0001
sex	F	−5.8933	0.6574	1367	−8.97	<0.0001
sex	M	0	.	.	.	.
agem		0.4158	0.04537	1367	9.17	<0.0001
aged		−0.6710	0.1013	1031	−6.63	<0.0001
bmic		0.6808	0.05154	1031	13.21	<0.0001
agem*bmic		−0.01257	0.006352	1031	−1.98	0.0481

Type 3 Tests of Fixed Effects

Effect	Num DF	Den DF	F Value	Pr > F
sex	1	1367	80.37	<0.0001
agem	1	1367	84.01	<0.0001
aged	1	1031	43.91	<0.0001
bmic	1	1031	174.49	<0.0001
agem*bmic	1	1031	3.92	0.0481

IX.3. Estimates of Individual Random Effects

Random Intercepts

The UNIVARIATE Procedure

Variable: Estimate

Moments

N	1370	Sum of weights	1370
Mean	0	Sum of observations	0
Standard deviation	7.06834366	Variance	49.9614822
Skewness	0.49675359	Kurtosis	0.52105557
Uncorrected SS	68397.2691	Corrected SS	68397.2691
Coefficient of variation	.	Standard error of mean	0.19096658

Basic Statistical Measures

Location		Variability	
Mean	0.00000	Standard deviation	7.06834
Median	−0.41782	Variance	49.96148
Mode	.	Range	45.58094
		Interquartile range	9.10450

Tests for Location: Mu0 = 0

Test		Statistic		p Value
Student's t	t	0	Pr > $|t|$	1.0000
Sign	M	−32	Pr > $|M|$	0.0887
Signed rank	S	−21231.5	Pr > $|S|$	0.1472

Quantiles (Definition 5)

Quantile	Estimate
100% Max	28.921164
99%	19.803465
95%	12.157012
90%	9.166159
75% Q3	4.211867
50% Median	−0.417823
25% Q1	−4.892630
10%	−8.709071
5%	−10.860915
1%	−14.057379
0% Min	−16.659780

Random Intercepts

```
                    Histogram                          #        Boxplot
    29+*                                                1           0
      .*                                                1           0
      .*                                                3           0
      .*                                                2           0
      .**                                               5           0
      .**                                               8           0
      .****                                            14           |
      .****                                            16           |
      .******                                          22           |
      .**********                                      42           |
      .**************                                  59           |
      .******************                              74           |
      .**************************                     110        +-----+
      .********************************               133        |     |
      .*******************************************    163        |  +  |
      .****************************************       149        *-----*
      .**********************************************  167        |     |
      .*******************************             127        +-----+
      .**************************                     111           |
      .******************                             73           |
      .************                                   45           |
      .********                                       31           |
      .***                                            11           |
   -17+*                                               3           |
       ----+----+----+----+----+----+----+--
       *May represent up to 4 counts
```

Random Slopes

The UNIVARIATE Procedure

Variable: Estimate

Moments

N	1370	Sum of weights	1370
Mean	0	Sum of observations	0
Standard deviation	0.54972217	Variance	0.30219446
Skewness	0.2619336	Kurtosis	3.73289701
Uncorrected SS	413.704214	Corrected SS	413.704214
Coefficient variation	.	Standard error of mean	0.01485193

Basic Statistical Measures

Location		Variability	
Mean	0.00000	Standard deviation	0.54972
Median	−0.00073	Variance	0.30219
Mode	.	Range	6.84861
		Interquartile range	0.54700

Tests for Location: Mu0 = 0

Test		Statistic		p Value
Student's t	t	0	Pr > |t|	1.0000
Sign	M	−1	Pr > |M|	0.9784
Signed rank	S	−6388.5	Pr > |S|	0.6629

Quantiles (Definition 5)

Quantile	Estimate
100% Max	3.738042849
99%	1.545551655
95%	0.898375686
90%	0.631162830
75% Q3	0.270318028
50% Median	−0.000733775
25% Q1	−0.276678880
10%	−0.603518420
5%	−0.888367817
1%	−1.475208166
0% Min	−3.110567508

Random Slopes

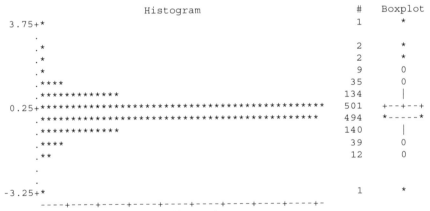

```
                 Histogram                               #    Boxplot
     3.75+*                                              1       *
         .
         . *                                             2       *
         . *                                             2       *
         . *                                             9       0
         .****                                          35       0
         .*************                                134       |
     0.25+*********************************************501    +--+--+
         .******************************************** 494    *-----*
         .*************                                140       |
         .****                                          39       0
         .**                                            12       0
         .
         .
     -3.25+*                                             1       *
          ----+----+----+----+----+----+----+----+----+-
          *May represent up to 11 counts
```

CHAPTER ELEVEN

The Normal Distribution and Likelihood Revisited

It is now time to address the generalization of regression analysis to the situation of non-normally distributed residuals. We start by placing our well-known normal distribution into the generalized context. This chapter introduces new terminology for maximum likelihood estimation for the normal distribution with equal variance and an alternative generalizable PROC for achieving it. The terminology arises from the context of generalized linear models further addressed in Chapter 12, where we consider the regression error to follow some non-normal distributions such as binomial and Poisson. For review, we return to likelihood equation (8.2).

In Chapter 2 and again via equation (8.5), we pointed out that when obtaining maximum likelihood estimators for ordinary regression, $\sum_{i=1}^{n}(y_i - \hat{\beta}_0 - \hat{\beta}_1 x_i)^2$ needs to be minimized, just as for least-squares estimation. We showed in Chapters 1 and 2 how this is done. Recall that $\log(L)$ is given by

$$\log(L) = -n\log(\hat{\sigma}_{y|x}\sqrt{2\pi}) - \frac{\sum_{i=1}^{n}(y_i - \hat{\beta}_0 - \hat{\beta}_1 x_i)^2}{2\hat{\sigma}_{y|x}^2} \tag{11.1}$$

and that the score equations for the regression parameters are

$$X'(Y - X\hat{\boldsymbol{\beta}}) = 0 \tag{11.2}$$

or

$$X'(Y - E(Y|X)) = 0$$

Quantitative Methods in Population Health, by Mari Palta
ISBN 0-471-45505-9   Copyright © 2003 John Wiley & Sons, Inc.

and the maximum likelihood estimator for the variance around the regression line is

$$\hat{\sigma}_{y|x}^2 = \frac{\sum_{i=1}^{n}(y_i - \hat{\beta}_0 - \hat{\beta}_1 x_i)^2}{n}$$

A whole host of new terminology is introduced to generalize the above development to situations with non-normally distributed regression errors. In the SAS outputs that follow and in the theory of generalized linear models [64] connected with it, $\sigma_{y|x}$ is called the *scale parameter*, while $\sigma_{y|x}^2$ is called the *dispersion parameter*. The sum $\sum_{i=1}^{n}(y_i - \hat{\beta}_0 - \hat{\beta}_1 x_i)^2$ is the *deviance*, while we previously called it the "residual" or "error" sum of squares. The change in terminology to "deviance" comes from viewing $\sum_{i=1}^{n}(y_i - \hat{\beta}_0 - \hat{\beta}_1 x_i)^2$ not as a sum of squared residuals, but as the difference in $(-2\log L)\sigma^2$ between two models with known σ^2: One model has β estimated and the other perfectly fits the data. Perfectly fitting the data means that

$$-2\log(L_P) = 2n\log(\sigma_{y|x}\sqrt{2\pi}) + \frac{\sum_{i=1}^{n}(y_i - y_i)^2}{\sigma_{y|x}^2} = 2n\log(\sigma_{y|x}2\pi)$$

while the $-2\log$ likelihood for the model is

$$-2\log(L_M) = 2n\log(\sigma_{y|x}\sqrt{2\pi}) + \frac{\sum_{i=1}^{n}(y_i - \hat{\beta}_0 - \hat{\beta}_1 x_i)^2}{\sigma_{y|x}^2}$$

the difference is

$$\frac{\sum_{i=1}^{n}(y_i - \hat{\beta}_0 - \hat{\beta}_1 x_i)^2}{\sigma_{y|x}^2}$$

and multiplying by $\sigma_{y|x}^2$ leads to the deviance being the error sum of squares.

11.1 PROC GENMOD

In the remaining chapters we will use PROC GENMOD in SAS to obtain estimators of regression parameters. This program is based on the theory of generalized linear models that uses maximum likelihood estimation for normal and non-normal distributions as a starting point. Because of the genesis of PROC GENMOD, it uses terminology that is different from what we have seen with PROC REG and PROC MIXED. Again, the strength of PROC GENMOD is that it can fit distributions other than the normal. This is important in population health research, where we often have binary variables or rates as outcomes. PROC MIXED, however, has more flexibility when the regression error is normally distributed. For example, PROC GENMOD does not fit random effects. PROC NLMIX, available from the SAS version (8.0 forward does this, but is beyond the scope of this text).

The example below compares PROC GENMOD with PROC REG and PROC MIXED.

11.1.1   Example

The output in OUTPUT PACKET X was produced for visit 1 blood pressure data from the Sleep Cohort, by the following statements:

PROC REG; MODEL SBP=AGE;
PROC MIXED METHOD=ML; SBP=AGE/S;
PROC GENMOD; MODEL SBP=AGE;

We first notice that PROC REG, PROC MIXED and PROC GENMOD have all produced the same estimates of the regression coefficients. The standard errors of these coefficients, on the other hand, are not identical, because PROC GENMOD and PROC MIXED used maximum likelihood estimation of $\hat{\sigma}^2_{y|x}$ while PROC REG used the unbiased approach of dividing the error sums of squares by the degrees of freedom $n - 2$. We may also note that PROC REG used t-tests for the regression parameters, founded in small sample theory, while PROC GENMOD used Wald χ^2-tests. We see that both PROC MIXED and PROC GENMOD provide the log likelihood.

Below the regression coefficients on the GENMOD output, we see the SCALE, which is estimated at 14.3298. This is close to the "Root MSE" on the PROC REG output of 14.34033. Again, PROC GENMOD divided the "deviance" or "error sum of squares" by 1365 rather than 1363 to obtain the ML-based SCALE. Further up on the outputs, we see that the "deviance" and "error sum of squares" are indeed the same. Finally, we see that PROC GENMOD does provide the "deviance" divided by the degrees of freedom after all, and that its value 205.6452 is the same as that of the "mean square error" provided by PROC REG.

For the normal distribution, the Pearson χ^2, which is more familiar from application to risks and rates, is defined to be the same as the deviance. Finally, the "scaled" values of the deviance and the Pearson chi-square are simply the deviance/degrees of freedom, divided by the maximum likelihood estimator of the dispersion. For the normal distribution, this is simply $(n - k)/n$.

The remainder of PACKET X is discussed in the next chapter.

OUTPUT PACKET X: INTRODUCING PROC GENMOD

X.1. Comparing PROC REG, PROC MIXED, and PROC GENMOD

SBP Versus Age REG, MIXED GENMOD—Wisconsin Sleep Cohort
Using PROC REG
  The REG Procedure

Model: MODEL1
Dependent Variable: SBP

Analysis of Variance

Source	DF	Sum of Squares	Mean Square	F Value	Pr > F
Model	1	11604	11604	56.43	<0.0001
Error	1363	**280294**	**205.64520**		
Corrected Total	1364	291898			

Root MSE		**14.34033**	R-square	0.0398	
Dependent mean		125.09145	Adjusted R-square	0.0390	
Coefficient of variation		11.46388			

Parameter Estimates

Variable	DF	Parameter Estimate	Standard Error	t Value	Pr > |t|
Intercept	1	107.98092	2.31066	46.73	<0.0001
Age	1	0.36605	0.04873	7.51	<0.0001

Using PROC MIXED with ML
  The Mixed Procedure

Model Information

Data set	WORK.A
Dependent variable	SBP
Covariance structure	Diagonal
Estimation method	ML
Residual variance method	Profile
Fixed effects SE method	Model-based
Degrees-of-freedom method	Residual

Dimensions

Covariance parameters	1
Columns in X	2
Columns in Z	0
Subjects	1
Maximum observation per subject	1370
Observations used	1365
Observations not used	5
Total observations	1370

Covariance Parameter Estimates

Covariance Parameter	Estimate
Residual	**205.34**

Fit Statistics

−2 Log likelihood	**11141.9**
AIC (smaller is better)	11147.9
AICC (smaller is better)	11147.9
BIC (smaller is better)	11163.6

Solution for Fixed Effects

Effect	Estimate	Standard Error	DF	t Value	Pr > $|t|$
Intercept	107.98	2.3090	1363	46.77	<0.0001
Age	0.3660	0.04869	1363	7.52	<0.0001

Using PROC GENMOD
   The GENMOD Procedure

Model Information

Data set	WORK.A
Distribution	Normal
Link function	Identity
Dependent variable	SBP
Observations used	1365
Missing values	13

Criteria for Assessing Goodness of Fit[a]

Criterion	DF	Value	Value/DF
Deviance	1363	**280294.4030**	**205.6452**
Scaled deviance	1363	1365.0000	1.0015
Pearson chi-square	1363	**280294.4030**	**205.6452**
Scaled Pearson X2	1363	1365.0000	1.0015
Log likelihood		**−5570.9493**	

[a] Algorithm converged.

Analysis of Parameter Estimates

Parameter	DF	Estimate	Standard Error	Wald 95% Confidence Limits		Chi-Square
Intercept	1	107.9809	2.3090	103.4554	112.5064	2187.05
Age	1	0.3660	0.0487	0.2706	0.4615	56.51
Scale	1	**14.3298**	0.2743	13.8022	14.8776	

Analysis of Parameter Estimates

Parameter	Pr > ChiSq
Intercept	<0.0001
Age	<0.0001
Scale	

Note: The scale parameter was estimated by maximum likelihood.

X.2. Changing the Relationship of Covariates to the Mean

SBP from Wisconsin Sleep Cohort with Identity and Log Link
Identity Link
   The GENMOD Procedure

Model Information

Data set	WORK.A
Distribution	Normal
Link function	**Identity**
Dependent variable	SBP
Observations used	1364
Missing values	14

Criteria for Assessing Goodness of Fit

Criterion	DF	Value	Value/DF
Deviance	1359	241336.0660	177.5836
Scaled deviance	1359	1364.0000	1.0037
Pearson chi-square	1359	241336.0660	177.5836
Scaled Pearson X2	1359	1364.0000	1.0037
Log likelihood		−5465.3065	

Analysis of Parameter Estimates

Parameter		DF	Estimate	Standard Error	Wald 95% Confidence Limits		Chi-Square
Intercept		1	127.4490	0.5241	126.4219	128.4761	59143.9
sex	F	1	−6.5731	0.7305	−8.0048	−5.1413	80.97
sex	M	0	0.0000	0.0000	0.0000	0.0000	.
agec		1	0.3691	0.0494	0.2724	0.4659	55.91
bmic		1	0.5945	0.0654	0.4663	0.7228	82.53
agec*bmic		1	−0.0189	0.0075	−0.0336	−0.0043	6.39
Scale		1	13.3016	0.2547	12.8117	13.8102	

Analysis of Parameter Estimates

Parameter		Pr > ChiSq
Intercept		<0.0001
sex	F	<0.0001
sex	M	.
agec		<0.0001
bmic		<0.0001
agec*bmic		0.0115

Note: The scale parameter was estimated by maximum likelihood.

Log Link
   The GENMOD Procedure

Model Information

Data set	WORK.A
Distribution	Normal
Link function	**Log**
Dependent variable	SBP
Observations used	1364
Missing values	14

Criteria for Assessing Goodness of Fit

Criterion	DF	Value	Value/DF
Deviance	1359	241924.2212	178.0164
Scaled deviance	1359	1364.0022	1.0037
Pearson chi-square	1359	241924.2212	178.0164
Scaled Pearson X2	1359	1364.0022	1.0037
Log likelihood		−5466.9666	

Analysis of Parameter Estimates

Parameter	DF		Estimate	Standard Error	Wald 95% Confidence Limits		Chi-Square
Intercept		1	4.8475	0.0041	4.8394	4.8555	1396599
sex	F	1	−0.0530	0.0059	−0.0645	−0.0414	80.57
sex	M	0	0.0000	0.0000	0.0000	0.0000	.
agec		1	0.0030	0.0004	0.0022	0.0038	55.52
bmic		1	0.0046	0.0005	0.0036	0.0056	83.75
agec*bmic		1	−0.0001	0.0001	−0.0003	−0.0000	6.92
Scale		1	13.3178	0.2550	12.8273	13.8270	

Analysis of Parameter Estimates

Parameter		Pr > ChiSq
Intercept		<0.0001
sex	F	<0.0001
sex	M	.
agec		<0.0001
bmic		<0.0001
agec*bmic		0.0085
Scale		

Note: The scale parameter was estimated by maximum likelihood.

Taking Log of Outcome
  The GENMOD Procedure

Model Information

Data set	WORK.A	
Distribution	Normal	
Link function	Identity	
Dependent variable	LSBP	(log of systolic blood pressure)
Observations used	1364	
Missing values	14	

Criteria for Assessing Goodness of Fit

Criterion	DF	Value	Value/DF
Deviance	1359	15.1214	0.0111
Scaled deviance	1359	1364.0000	1.0037
Pearson chi-square	1359	15.1214	0.0111
Scaled Pearson X2	1359	1364.0000	1.0037
Log likelihood		1134.9763	

Analysis of Parameter Estimates

Parameter	DF		Estimate	Standard Error	Wald 95% Confidence Limits		Chi-Square
Intercept		1	4.8417	0.0041	4.8336	4.8498	1362269
sex	F	1	−0.0542	0.0058	−0.0655	−0.0428	87.77
sex	M	0	0.0000	0.0000	0.0000	0.0000	.
agec		1	0.0029	0.0004	0.0021	0.0037	55.23
bmic		1	0.0048	0.0005	0.0037	0.0058	84.18
agec*bmic		1	−0.0001	0.0001	−0.0003	−0.0000	6.31
Scale		1	0.1053	0.0020	0.1014	0.1093	

Analysis of Parameter Estimates

Parameter		Pr > ChiSq
Intercept		<0.0001
sex	F	<0.0001
sex	M	.
agec		<0.0001
bmic		<0.0001
agec*bmic		0.0120
Scale		

Note: The scale parameter was estimated by maximum likelihood.

CHAPTER TWELVE

The Generalization to Non-normal Distributions

Among regression analyses with non-normally distributed outcome, logistic regression is perhaps the most well known and widely used. There are many ways to motivate, derive, and interpret logistic regression. In the last decade or so, the most common framework for linking logistic and ordinary regression, as well as regression analyses for other distributions of the outcome, has been the approach of generalized linear models [64]. The approach starts with the realization that the score equations for estimating regression parameters for many distributions for the outcome can be written in a form similar to (11.2). To see this generality, it is useful to be aware that the probability or probability density of many commonly used distributions can be expressed by a single formula. This formula, discussed briefly below, describes the so-called exponential family of distributions, which includes (among others) the normal, the binomial, and the Poisson distribution.

12.1 THE EXPONENTIAL FAMILY

Statisticians have found that many distributions we are interested in, such as the normal, binomial, and Poisson, have probability (density) that can be written

$$f(y) = \exp\{(y\theta - b(\theta))/a(\phi) + c(y, \phi)\} \qquad (12.1)$$

Here, a, b, and c are functions that determine what type of distribution (12.1) describes. There are two parameters θ and ϕ. Usually ϕ, which is labeled the "dispersion parameter," is assumed "known." As indicated in Chapter 11, the dispersion parameter is σ^2 for the normal distribution, so this is a stretch in that case. However, as we saw there and earlier, σ^2 can be estimated almost as an

Quantitative Methods in Population Health, by Mari Palta
ISBN 0-471-45505-9   Copyright © 2003 John Wiley & Sons, Inc.

afterthought, so it can be considered "temporarily" known. The parameter θ is the center of attention, because it is related to the mean μ of the distribution. As we have seen, regression analysis usually focuses on estimating the mean of y conditionally on x. The parameter θ is known as the *canonical parameter*; and for the normal distribution, actually $\theta = \mu$. To see this, the normal probability density can be expressed as

$$f(y) = \frac{1}{\sigma\sqrt{2\pi}} \exp\left(-\frac{(y-\mu)^2}{2\sigma^2}\right)$$

$$= \exp\{(y\mu - \mu^2/2)/\sigma^2 - \frac{1}{2}[y^2/\sigma^2 + \log(2\pi\sigma^2)]$$

To verify remember that $\exp[-1/2\log(2\pi\sigma^2)] = \frac{1}{\sigma\sqrt{2\pi}}$ and that $(y-\mu)^2 = (y^2 + \mu^2 - 2y\mu)$. Identifying the above expression with (12.1), one finds that

$$a(\phi) = \phi = \sigma^2$$

$$b(\theta) = \theta^2/2$$

$$c(y, \theta) = -\frac{1}{2}\{y^2/\sigma^2 + \log(2\pi\sigma^2)\}$$

for the normal distribution.

Although the general formula for the exponential family has the parameters θ and ϕ, these themselves do not usually hold any particular interest in statistical applications. Typically, we are focusing on the mean and variance of y. It can be shown that the mean and variance are related to functions of the canonical parameter θ. The relevant functions are derivatives of the function b in the definition of the distribution:

$$E(y) = \mu = \frac{d}{d\theta}b(\theta) = b'(\theta)$$

$$\text{Var}(y) = \left[\frac{d^2}{d\theta^2}b(\theta)\right]a(\phi) = b''(\theta)a(\phi)$$

In the above, μ is expressed as a function of θ. It also follows that if we want to obtain θ from μ, $\theta(\mu) = b'^{-1}(\mu)$, so θ can also be expressed in terms of μ. The relationships can be verified for the normal distribution because the derivative of $b(\theta) = \theta^2/2$ is $b'(\theta) = \theta$, which we already saw was $= \mu$, and the second derivative of $b(\theta)$ is $b''(\theta) = 1$, so that the variance is $a(\phi)$, which is $\phi = \sigma^2$. Most often, the function a is assumed to be of form

$$a(\phi) = \phi/\omega$$

The other part of Var(y) is $b''(\theta)$, known as the *variance function*. It is given in Table 12.1 as a function of the mean μ. For the normal distribution, the function a is just a constant $= 1$.

Table 12.1   Characteristics of Three Distributions in the Exponential Family

	Normal	Binomial	Poisson
Outcome y	Continuous measurement	Proportion in m trials	# of events during t
Parameters	μ, σ^2	$\mu = \pi, m$	$\mu = \lambda t$
$a(\phi)$	σ^2	$1/m$	1
$b(\theta)$	$\theta^2/2$	$\log(1 + \exp(\theta))$	$\exp(\theta)$
$c(y, \phi)$	$-\frac{1}{2}(y^2/\phi + \log(2\pi\phi))$	$\log\begin{pmatrix} m \\ my \end{pmatrix}$	$-\log y!$
$\mu(\theta) = b'(\theta)$	θ	$\frac{\exp(\theta)}{1+\exp(\theta)}$	$\exp(\theta)$
$\theta(\mu) = b'^{-1}(\mu)$	μ	$\log\left(\frac{\mu}{1-\mu}\right)$	$\log(\mu)$
Canonical link	identity	logit	log
$V(\mu) = b''(\theta(\mu))$	1	$\mu(1-\mu)$	μ

Table 12.1 provides the functions a, b, and c, as well as some additional information we will use later for the three distributions we consider in this text.

12.1.1   The Binomial Distribution

You will recall that the usual formulation of the **binomial** distribution is for the probability of "number of successes s in m independent trials." For population health, an application of the binomial distribution may be to compute the probability of a certain number of people developing a disease in a cohort. A binary (or Bernoulli, as it is also called) outcome, is just the binomial with $m = 1$. The usual way to write the binomial probability is

$$\text{Prob}(s|m) = \begin{pmatrix} m \\ s \end{pmatrix} \pi^s (1 - \pi)^{m-s}$$

where s is the number of successes. The mean of this distribution is $E(s) = m\pi$, so that when there is only one trial and s is either 0 or 1, $E(s) = \pi$. The variance is $\text{Var}(s) = m\pi(1 - \pi)$. For easier transition between the exponential family functions for $m > 1$ to $m = 1$ trials, the information in Table 12.1 is given not for s; but for the outcome $y = s/m$, the proportion of successes in m trials. Clearly, then $s = my$. Focusing on the proportion being the outcome has the advantage of the mean μ being equal to the probability of success for both binary and binomial outcomes.

Applying the functions from Table 12.1 and some facility with exponentials and logarithms leads to

$$\text{Prob}(y|m) = f(y) = \exp\left\{\left(y\log\left(\frac{\mu}{1-\mu}\right) - \log\left(\frac{1}{1-\mu}\right)\right)m + \log\binom{m}{my}\right\}$$

$$= \binom{m}{my}\exp\left(\log\left[\left(\frac{\mu}{1-\mu}\right)^{ym}\left(\frac{1}{1-\mu}\right)^{-m}\right]\right)$$

$$= \binom{m}{my}\mu^{ym}(1-\mu)^{m-ym}$$

The binomial distribution makes the assumption that the events are independent. This assumption is most commonly violated by trials falling into clusters with different π, or by an event in one person leading to an event in another person.

12.1.1.1 *Example*

In the sleep survey at five state agencies, the overall percentage of subjects reporting habitual snoring was 32.7%. Hence among state workers the probability of being a habitual snorer is estimated at 0.327. This means that the probability of finding 4 to be habitual snorers in a sample of 10 state workers is

$$\text{Prob}(4|10) = \binom{10}{4}0.327^4(1-0.327)^6$$

$$= \frac{10 \times 9 \times 8 \times 7}{1 \times 2 \times 3 \times 4}0.327^4(1-0.327)^6 = 0.223$$

The mean of the distribution of the number of snorers in the sample is 3.27, and the variance is $10 \times 0.327(1 - 0.327) = 2.2$. The independence assumption is likely to hold here, if the sample is obtained randomly. Independence could be violated if individuals discussed the question and influenced each other's answers.

12.1.2 The Poisson Distribution

Another important distribution in population health research is the **Poisson**. This distribution is used to obtain the number of events in a population in a given time period or per person years of event-free observation. It is different from the binomial in several ways. First of all, it is assumed that the population size is infinite compared to the number of events. Hence no upper limit m for the number of events is imposed. Second, by introducing the concept of "per time period" or "per person year," varying follow-up times are allowed. In fact, the mean of the Poisson distribution per follow-up unit (time or person year) is known as a rate. The probability of y events during a time period t (say) from the Poisson distribution is given as

$$\text{Prob}(y) = \frac{(\lambda t)^y \exp(-\lambda t)}{y!}$$

Here λ is the rate per whatever time unit t is measured in. Both the mean and variance of the Poisson distribution are equal to $\mu = \lambda t$. When the population size n is large, and the probability π of an event is small as often happens in population health, the binomial distribution and the Poisson distribution give very similar probabilities for observing y events. In that case $\lambda t \approx \pi$, which is a statement of the well-known fact that when the risk is low, the rate and the risk are approximately equal (see, e.g., Ref. 65). Because of this, the Poisson distribution is also used for situations such as "prevalence" of a disease, which do not refer to a time period. In these situations, t represents the size of the population from which the prevalence arose.

The Poisson distribution makes the assumption that events are independent, that the rate is constant, and that the probability of an event goes to 0 when the time period becomes small The independence assumption is often violated, but is more likely to hold for small t.

The formula for the Poisson distribution can again be obtained by inserting functions from Table 12.1 into the exponential distribution and applying rules for exponentials and logarithms.

12.1.3 Example

The rate of hospitalization of children aged 0–2 in Wisconsin is 90 per 1000 person years (i.e., 0.09 year $^{-1}$) [66]. Then, if the population between these ages in an area is 100, the mean number of hospitalizations in a year is $100 \times 0.09 = 9$, and the variance is 9 as well. The probability of no hospitalizations in the age group during a year is

$$\text{Prob}(0) = \frac{(0.09 \times 100)^0 \exp(-0.09 \times 100)}{0!} = 0.00012$$

The Poisson distribution may be violated, because some children have multiple hospitalization due to some underlying chronic condition. Also outbreaks of infectious diseases may lead to clusters of cases.

12.2 SCORE EQUATIONS FOR THE EXPONENTIAL FAMILY AND THE CANONICAL LINK

Because of the "exponential nature" of the exponential family, it's quite easy to obtain that

$$\log(L) = \sum_{i=1}^{n} L(\{y_i\theta - b(\theta)\}/a(\phi) + c(y_i, \phi))$$

If the purpose were to estimate θ (ϕ is considered "known"), one can easily obtain the relevant score equation (see Chapter 11 for the definition of a score)

$$\sum_{i=1}^{n} \{y_i - b'(\hat{\theta})\}/a(\phi) = 0 \tag{12.2}$$

This is based on taking the derivative with respect to $\hat{\theta}$. However, we are not usually interested in estimating θ per se. Rather, our purpose is regression analysis relating parameters to covariates. If we set

$$\theta = \beta_0 + \beta_1 x_{1i} + \cdots$$

the chain rule would apply as in Chapter 1, and we obtain equations

$$\sum_{i=1}^{n}\{y_i - b'(\hat{\beta}_0 + \hat{\beta}_1 x_{1i} + \cdots)\}/a(\phi) = 0$$

$$\sum_{i=1}^{n} x_{1i}\{y_i - b'(\hat{\beta}_0 + \hat{\beta}_1 x_{1i} + \cdots)\}/a(\phi) = 0 \qquad (12.3)$$

$$\cdots$$

Remembering that $b'(\theta)$ equals the mean and realizing that $a(\phi)$ can be canceled, equation (12.3) can also be written

$$X'(Y - \hat{\mu}_{y|x}) = 0$$

$$\text{or} \quad X'(Y - \hat{E}(Y|X)) = 0 \qquad (12.4)$$

identically to the score equations (11.2) for the normal distribution. However, formula (12.4) hides a generalization, because if the canonical parameter θ is linear in the predictors, then the mean $\mu_{y|x}$ is related to the predictors through

$$\mu_{y|x} = b'(\beta_0 + \beta_1 x_{1i} + \cdots \beta_0 + \beta_1 x_{1i} + \cdots) \qquad (12.5)$$

which implies linearity in the mean

$$\mu_{y|x} = \beta_0 + \beta_1 x_{1i} + \cdots \beta_0 + \beta_1 x_{1i} + \cdots$$

only for the normal distribution. In contrast to the normal distribution case, we know from Table 12.1 that for a binomial outcome y, the quantity $\hat{E}(Y|X)$ resulting from b' in equation (12.4) is

$$\mu_{y|x} = \frac{\exp(\hat{\beta}_0 + \hat{\beta}_1 x_{1i} + \cdots)}{1 + \exp(\hat{\beta}_0 + \hat{\beta}_1 x_{1i} + \cdots)}$$

and for Poisson outcome

$$\mu_{y|x} = \exp(\beta_0 + \beta_1 x_{1i} + \cdots \beta_0 + \beta_1 x_{1i} + \cdots)$$

These equations can be rewritten as

$$\log\left(\frac{\mu_{y|x}}{1 - \mu_{y|x}}\right) = \log\left(\frac{\pi}{1 - \pi}\right) = \beta_0 + \beta_1 x_{1i} + \cdots$$

and

$$\log(\mu_{y|x}) = \beta_0 + \beta_1 x_{1i} + \cdots$$

respectively. A transformation applied this way to the mean, and set equal to a linear expression in β's, is referred to as a link function. In the above, after we set θ equal to a linear expression, $b'^{-1}(\mu) = \theta$ was automatically linearly related to the predictors. This link function is referred to as the *canonical link*. It is the canonical link that yields equation (12.4) for estimating β. It should also be noted that, although equation (12.4) looks simple, because of what is hidden in $\hat{\mu}_{y|x}$, it can generally be solved only through iterative numerical methods (see McCullagh and Nelder [64]). The names of the three canonical link functions we have addressed are in Table 12.1.

12.3   OTHER LINK FUNCTIONS

Further generalization is possible, because we can apply functions other than the canonical link b'^{-1} to $\mu_{y|x}$. We denote a general link function by h (either h or g is used in the literature). Then the canonical link means $h = b'^{-1}$; that is, h is the inverse of the function b'. If h is not the canonical link, we have the more complicated relationship where θ is not linear

$$\theta = b'^{-1}(\mu_{y|x}) = b'^{-1}[h^{-1}(\beta_0 + \beta_1 x_1 + \cdots)]$$

and obtaining the score equations for $\hat{\beta}$ involves applying the chain rule not once, but twice. For example,

$$\frac{\partial \theta}{\partial \beta_1} = \frac{d\theta}{d\mu_{y|x}} \frac{\partial \mu_{y|x}}{\partial \beta_1} = \frac{1}{b''(\mu_{y|x})} \frac{\partial \mu_{y|x}}{\partial \beta_1}$$

where we have also used the rule for a derivative of an inverse. The corresponding score equation element becomes

$$\sum \left(\frac{d\mu_{y|x}}{d\beta_1} \times \frac{1}{V(\mu_y|x)} \{y_i - \hat{\mu}_{y|x}\} \right) = 0$$

where we have incorporated that b'' is the variance function $V(\theta)$ from Table 12.1. Initially we expressed the variance as a function of θ and ϕ, but as shown in Table 12.1, the part that depends on θ can also be expressed in terms of $\mu_{y|x}$. Putting together all the score equations for the regression parameters in matrix form, most books and papers express the score equation as

$$D'V^{-1}(Y - \mu) = 0 \qquad (12.6)$$

where D' has a row for each subject $i = 1, \ldots, n$, and the columns of D' are derivatives of $\mu_{y|x}$ with respect to the respective regression coefficient. V^{-1} is the diagonal matrix with the inverse of the variance of each observation expressed as a function of the mean on the main diagonal. Hence expression (12.6) is in longhand:

$$\begin{pmatrix} \frac{\partial h^{-1}(\beta_0+\beta_1 x_{11}\cdots)}{\partial \beta_0} & \frac{\partial h^{-1}(\beta_0+\beta_1 x_{12}\cdots)}{\partial \beta_0} & \cdots \\ \frac{\partial h^{-1}(\beta_0+\beta_1 x_{11}\cdots)}{\partial \beta_1} & \frac{\partial h^{-1}(\beta_0+\beta_1 x_{12}\cdots)}{\partial \beta_1} & \cdots \\ \vdots & \vdots & \ddots \end{pmatrix}$$

$$\times \begin{pmatrix} 1/\mathrm{Var}[h^{-1}(\beta_0 + \beta_1 x_{11}\cdots)] & 0 & \cdots \\ 0 & 1/\mathrm{Var}[h^{-1}(\beta_0 + \beta_1 x_{12}\cdots)] & \cdots \\ \vdots & \vdots & \ddots \end{pmatrix}$$

$$\times \left(\begin{pmatrix} y_1 \\ \vdots \\ y_n \end{pmatrix} - \begin{pmatrix} h^{-1}(\beta_0 + \beta_1 x_{11}\cdots) \\ \vdots \\ h^{-1}(\beta_0 + \beta_1 x_{1n}\cdots) \end{pmatrix} \right) = 0$$

The information above is provided to facilitate further reading on this topic and to recognize mathematical expressions often presented in papers on regression analysis of non-normally distributed data. PROC GENMOD can painlessly fit an array of link functions, but assumes the canonical link for each distribution as the default.

12.3.1 Example

Looking back at the GENMOD output in OUTPUT PACKET X, we see that the link is listed as IDENTITY, and the distribution is listed as NORMAL. This is the default if no other distribution or link is specified to GENMOD. If, for some reason we do not want the identity link for the normal distribution, we must specify that. Output from the following is also in OUTPUT PACKET X. Consider a regression equation

$$\log(\mu_{y|x}) = \beta_0 + \beta_1 x_{1i} + \cdots$$

which may be relevant if the dependence of the mean on covariates is stronger than linear. We consider fitting this model to the visit 1 blood pressure data from the sleep study. The following statements produce regression analyses, where we predict the logarithm of the mean blood pressure from age, and another analysis predicting the mean of the log blood pressure from age:

LSBP=LOG(SBP);
PROC GENMOD; CLASS SEX;
MODEL SBP=SEX AGEC BMIC AGEC*BMIC/LINK=LOG DIST=NORMAL;
PROC REG; MODEL LSBP=AGE;

We see that PROC GENMOD, like PROC MIXED, has the ability to create CLASS variables and interactions. In OUTPUT PACKET X we see that the link function is indeed now listed as log. We notice that the deviance is slightly larger for the log link, however, indicating that this structure for the mean fits less well. For comparison, output packet X provides an ordinary regression analysis using log (SBP) as the outcome. The coefficients are very similar. However, one soon notices that the two approaches do not really represent the same analysis. The difference comes in the fact that the error term has not been transformed by PROC GENMOD. In fact, GENMOD has transformed only the mean and has fit the model

$$y_i = \exp(\beta_0 + \beta_1 \text{sex}_i + \beta_2 \text{agec}_i \cdots) + \epsilon_i$$

where ϵ_i has a normal distribution with variance $\sigma^2 (= \phi)$ along the whole curve. In fact, we see that the scale parameter using the log link is not too different from that using the identity link. PROC REG, on the other hand, has fit the regression

$$y_i = \exp(\beta_0 + \beta_1 \text{sex}_i + \beta_2 \text{age}_i \cdots + \epsilon_i)$$

PROC REG makes the assumption that it is the error term of $\log(y_i)$ that has equal variance.

CHAPTER THIRTEEN

Modeling Binomial and Binary Outcomes

Readers are probably already familiar with logistic regression for binary data. As mentioned above, the goal with such data is to model the response probability π of having a certain outcome. In epidemiology and population health, logistic regression is chosen for several reasons. First of all, it is a transformation that spreads the originally limited value of π across the whole range of real numbers. This makes predicted values of $\hat{\pi}$ resulting from the regression realistic. Second, the regression coefficients have very desirable interpretation as logs of odds ratios. With this comes not only convenience, but all the favorable properties of the odds ratio. These include the applicability of the regression analysis to case-control studies. As we saw, the formulation of the exponential family also singles out the logit transform as a natural one from a mathematical perspective.

The framework of generalized linear models does not change logistic regression. By placing logistic regression in a larger context, though, it allows us to express the regression equation, the likelihood, and the score equations in more general notation. The framework seamlessly incorporates transformations other than the logit (i.e., other link functions h) and creates the bridge to the analysis of correlated data (see Chapter 15).

13.1 A BRIEF REVIEW OF LOGISTIC REGRESSION

Logistic regression is based on the transformation $\log(\frac{\pi}{1-\pi})$, which is set equal to the linear regression $\beta_0 + \beta_1 x_{1i} + \cdots$. Traditionally, instead of relying on the likelihoods and score equations presented in Chapter 12 for the exponential family, results for logistic regression have been be derived directly by specifying

Quantitative Methods in Population Health, by Mari Palta
ISBN 0-471-45505-9   Copyright © 2003 John Wiley & Sons, Inc.

the logistic response probability to be [65]

$$\pi_i = \frac{\exp(\beta_0 + \beta_1 x_{1i} + \cdots)}{1 + \exp(\beta_0 + \beta_1 x_{1i} + \cdots)}$$

and the nonresponse probability to be

$$(1 - \pi_i) = \frac{1}{1 + \exp(\beta_0 + \beta_1 x_{1i} + \cdots)}$$

then multiplying these together according to the observed data. The observed data can be either individual binary outcomes, or a set of y_i indicating the proportion of successes in m_i trials. Formulating the likelihood in terms of binary outcomes and letting s be the number of successes, one obtains

$$L = \prod_{i=1}^{s} \hat{\pi}_i \prod_{i=s+1}^{n} (1 - \hat{\pi}_i) \tag{13.1}$$

which is

$$L = \prod_{i=1}^{s} \frac{\exp(\hat{\beta}_0 + \hat{\beta}_1 x_{1i} + \cdots)}{1 + \exp(\hat{\beta}_0 + \hat{\beta}_1 x_{1i} + \cdots)} \prod_{i=s+1}^{n} \frac{1}{1 + \exp(\hat{\beta}_0 + \hat{\beta}_1 x_{1i} + \cdots)}$$

One then proceeds by taking derivatives of $\log(L)$ directly with respect to the β's. We can use PROC GENMOD to fit logistic regression for both binary and binomial ($m_i > 1$) outcomes. An example is given in OUTPUT PACKET XI.

PROC LOGIST requires a DESCENDING option to be specified for the coefficients to predict $\log(\frac{\pi}{1-\pi})$ rather than $\log(\frac{1-\pi}{\pi})$. (The same feature has been added to version 8.2 of GENMOD for the binary data situation.) This convention arose through the genesis of PROC LOGIST from an older weighted least-squares solution that preceded the generalized linear model framework as presented in Chapter 12 [67]. PROC LOGIST has the advantage of many features in the output and options that are useful in population health research. Among these is the fact that PROC LOGIST painlessly provides odds ratios and their confidence intervals. PROC LOGIST also provides several likelihood-based statistics; and through the/LACKFIT option, the Hosmer and Lemeshow [68] goodness-of-fit test Version 8 of SAS allows categorical variables to be introduced directly into the model by the CLASS statement and allows interaction effects to be created by the variablea*variableb notation. Because the purpose here is to discuss logistic regression from the generalized models perspective, we will emphasize the application of PROC GENMOD below. However, many analyses involving logistic regression specifically are better served by PROC LOGIST.

13.1.1 Example: Review of the Output from PROC LOGIST

In the Newborn Lung Project, we modeled the probability of a very-low-birth-weight infant dying before one month of age (DEATH=1 if died DEATH=0 if survived [22]). The data set includes all babies admitted to the 6 NICU's. Predictors INDYR and SURFYR are indicator variables for time periods of birth (just as in Chapter 7). The importance of these time periods derives from the fact that INDYR=1 represents the year (8/1/89–7/31/90) when exogenous surfactant therapy was first available as an investigational new drug (IND). SURFYR represents the period after 7/31/90 when surfactant was generally available. INDYR=SURFYR=0 represents the year 8/1/88–7/31/89 when surfactant was available only to a very small group of infants participating in randomized trials.

The following commands were run:

PROC LOGIST DESCENDING; MODEL DEATH=INDYR SURFYR;

Referring to OUTPUT PACKET XI, we see that PROC LOGIST provides the $-2\log(L)$ and two other likelihood-based tests for the model at hand versus one with an intercept only. Equivalently, these test the significance of all the covariates together (i.e., of whether there are mortality differences between the time periods). The three tests are the likelihood ratio test, formed as $-2\log(L_1) + 2\log(L_2)$, the score test based on the first derivatives of $\log(L)$, and their variance matrix evaluated under the null hypothesis, and the Wald statistic-based estimated coefficients and their variance matrix under the fitted model. In the case at hand, they yield similar results ($\chi^2(2) = 8.19$, 8.12, and 8.02, respectively) and are all statistically significant. These tests tell us that the model with different mortality risk for the three time periods fits the data significantly better than a model which assumed constant mortality throughout the three years. You may also note the AIC, which in this case is the $-2\log(L)$ adjusted for the three fixed parameters (so $-2\log(L)+2\times3$).

Turning to the regression coefficients, recall that we created the indicator variables for the time periods, so that each coefficient is the difference in $\log(\frac{\pi}{1-\pi})$ of that time period from the pre-surfactant era. Hence the coefficients and corresponding odds ratios obtained by $\exp(\beta_1) = \exp(-0.572) = 0.565$ and $\exp(\beta_2) = \exp(-0.246) = 0.782$ are those of death during the two post-surfactant time periods versus the pre-surfactant time period. The odds ratios and their (Wald) confidence intervals, which would otherwise be obtained by calculating $\exp[\hat{\beta} \pm 1.96\text{se}(\hat{\beta})]$, are automatically provided by PROC LOGIST. From Chapter 5, we know that the standard error in this expression is obtained from the inverse of minus the matrix of second derivatives of $\log(L)$, known as the information matrix. The χ^2s of the coefficients were obtained by $[\frac{\hat{\beta}}{\text{se}(\hat{\beta})}]^2$ and are Wald chi-squares. We know that both the confidence intervals and good only in large samples. If the sample size were small, we should have turned to "exact" procedures similar to Fisher's exact test, some of which are available in version 8 of SAS as part of PROC LOGIST and PROC FREQ.

For the sake of completeness, it should be pointed out that (just as in PROC GENMOD below) we could have used a categorical variable BIRTHYR coded 0, 1, 2 for the three time periods directly. Including the statement CLASS BIRTHYR; would have created indicator variables with the last year serving as the default baseline category. Also, if the data had been provided in a binomial fashion as

number of births NUMB and number of deaths NDTHS, the same model could
have been fit by the command

PROC LOGIST; MODEL NDTHS/NUMB=INDYR SURFYR;

Because the model with indicator variables for the years makes no linearity
assumptions, the only manner in which it would not fit is lack of independence
between outcomes so that the correct likelihood is not the product of individual
probabilities. Such violation could enter via clustering of deaths and would lead to
standard errors being underestimated just as in the correlated normal residual case.
We have seen little evidence, however, that clustering (e.g., caused by multiple
births or hospital of admission) has influenced results emerging from this data set.

13.2 ANALYSIS OF BINOMIAL DATA IN THE GENERALIZED LINEAR MODELS FRAMEWORK

In the exponential family notation,

$$\mu = \pi = \frac{\exp(\theta)}{1 + \exp(\theta)}$$

is the function b' in Chapter 12 for binomial outcome. Table 12.1 shows that the
scale parameter ϕ is 1 for the binomial distribution with the number of trials $m = 1$.
This is because the variance of the binary outcome is $\pi(1 - \pi)$, hence completely
determined by the mean $\mu = \pi$, or in exponential family notation because $a(\phi) = 1$
and $b'(\theta) = \frac{\exp(\theta)}{1+\exp(\theta)} = \pi$ we have

$$Var(y) = b''(\theta)a(\phi) = b''(\theta) = \frac{d}{d\theta} \frac{\exp(\theta)}{1 + \exp(\theta)}$$

$$= \frac{\exp(\theta)}{1 + \exp(\theta)} - \left[\frac{\exp(\theta)}{1 + \exp(\theta)} \right]^2 = \pi(1 - \pi)$$

Another important feature of a generalized linear model is the deviance function,
briefly mentioned in Chapter 11. It was not addressed in Chapter 12, because the
interpretation of the deviance is somewhat specific to the distribution at hand and
generalization is not as helpful as it is for the score equations. The deviance is the
difference in $-2\log(L)\phi$ between two models with the same dispersion parameter,
the one at hand and the one that fits the data perfectly. It is the latter part that
turns out to be very specific, as we will see in examples below. We first rewrite
the likelihood (13.1) in some helpful ways.

If the data have been ordered so that the first s observations have $y = 1$,
equation (13.1) for the likelihood can be written

$$\log(L) = \sum_{i=1}^{k} \log(\hat{\pi}_i) + \sum_{i=s+1}^{n} \log(1 - \hat{\pi}_i) \tag{13.2}$$

or (switching notation to be more generic)

$$\log(L) = \sum_{i=1}^{n} [y_i \log(\hat{\mu}_i) + (1 - y_i) \log(1 - \hat{\mu}_i)] \qquad (13.3)$$

where, since y_i is coded 0, 1, the first part of the expression is nonzero only for the first observations and vice versa. For the general binomial case, where y_i is the proportion of positive responses in m_i trials and $m_i y_i$ is the number of positive responses, we have a grouped version of (13.3)

$$\log(L) = \sum_{i=1}^{n} m_i y_i \log(\hat{\pi}_i) + \sum_{1}^{n} (m_i - m_i y_i) \log(1 - \hat{\pi}_i)$$

which can also be written

$$\log(L) = \sum_{i=1}^{n} m_i [y_i \log(\hat{\mu}_i) + (1 - y_i) \log(1 - \hat{\mu}_i)]$$

This latter expression simplifies to (13.3) when $m_i = 1$. Note that the above formulations of $\log(L)$ do not involve any link function. The construction of this likelihood only assumes the observations to be independent. However, in a regression situation, a link function is hidden in

$$\hat{\mu}_i = h^{-1}(\hat{\beta}_0 + \hat{\beta}_1 x_{1i} + \cdots)$$

It is when this specific expression linking $\pi_i (= \mu_i)$ to a linear regression is inserted, and derivatives $\frac{\partial \mu}{\partial \beta}$ taken with respect to β, that the link function begins to matter.

Returning to the derivation of the deviance, the perfect fit for binary data produces a likelihood $L = 1$ because "perfect fit" means that $\pi_i = 1$ for "successes" and $(1 - \pi_i) = 1$ for "failures," so the likelihood is a product of 1's. Then the $\log(L) = 0$ for that model. Hence the deviance for binary outcome just equals $-2 \log(L)$. However, for binomial outcome the deviance turns out differently. Then, "perfect fit" implies

$$\log(L) = \sum_{i=1}^{n} m_i [y_i \log(y_i) + (1 - y_i) \log(1 - y_i)]$$

so the difference in $-2 \log(L)$ between the fitted and the perfect model becomes

$$-2 \sum_{i=1}^{n} m_i [y_i \log(\hat{\mu}_i) + (1 - y_i) \log(1 - \hat{\mu}_i)]$$

$$+ 2 \sum_{i=1}^{n} m_i [y_i \log(y_i) + (1 - y_i) \log(1 - y_i)]$$

$$= 2 \sum_{i=1}^{n} [m_i y_i \log(y_i / \hat{\mu}_i) + m_i (1 - y_i) \log[(1 - y_i)/(1 - \hat{\mu}_i)] \qquad (13.4)$$

Equation (13.4) is the usual expression for the deviance of the binomial distribution (where we have retained the notation that y_i denotes the *proportion* of successes.) Multiplying denominators and numerators inside the logs by m_i leads to

$$\text{deviance} = 2\sum_{i=1}^{n}\{m_i\,y_i\,\log(m_i\,y_i/m_i\hat{\mu}_i) + m_i(1-y_i)\log[m_i(1-y_i)/(m_i(1-\hat{\mu}_i))]\}$$

which is sometimes written [65]

$$\text{deviance} = 2\sum_{l=1}^{2n} O_l \log(O_l/E_l) \tag{13.5}$$

where O_l is the observed and E_l the expected (from the model) number of observations falling in each cell of the $n \times 2$ table formed by the binomial group by outcome classification. Because of the way the deviance was constructed, it follows a χ^2-distribution with degrees of freedom equal to n minus the number of parameters estimated in obtaining E_l. Obviously, only group level covariates can be included with grouped data, so the maximum number of parameters is n. Fitting n parameters produces the perfect fit and is referred to as a "saturated" model. The upper limit on the number of parameters with grouped data allows the saturated model to have a restricted number of parameters, and it leads to the deviance approximately following a χ^2-distribution when the $m_i\pi_i$ and $m_i(1-\pi_i)$ are reasonably large. Obviously this condition cannot hold for individual level binary data.

Another common measure of goodness of fit for grouped data is the Pearson statistic [65]. For the normal distribution, we saw that this statistic equals the deviance. For binomial outcome, it is given by

$$\sum_{l=1}^{2n}(O_l - E_l)^2/E_l$$

with quantities defined as above. It is of interest that the Pearson statistics can also be written

$$\sum_{i=1}^{n}(y_i - \hat{\pi}_i)^2/[\hat{\pi}_i(1-\hat{\pi}_i)/n_i]$$

so it is a direct comparison of (a) the variability in the proportion "with success" observed between groups and (b) the variability predicted in that proportion based on the model and the binomial distribution. For grouped data the statistic has a limiting χ^2-distribution, when cell sizes become large.

Note that the deviance and Pearson statistics in GENMOD are not the same as the χ^2-tests automatically provided by PROC LOGIST. The latter test whether the model does any good for prediction (compared to a model with no predictors).

PROC GENMOD can produce similar likelihood ratio statistics that test the benefit of adding variables via the TYPE1 and TYPE3 options in the MODEL statement. The default GENMOD chi-squares are for testing the reverse, namely how much lack of prediction there is compared to a saturated model. Unfortunately these goodness-of-fit chi-squares can only be used when the data fall into a finite number of predetermined groups. Otherwise, we again have the problem that the degrees of freedom go up together with the sample size, and the large sample distribution properties break down. The limited number of parameters arises from the fact that the binomial (grouped) model only can accommodate group level variables. In our example, however, a variable such as birth weight can be properly adjusted for only in the binary outcome model.

For data that are not grouped, a grouping of some kind has to be imposed before performing tests for lack of fit. This can be done, for example, by the /LACKFIT option in PROC LOGIST, which forms deciles of predicted risk groups. The LACKFIT χ^2 is similar to the Pearson lack-of-fit test, and it pertains to a situation where the data have been grouped into an arbitrary number of risk groups. Hosmer and Lemeshow [68] showed that assuming the test has degrees of freedom two less than the number of groups (i.e., usually 8) works well. All goodness-of-fit tests discussed are sensitive to (a) misspecification of the relationship of covariates to the mean [including linearity (etc.) assumptions and choice of link function] and (b) lack of independence between observations.

From the generalized linear model framework, the transformation $\log(\frac{\pi}{1-\pi})$ of π was the most natural choice of link function h. It is a link function, because π is the mean of the distribution of the binary outcome y or of the proportion of "successes" in the binomial case. The logistic link is the canonical link b'^{-1}, resulting in the simplified score or "estimating" equations (12.4)

$$X'(Y - E(Y|X)) = 0$$

which in this case translate into

$$
\begin{pmatrix} 1 & 1 & \cdots & 1 \\ x_{11} & x_{12} & \cdots & x_{1n} \\ \cdots & \cdots & \cdots & \cdots \end{pmatrix}
\left(\begin{pmatrix} y_1 \\ \vdots \\ y_n \end{pmatrix} - \begin{pmatrix} \dfrac{\exp(\beta_0 + \beta_1 x_{11} \cdots)}{1 + \exp(\beta_0 + \beta_1 x_{11} \cdots)} \\ \vdots \\ \dfrac{\exp(\beta_0 + \beta_1 x_{1n} \cdots)}{1 + \exp(\beta_0 + \beta_1 x_{1n} \cdots)} \end{pmatrix} \right) = 0
$$

These cannot be solved directly. However, the technique used to obtain an iterative solution (known as Fisher scoring) is beyond the scope here. It is described in the book by McCullagh and Nelder [64]. PROC GENMOD, of course, does this for us (as does PROC LOGIST). We will first discuss our example as analyzed with the logit link, but will introduce some alternative link functions in Section 13.3.

13.2.1 Example of Logistic Regression with Binary Outcome

OUTPUT PACKET XI contains the analysis of the neonatal mortality data with PROC GENMOD. GENMOD was applied in several ways to illustrate different aspects of how it works. We first consider the result of the following basic statements.

PROC GENMOD DESCENDING;
MODEL DEATH=INDYR SURFYR/DIST=BINOMIAL;

We did not need to specify the link, because GENMOD automatically chooses the canonical link, which is logit for the binomial. Comparison of the first output from GENMOD with that of LOGIST confirms that coefficients and standard errors are the same. The scale parameter is given as 1, as expected. We also see that the deviance from PROC GENMOD is indeed identical to the $-2\log(L) = 983.735$ provided by LOGIST.

Without additional options and special statements, PROC GENMOD output is a bit thin as compared to that of PROC LOGIST. We added odds ratios and their confidence intervals by the statements below. The output is on the next page of OUTPUT PACKET XI. We also added a TYPE1 option to the model statement.

PROC GENMOD DESCENDING;
MODEL DEATH=INDYR SURFYR/DIST=BINOMIAL TYPE1;
ESTIMATE 'OR INDYR' INDYR 1/EXP;
ESTIMATE 'OR SURFYR' SURFYR 1/EXP;
ESTIMATE 'OR SURF VS IND' INDYR -1 SURFYR 1/EXP;

The ESTIMATE commands tell GENMOD to exponentiate the coefficients of INDYR and SURFYR and give the resulting odds ratios the names in quotes. The quantity "1" indicates that the odds ratio will be for one unit change. Other constants could have been chosen. The last statement leads to an estimate of the odds ratio between the last two time periods, as the coefficient of INDYR is multiplied by -1 and added to the coefficient of SURFYR. We see that the resulting odds ratios and 95% confidence intervals are 0.565 [0.380, 0.930], 0.782 [0.540, 1.13] and 1.38 [0.925, 2.07], respectively. In addition, we created a sequential (Type 1) likelihood ratio analysis, which shows that INDYR added to the model by itself had $\chi^2(1) = 6.48$ ($p = 0.011$) and that adding SURFYR to the model with intercept and INDYR led to likelihood ratio $\chi^2(1) = 1.71$ ($p = 0.190$). Part of the upturn in neonatal mortality after the IND period and lack of significance of the coefficient of SURFYR is explained by admission of ever smaller neonates to the NICU's. We show some birth weight adjusted analyses in Section 13.2.3 below.

To have GENMOD create the indicator variables, we can use the original 0, 1, 2 birth year variable BIRTHYR in a CLASS statement. This statement will, as a default, choose the last category as the comparison group. However, we can craft the ESTIMATE statements to compute odds ratios to reflect any comparisons we want. Below, we see that this involves setting up a so-called "contrast" [69] that tells the procedure how the comparison between the three years is to be made.

```
PROC GENMOD DESCENDING; CLASS BIRTHYR;
MODEL DEATH=BIRTHYR/DIST=BINOMIAL;
ESTIMATE 'OR INDYR' BIRTHYR -1 1 0/EXP;
ESTIMATE 'OR SURFYR' BIRTHYR -1 0 1/EXP;
ESTIMATE 'SURF VS IND' BIRTHYR 0 -1 1/EXP;
```

We see that the ESTIMATE statements result in the same odds ratios as above. It is also important to know that the specific way indicator variables are created does not affect overall tests for the model, nor does it affect goodness-of-fit statistics.

Finally, we run an analysis without the CLASS statement. The commands used were

```
PROC GENMOD DESCENDING;
MODEL DEATH=BIRTHYR/DIST=BINOMIAL;
ESTIMATE 'OR INDYR' BIRTHYR 1/EXP;
ESTIMATE 'OR SURFYR' BIRTHYR 2/EXP;
ESTIMATE 'SURF VS IND' BIRTHYR 1/EXP;
```

The important difference between this analysis and the previous one is the assumption here that the odds ratio is constant between subsequent years. When we duplicate the comparisons we made above in the ESTIMATE commands, the assumption is reflected in the 'OR INDYR' and 'SURF VS IND' odds ratios being estimated the same way—that is, as the exponential of a one-unit change in year 0.878 [0.724, 1.06]. The odds ratio between the surfactant year and baseline is estimated as the exponential of a two-year change 0.771 [0.525, 1.13]. Because all three odds ratios are based on the same regression coefficient, they all have the same $\chi^2(1)$ statistic.

We have touched upon the fact that different ways of choosing indicator variables do not affect the overall $-2\log(L)$. The linear trend in the latest model can actually be framed as another choice of one indicator variable (with the other indicator to completely capture all differences between years being a quadratic trend), so the linear trend model is nested in all two indicator models. This means that we can compare the deviance 990.1765 for the latest model with that for the indicator variable model of 983.735. The deviance difference (which is the same as the difference in $-2\log(L)$) is quite significant ($\chi^2_{0.95}(1) = 3.84$), indicating that the differences between years cannot be well captured by a linear trend.

13.2.2 Example with Binomial Outcome

Sometimes data on binary outcomes are more conveniently obtainable as counts y of the number of deaths (say) and population sizes, rather than as individual binary outcomes. This can happen when data are not specifically collected for research, but are acquired from official or government sources, say, or when individual level data cannot be obtained due to human subject confidentiality considerations. Of course, a major disadvantage in modeling such a data set is the lack of individual level information.

To illustrate the analysis of grouped data, the mortality data from the NICU's were collapsed into numbers of admissions and numbers of deaths each year. (This was done only to show how GENMOD works in this situation, as the natural choice for our data was the analysis given above.) The collapsing was performed by the statements

PROC SORT; BY BIRTHYR;
PROC MEANS N MEAN SUM; BY BIRTHYR; VAR DEATH;
OUTPUT OUT=COLL SUM=NDTHS N=NUMB;

OUTPUT PACKET XII contains some output from these statements. The tabulation includes the number of births (the risk denominator, obtained through the N option), the proportion of deaths in each deaths in each time period (i.e., risks, obtained by the MEAN option), and the number of deaths in each time period (obtained by the SUM option). The new SAS data set is named COLL and contains the number of deaths NDTHS for each BIRTHYR, along with the number of births NUMB in the same time period. The data set COLL has only three observations—one for each time period (and three variables BIRTHYR NDTHS NUMB).

Now, to obtain the logistic regression on these data, we run

DATA NEW; SET COLL;
PROC GENMOD;
CLASS BIRTHYR;
MODEL NDTHS/NUMB= BIRTHYR/DIST=BINOMIAL;

Here, we have told GENMOD that the binomial numbers of outcomes arose from the number NUMB of "trials." Note that the DESCENDING option is not used in this case. The output is in OUTPUT PACKET XII.

Looking at the output, we see that the regression coefficients and their standard errors are identical to those obtained by the binary outcome analysis. The $\log(L)$ is also identical. However, the deviance has turned out to be 0 in this case. This is because, for the grouped data, the model fits perfectly. It is a so-called "saturated model." (Chapter 7 in Selvin [70] has further discussion of saturated models.) There are three "means" to be fitted (the three probabilities of death); there are also three parameters, one for each mean. A saturated model just reproduces the observed probabilities. The deviance was not 0 when the data were left as binary, because the death or survival of each single baby was not exactly predicted.

To illustrate further how the deviance works, we run the logistic analysis.

PROC GENMOD; MODEL NDTHS/NUMB=BIRTHYR/DIST=BINOMIAL;

The output is in OUTPUT PACKET XII. Here, we are forcing a linear trend across risks of death in the three time periods. Hence the model is no longer saturated. We see that the deviance is now 6.44, the difference in $-2\log(L)$ between this model and the previous model. It is identical to the likelihood ratio test result we obtained when comparing the saturated and trend models with binary outcome in the previous section. The models with binary and binomial data are the same; only the deviances are computed differently.

13.2.3   Some More Examples of Goodness-of-Fit Tests

In the above example it is not necessary to group the entire data set to compute the grouped deviance. The deviance and Pearson χ^2-tests for the model with trend can be obtained by

PROC GENMOD DESCENDING;
MODEL DEATH=BIRTHYR/DIST=BINOMIAL AGGREGATE=BIRTHYR;

The output from this statement is in OUTPUT PACKET XIII. We see that the deviance $\chi^2(1)$ is 6.44 and that the Pearson $\chi^2(1)$ is similar at 6.22, as before. It is a limitation that the AGGREGATE option can be used only with categorical variables that are in the model. Hence it is most useful to test for trends across levels of ordinal variables (as we did here), or for more complex models with interactions between categorical variables.

For testing the fit of models with continuous predictors, we revert to PROC LOGIST. As indicated above, birth weight of those admitted to the NICU's changed across the study period. We therefore include birth weight as a continuous variable, and we assess the fit of the model by statements

PROC LOGIST DESCENDING;
MODEL DEATH=BW INDYR SURFYR/LACKFIT;

Outputs are in OUTPUT PACKET XIII. We see that the model does not appear to fit very well as the Hosmer and Lemeshow test yields $p = 0.0155$ for goodness of fit. We also notice that there tend to be too few deaths expected in the low-risk deciles, whereas there tend to be too many in the high-risk deciles. We add (BW-1000)**2 to the model and find the fit to be very good with $p = 0.89$ and good agreement between observed and expected values. The odds ratios are now more similar for the IND year versus baseline of 0.507 [0.326, 0.789] and for the surfactant year versus baseline of 0.645 [0.423, 0.983], respectively. After adjustment for birth weight, the neonatal mortality after surfactant became generally available is significantly lower than presurfactant.

13.3   OTHER LINKS FOR BINARY AND BINOMIAL DATA

Although the logit link is the canonical link and, for good reasons, most favored by epidemiologist, there are at least three other traditional links (or transformations) of $\pi = \mu$ or of the observed proportion y (with grouped data) used in various fields of application. The first, and currently perhaps least important, one stems from randomized experiments and the tradition of analysis of variance. In the days when software was nonexistent, people were eager to transform proportions into quantities that had equal variance, so that they could perform the usual ANOVA and regression tests. They found that, as long as the sample size m is the same in each group, the transformation $\sin^{-1}\sqrt{y}$, achieves this [71]. The transformation, of course, was applied to the observed proportions, as the whole point was to affect the variance of the error term. In contrast, a link function is applied to the true underlying mean, leaving the error term to follow the binomial distribution.

From the fields of pharmacology [72] and psychometrics [73] comes the probit (sometimes also called the normit) link. The origin of the probit link is in so-called latent variable analysis. One imagines (or—in some cases—knows) that there is a normally distributed variable underlying the response. There may be a continuous variable Y that represents "true health" of individuals in the population. When asked, people may say they are in "good health" if their health level is above a threshold D. Then, the probability of a positive response $y_i = 1$ for a person is given by

$$\text{Prob}(y_i = 1) = \text{Prob}(D < Y_i)$$

If Y is normally distributed with mean μ_Y and variance σ_Y^2 in the population, we have that

$$\text{Prob}\left(\frac{D - \mu_Y}{\sigma_Y} < \frac{Y_i - \mu_Y}{\sigma_Y}\right) = \text{Prob}\left(Z_i < -\frac{D - \mu_Y}{\sigma_Y}\right) = \Phi\left(-\frac{D - \mu_Y}{\sigma_Y}\right)$$

where Φ denotes the standard normal cumulative probability distribution (e.g., $\Phi(-1.96) = 0.025$). If, in addition, the true health of a person depends on characteristics x, we may have a linear regression equation

$$\mu_{Y|x} = \beta_0 + \beta_1 x_1 + \cdots$$

where Y has variability $\sigma_{Y|x}^2$ around the regression line. The probability a person will say they are in good health is then

$$\text{Prob}(y_i = 1|D, x_1 \cdots) = \mu_y = \pi_y$$
$$= \Phi\left(-\frac{D - \beta_0 + \beta_1 x_{1i} + \cdots}{\sigma_{Y|x}}\right)$$
$$= \Phi\left(\frac{\beta_0}{\sigma_{Y|x}} - \frac{D}{\sigma_{Y|x}} + \frac{\beta_1}{\sigma_{Y|x}} x_{ii} + \cdots\right)$$

We see that the cumulative normal probability serves as link function to model the probability of response linearly on covariates. This is the probit link and can be specified in GENMOD as such (LINK=PROBIT). Standardization of the coefficients must occur, because we would not know what standard deviation to use just from the binary outcome. Hence, the coefficients estimated are $\beta_1/\sigma_{Y|x}$, and so on.

A final link that is somewhat popular with binary or binomial outcomes is the complementary log($-$log) defined as $h(\pi) = \log[-\log(1-\pi)]$. A less well known feature of this link is the fact that if events are imagined as arising from underlying rates λ_i where $\log(\lambda_i)$ depends linearly on the risk factors, the complementary log($-$log) will produce the coefficients of that regression. In other words, the coefficients from this link can be interpreted as logarithms of *rate ratios* (or hazard ratios). In this sense, it is the $\log(-\log)$ link that generalizes into Poisson regression and into models for censored data such as the proportional hazards model (not covered in this text). For more information on survival analysis, the reader is referred to the book by Klein and Moeschberger [74].

Of course, linearity with the logit link does not imply linearity with either of the other two links—quite the opposite. In the strict sense, at most one of these links can produce a truly linear relationship between $h(\pi)$ and the risk factors. However, in practice they are usually so close that the difference can be ignored. When the response probability is low, the logit and complementary $\log(-\log)$ are almost indistinguishable, which is a result of rates, risks, and odds being similar in that situation. The probit and logit are close in their predictions and in significance of the coefficients, except for very high or very low outcome probabilities.

Due to the latent variable framework described above under the probit link, it can be shown that: (a) If there is indeed a continuous normally distributed underlying variable, the coefficients from the probit will be the same as coefficients from ordinary regression of that variable- standardized to $\sigma_{Y|x}$ units. (b) The coefficients from the logit link will be approximately 1.8 times as large as those from the probit link. This is because 1/1.8 represents the standard deviation of the logistic distribution that may be imagined to hold for the continuous latent scale. (The logistic distribution has shape very similar to the normal.) It is reassuring to know that when a normally distributed variable is dichotomized, the results of regression analyses using the probit or logit link will yield parallel or almost parallel results to those that could have been obtained from the original continuous scale. Of course, statistical efficiency will be lost by the dichotomization. The advantage of dichotomizing is that if the continuous variable is not normally distributed, the dichotomized results are still valid as referring to the probability of response. In that case, the coefficients of the probit and logit regressions can be seen as related to those of an underlying variable that is a transformation of the original scale to make it normally distributed. The transformation, however, is not explicitly specified.

13.3.1 Example

OUTPUT PACKET XIV contains outputs from the logit, probit, and complementary $\log(-\log)$ links from the neonatal death data. The commands used were

PROC GENMOD DESCENDING;
MODEL DEATH=INDYR SURFYR/DIST=BINOMIAL TYPE3;
PROC GENMOD DESCENDING;
MODEL DEATH=INDYR SURFYR/DIST=BINOMIAL LINK=PROBIT TYPE3;
PROC GENMOD DESCENDING;
MODEL DEATH=INDYR SURFYR/DIST=BINOMIAL LINK=CLL TYPE3;

Because no linearity assumptions have been made in these saturated models, the likelihoods and deviances are identical. All three models produce the same $\hat{\mu}_i$ but differ in, for example, $\hat{\beta}_{\text{INDYR}} = h(\hat{\mu}_{\text{INDYR}}) - h(\hat{\mu}_{\text{BASELINE}})$. The difference in coefficients is to be interpreted simply as different choices of measure of association in this case. The link function, in fact, dictates the measure of association produced. As expected, the ratio between the INDYR coefficient from the logit model (-0.5715) to the coefficient from the probit model (-0.3212) is 1.80. The probit coefficient can be interpreted as a standardized improvement with surfactant in the underlying (latent) continuous illness level of the neonate. It is assumed in this way of thinking that when that illness level crosses a threshold, the neonate dies. The complementary log($-$log) coefficient can be thought of as the log of a ratio of underlying mortality operating on month-old infants, so the ratio between the IND and baseline periods is 0.596, fairly similar to the odds ratio of 0.565.

A somewhat disturbing result is the difference in the Wald χ^2's for the coefficients for the different link function. However, we see that the more reliable likelihood ratio tests produced by the TYPE3 option are the same.

Finally we fit models that include birth weight and birth weight squared. Theoretically, we know that not all three link functions can fit the birth weight relationship correctly. We see that the models are not exactly the same now, but the deviances are quite similar, with the lowest deviance for the logit link. The significance of the birth year comparison is also strongest for the logit link, perhaps indicating that birth weight was the most appropriately adjusted for with this link function.

OUTPUT PACKET XI: LOGISTIC REGRESSION ANALYSIS WITH PROC LOGIST AND PROC GENMOD

XI.1 Basic PROC LOGIST and PROC GENMOD Outputs

Analysis of Binary Infant Death Data by PROC LOGIST and PROC GENMOD
PROC LOGIST with Indicators for Birthyr
   The LOGISTIC Procedure

Model Information	
Data set	WORK.A
Response variable	death
Number of response levels	2
Number of observations	1040
Model	**binary logit**
Optimization technique	Fisher's scoring

Response Profile

Ordered Value	Death	Total Frequency
1	1	191
2	0	849

Probability modeled is death = 1.

Model Convergence Status

Convergence criterion (GCONV=1E-8) is satisfied.

Model Fit Statistics

Criterion	Intercept Only	Intercept and Covariates
AIC	993.929	989.735
SC	998.876	1004.576
$-2 \log L$	991.929	**983.735**

Testing Global Null Hypothesis: BETA = 0

Test	Chi-Square	DF	Pr > ChiSq
Likelihood ratio	8.1937	2	0.0166
Score	8.1163	2	0.0173
Wald	8.0164	2	0.0182

Analysis of Maximum Likelihood Estimates

Parameter	DF	Estimate	Standard Error	Wald Chi-Square	Pr > ChiSq
Intercept	1	−1.2338	0.1303	89.5993	<40.0001
indyr	1	−0.5715	0.2019	8.0140	0.0046
surfyr	1	−0.2464	0.1887	1.7065	0.1914

Odds Ratio Estimates

Effect	Point Estimate	95% Wald Confidence Limits	
indyr	**0.565**	**0.380**	**0.839**
surfyr	**0.782**	**0.540**	**1.131**

Association of Predicted Probabilities and Observed Responses

Percent concordant	39.7	Somers' D	0.124
Percent discordant	27.3	Gamma	0.185
Percent tied	33.0	Tau-a	0.037
Pairs	162159	c	0.562

Default GENMOD Output for Binary Data
  The GENMOD Procedure

Model Information

Data set	WORK.A
Distribution	**Binomial**
Link function	**Logit**
Dependent variable	death
Observations used	1040

Response Profile

Ordered Value	Death	Total Frequency
1	1	191
2	0	849

PROC GENMOD is modeling the probability that death = '1'.

Criteria for Assessing Goodness of Fit[a]

Criterion	DF	Value	Value/DF
Deviance	1037	983.7354	0.9486
Scaled deviance	1037	983.7354	0.9486
Pearson chi-square	1037	1040.0000	1.0029
Scaled Pearson X2	1037	1040.0000	1.0029
Log likelihood		**−491.8677**	

[a] Algorithm converged.

Analysis of Parameter Estimates

Parameter	DF	Estimate	Standard Error	Wald 95% Confidence Limits		Chi-Square
Intercept	1	−1.2338	0.1303	−1.4893	−0.9783	89.60
surfyr	1	−0.2464	0.1887	−0.6162	0.1233	1.71
indyr	1	−0.5715	0.2019	−0.9672	−0.1758	8.01
Scale	0	1.0000	0.0000	1.0000	1.0000	

Analysis of Parameter Estimates

Parameter	Pr > ChiSq
Intercept	<0.0001
surfyr	0.1914
indyr	0.0046
Scale	

XI.2. Adding Information to the PROC GENMOD Output

Analysis of Binary Infant Death Data by PROC LOGIST and PROC GENMOD
PROC GENMOD with Options Giving Odds Ratios and Type 1 LR Tests
  The GENMOD Procedure

Model Information

Data set	WORK.A
Distribution	**Binomial**
Link function	**Logit**
Dependent variable	death
Observations used	1040

Response Profile

Ordered Value	Death	Total Frequency
1	1	191
2	0	849

PROC GENMOD is modeling the probability that death = '1'.

Criteria for Assessing Goodness of Fit[a]

Criterion	DF	Value	Value/DF
Deviance	1037	983.7354	0.9486
Scaled deviance	1037	983.7354	0.9486
Pearson chi-square	1037	1040.0000	1.0029
Scaled Pearson X2	1037	1040.0000	1.0029
Log likelihood		−491.8677	

[a] Algorithm converged.

Analysis of Parameter Estimates

Parameter	DF	Estimate	Standard Error	Wald 95% Confidence Limits		Chi-Square
Intercept	1	−1.2338	0.1303	−1.4893	−0.9783	89.60
indyr	1	−0.5715	0.2019	−0.9672	−0.1758	8.01
surfyr	1	−0.2464	0.1887	−0.6162	0.1233	1.71
Scale	0	1.0000	0.0000	1.0000	1.0000	

Analysis of Parameter Estimates

Parameter	Pr > ChiSq
Intercept	<0.0001
indyr	0.0046
surfyr	0.1914
Scale	

Note: The scale parameter was held fixed.

LR Statistics for Type 1 Analysis

Source	Deviance	DF	Chi-Square	Pr > ChiSq
Intercept	991.9291			
indyr	985.4462	1	6.48	0.0109
surfyr	983.7354	1	1.71	0.1909

Contrast Estimate Results

Label	Estimate	Standard Error	Alpha	Confidence Limits	
OR indyr	−0.5715	0.2019	0.05	−0.9672	−0.1758
Exp (OR indyr)	**0.5647**	0.1140	0.05	**0.3802**	**0.8388**
OR surfyr	−0.2464	0.1887	0.05	−0.6162	0.1233
Exp (OR surfyr)	**0.7816**	0.1474	0.05	**0.5400**	**1.1312**
OR surf vs. ind	0.3250	0.2058	0.05	−0.0784	0.7285
Exp (OR surf vs. ind)	**1.3841**	0.2849	0.05	**0.9246**	**2.0719**

Contrast Estimate Results

Label	Chi-Square	Pr > ChiSq
OR indyr	8.01	0.0046
Exp (OR indyr)		
OR surfyr	1.71	0.1914
Exp (OR surfyr)		
OR surf vs. ind	2.49	0.1143
Exp (OR surf vs. ind)		

XI.3. Other Ways of Coding Birth Year

Analysis of Binary Infant Death Data by PROC LOGIST and PROC GENMOD
Using the Indicator Variables GENMOD Generates
  The GENMOD Procedure

Model Information

Data set	WORK.A
Distribution	Binomial
Link function	Logit
Dependent variable	death
Observations used	1040

Class Level Information

Class	Levels	Values
birthyr	3	0 1 2

Response Profile

Ordered Value	Death	Total Frequency
1	1	191
2	0	849

PROC GENMOD is modeling the probability that death = '1'.

Parameter Information

Parameter	Effect	Birthyr
Prm1	Intercept	
Prm2	birthyr	0
Prm3	birthyr	1
Prm4	birthyr	2

Criteria for Assessing Goodness of Fit[a]

Criterion	DF	Value	Value/DF
Deviance	1037	983.7354	0.9486
Scaled deviance	1037	983.7354	0.9486
Pearson chi-square	1037	1040.0000	1.0029
Scaled Pearson X2	1037	1040.0000	1.0029
Log likelihood		−491.8677	

[a] Algorithm converged.

Analysis of Parameter Estimates

Parameter	DF		Estimate	Standard Error	Wald 95% Confidence Limits		Chi-Square
Intercept		1	−1.4802	0.1364	−1.7475	−1.2129	117.80
birthyr	**0**	1	**0.2464**	0.1887	−0.1233	0.6162	1.71
birthyr	**1**	1	**−0.3250**	0.2058	−0.7285	0.0784	2.49
birthyr	**2**	0	**0.0000**	0.0000	0.0000	0.0000	.
Scale		0	1.0000	0.0000	1.0000	1.0000	

Analysis of Parameter Estimates

Parameter		Pr > ChiSq
Intercept		<0.0001
birthyr	0	0.1914
birthyr	1	0.1143
birthyr	2	.
Scale		

Note: The scale parameter was held fixed.

Contrast Estimate Results

Label	Estimate	Standard Error	Alpha	Confidence Limits	
OR indyr	−0.5715	0.2019	0.05	−0.9672	−0.1758
Exp (OR indyr)	**0.5647**	0.1140	0.05	0.3802	0.8388
OR surfyr	−0.2464	0.1887	0.05	−0.6162	0.1233
Exp (OR surfyr)	**0.7816**	0.1474	0.05	0.5400	1.1312
OR surf vs. ind	0.3250	0.2058	0.05	−0.0784	0.7285
Exp (OR surf vs. ind)	**1.3841**	0.2849	0.05	0.9246	2.0719

Contrast Estimate Results

Label	Chi-Square	Pr > ChiSq
OR indyr	8.01	0.0046
Exp (OR indyr)		
OR surfyr	1.71	0.1914
Exp (OR surfyr)		
OR surf vs. ind	2.49	0.1143
Exp (OR surf vs. ind)		

Fitting Birth Year as Trend
   The GENMOD Procedure

Model Information

Data set	WORK.A
Distribution	Binomial
Link function	Logit
Dependent variable	death
Observations used	1040

Response Profile

Ordered Value	Death	Total Frequency
1	1	191
2	0	849

PROC GENMOD is modeling the probability that death = '1'.

Parameter Information

Parameter	Effect
Prm1	Intercept
Prm2	birthyr

Criteria for Assessing Goodness of Fit[a]

Criterion	DF	Value	Value/DF
Deviance	1038	990.1765	0.9539
Scaled deviance	1038	990.1765	0.9539
Pearson chi-square	1038	1040.5245	1.0024
Scaled Pearson X2	1038	1040.5245	1.0024
Log likelihood		−495.0882	

[a] Algorithm converged.

Analysis of Parameter Estimates

Parameter	DF	Estimate	Standard Error	Wald 95% Confidence Limits		Chi-Square
Intercept	1	−1.3630	0.1241	−1.6062	−1.1198	120.65
birthyr	**1**	**−0.1300**	0.0983	−0.3227	0.0627	1.75
Scale	0	1.0000	0.0000	1.0000	1.0000	

Analysis of Parameter Estimates

Parameter	Pr > ChiSq
Intercept	<0.0001
birthyr	0.1860
Scale	

Note: The scale parameter was held fixed.

Contrast Estimate Results

Label	Estimate	Standard Error	Alpha	Confidence Limits	
OR indyr	−0.1300	0.0983	0.05	−0.3227	0.0627
Exp (OR indyr)	**0.8781**	0.0863	0.05	0.7242	1.0647
OR surfyr	−0.2600	0.1966	0.05	−0.6454	0.1254
Exp (OR surfyr)	**0.7710**	0.1516	0.05	0.5245	1.1335
OR surf vs. ind	−0.1300	0.0983	0.05	−0.3227	0.0627
Exp (OR surf vs. ind)	**0.8781**	0.0863	0.05	0.7242	1.0647

Contrast Estimate Results

Label	Chi-Square	Pr > ChiSq
OR indyr	1.75	0.1860
Exp (OR indyr)		
OR surfyr	1.75	0.1860
Exp (OR surfyr)		
OR surf vs. ind	1.75	0.1860
Exp (OR surf vs. ind)		

OUTPUT PACKET XII: ANALYSIS OF GROUPED BINOMIAL DATA

Analysis of Grouped Binomial Data by GENMOD
Number at Risk, Risk, and Number of Deaths Each Year
   The MEANS Procedure

Analysis Variable: death

N	Mean	Sum
birthyr = 0		
337	0.2255193	76.0000000
birthyr = 1		
347	0.1412104	49.0000000
birthyr = 2		
356	0.1853933	66.0000000

Saturated Model
   The GENMOD Procedure

Model Information

Data set	WORK.COLL
Distribution	Binomial
Link function	Logit
Response variable (events)	**ndths**
Response variable (trials)	**numb**
Observations used	3
Number of events	191
Number of trials	1040

Class Level Information

Class	Levels	Values
birthyr	3	0 1 2

Criteria for Assessing Goodness of Fit[a]

Criterion	DF	Value	Value/DF
Deviance	0	0.0000	.
Scaled deviance	0	0.0000	.
Pearson chi-square	0	0.0000	.
Scaled Pearson X2	0	0.0000	.
Log likelihood		−491.8677	

[a] Algorithm converged.

Analysis of Parameter Estimates

Parameter	DF		Estimate	Standard Error	Wald 95% Confidence Limits		Chi-Square
Intercept		1	−1.4802	0.1364	−1.7475	−1.2129	117.80
birthyr	0	1	0.2464	0.1887	−0.1233	0.6162	1.71
birthyr	1	1	−0.3250	0.2058	−0.7285	0.0784	2.49
birthyr	2	0	0.0000	0.0000	0.0000	0.0000	.
Scale		0	1.0000	0.0000	1.0000	1.0000	

Analysis of Parameter Estimates

Parameter		Pr > ChiSq
Intercept		<0.0001
birthyr	0	0.1914
birthyr	1	0.1143
birthyr	2	.

Note: The scale parameter was held fixed.

Trend Across Birth Years
  The GENMOD Procedure

Model Information

Data set	WORK.COLL
Distribution	Binomial
Link function	Logit
Response variable (events)	**ndths**
Response variable (trials)	**numb**
Observations used	3
Number of events	191
Number of trials	1040

Criteria for Assessing Goodness of Fit[a]

Criterion	DF	Value	Value/DF
Deviance	1	6.4411	6.4411
Scaled deviance	1	6.4411	6.4411
Pearson chi-square	1	6.2187	6.2187
Scaled Pearson X2	1	6.2187	6.2187
Log likelihood		−495.0882	

[a] Algorithm converged.

Analysis of Parameter Estimates

Parameter	DF	Estimate	Standard Error	Wald 95% Confidence Limits		Chi-Square
Intercept	1	−1.3630	0.1241	−1.6062	−1.1198	120.65
birthyr	1	−0.1300	0.0983	−0.3227	0.0627	1.75
Scale	0	1.0000	0.0000	1.0000	1.0000	

Analysis of Parameter Estimates

Parameter	Pr > ChiSq
Intercept	<0.0001
birthyr	0.1860
Scale	

Note: The scale parameter was held fixed.

OUTPUT PACKET XIII: SOME GOODNESS-OF-FIT TESTS FOR BINOMIAL OUTCOME

XIII.1. Grouped Data

Some Goodness-of-Fit Tests for Infant Death Data
PROC GENMOD Testing with the Aggregate Option
  The GENMOD Procedure

Model Information

Data set	WORK.A
Distribution	Binomial
Link function	Logit
Dependent variable	death
Observations used	1040

Response Profile

Ordered Value	Death	Total Frequency
1	1	191
2	0	849

PROC GENMOD is modeling the probability that death = '1'.

Criteria for Assessing Goodness of Fit[a]

Criterion	DF	Value	Value/DF
Deviance	**1**	**6.4411**	6.4411
Scaled deviance	1	6.4411	6.4411
Pearson chi-square	**1**	**6.2187**	6.2187
Scaled Pearson X2	1	6.2187	6.2187
Log likelihood		**−495.0882**	

[a] Algorithm converged.

Analysis of Parameter Estimates

Parameter	DF	Estimate	Standard Error	Wald 95% Confidence Limits		Chi-Square
Intercept	1	−1.3630	0.1241	−1.6062	−1.1198	120.65
birthyr	1	−0.1300	0.0983	−0.3227	0.0627	1.75
Scale	0	1.0000	0.0000	1.0000	1.0000	

Analysis of Parameter Estimates

Parameter	Pr > ChiSq
Intercept	<0.0001
birthyr	0.1860
Scale	

XIII.2. The Hosmer and Lemeshow Test with Continuous Covariates

Some Goodness-of-Fit Tests for Infant Death Data
PROC LOGIST with the Lackfit Option
  The LOGISTIC Procedure

Model Information

Data set	WORK.A
Response variable	death
Number of response levels	2
Number of observations	1040
Model	binary logit
Optimization technique	Fisher's scoring

Response Profile[a]

Ordered Value	Death	Total Frequency
1	1	191
2	0	849

Probability modeled is death = 1.

Model Convergence Status

Convergence criterion (GCONV=1E-8) is satisfied.

Model Fit Statistics

Criterion	Intercept Only	Intercept and Covariates
AIC	993.929	824.187
SC	998.876	843.975
$-2 \log L$	991.929	816.187

Testing Global Null Hypothesis: BETA = 0

Test	Chi-Square	DF	Pr > ChiSq
Likelihood ratio	175.7425	3	<0.0001
Score	167.4647	3	<0.0001
Wald	133.4080	3	<0.0001

Analysis of Maximum Likelihood Estimates

Parameter	DF	Estimate	Standard Error	Wald Chi-Square	Pr > ChiSq
Intercept	1	2.8372	0.3660	60.0796	<0.0001
bw	1	−0.00407	0.000359	128.3807	<0.0001
indyr	1	−0.7221	0.2220	10.5757	0.0011
surfyr	1	−0.4645	0.2106	4.8656	0.0274

Odds Ratio Estimates

Effect	Point Estimate	95% Wald Confidence Limits	
bw	0.996	0.995	0.997
indyr	0.486	0.314	0.751
surfyr	0.628	0.416	0.950

Association of Predicted Probabilities and Observed Responses

Percent concordant	77.9	Somers' D	0.562
Percent discordant	21.7	Gamma	0.565
Percent tied	0.4	Tau-a	0.169
Pairs	162159	c	0.781

Partition for the Hosmer and Lemeshow Test

Group	Total	death = 1 Observed	death = 1 Expected	death = 0 Observed	death = 0 Expected
1	104	3	2.60	101	101.40
2	105	10	3.99	95	101.01
3	104	6	5.50	98	98.50
4	105	10	7.92	95	97.08
5	104	5	11.09	99	92.91
6	104	16	15.86	88	88.14
7	105	17	21.60	88	83.40
8	106	25	28.95	81	77.05
9	104	36	38.70	68	65.30
10	99	63	54.78	36	44.22

Hosmer and Lemeshow Goodness-of-Fit Test

Chi-Square	DF	Pr > ChiSq
18.8901	8	0.0155

Adding a Squared Term of Birth Weight
  The LOGISTIC Procedure

Model Information

Data set	WORK.A
Response variable	death
Number of response levels	2
Number of observations	1040
Model	binary logit
Optimization technique	Fisher's scoring

Response Profile[a]

Ordered Value	Death	Total Frequency
1	1	191
2	0	849

[a] Probability modeled is death = 1.

Model Convergence Status

Convergence criterion (GCONV=1E-8) is satisfied.

Model Fit Statistics

Criterion	Intercept Only	Intercept and Covariates
AIC	993.929	816.664
SC	998.876	841.399
$-2 \log L$	991.929	806.664

Testing Global Null Hypothesis: BETA = 0

Test	Chi-Square	DF	Pr > ChiSq
Likelihood ratio	185.2651	4	<0.0001
Score	208.4817	4	<0.0001
Wald	148.3246	4	<0.0001

Analysis of Maximum Likelihood Estimates

Parameter	DF	Estimate	Standard Error	Wald Chi-Square	Pr > ChiSq
Intercept	1	2.3158	0.3847	36.2421	<0.0001
bw	1	−0.00382	0.000340	126.1807	<0.0001
bwsq	1	3.728E-6	1.208E-6	9.5161	0.0020
indyr	1	−0.6796	0.2258	9.0545	0.0026
surfyr	1	−0.4381	0.2150	4.1532	0.0416

Odds Ratio Estimates

Effect	Point Estimate	95% Wald Confidence Limits	
bw	0.996	0.996	0.997
bwsq	1.000	1.000	1.000
indyr	0.507	0.326	0.789
surfyr	0.645	0.423	0.983

Association of Predicted Probabilities and Observed Responses

Percent concordant	78.0	Somers' D	0.566
Percent discordant	21.4	Gamma	0.569
Percent tied	0.6	Tau-a	0.170
Pairs	162159	c	0.783

Partition for the Hosmer and Lemeshow Test

Group	Total	death = 1 Observed	Expected	death = 0 Observed	Expected
1	105	4	4.50	101	100.50
2	104	6	5.59	98	98.41
3	107	9	7.34	98	99.66
4	103	8	8.27	95	94.73
5	104	7	9.90	97	94.10
6	104	17	13.10	87	90.90
7	104	15	17.66	89	86.34
8	104	24	24.74	80	79.26
9	104	40	37.60	64	66.40
10	101	61	62.29	40	38.71

Hosmer and Lemeshow Goodness-of-Fit Test

Chi-Square	DF	Pr > ChiSq
3.5940	**8**	**0.8918**

OUTPUT PACKET XIV: THREE LINK FUNCTIONS FOR BINARY OUTCOME

XIV.1. Saturated Models

Fitting Different Link Functions to Binary Outcome
Logit Link
  The GENMOD Procedure

Model Information

Data set	WORK.A
Distribution	Binomial
Link function	**Logit**
Dependent variable	death
Observations used	1040

PROC GENMOD is modeling the probability that death = '1'.

Criteria for Assessing Goodness of Fit

Criterion	DF	Value	Value/DF
Deviance	1037	**983.7354**	0.9486
Scaled deviance	1037	983.7354	0.9486
Pearson chi-square	1037	1040.0000	1.0029
Scaled Pearson X2	1037	1040.0000	1.0029
Log likelihood		−491.8677	

Analysis of Parameter Estimates

Parameter	DF	Estimate	Standard Error	Wald 95% Confidence Limits		Chi-Square
Intercept	1	−1.2338	0.1303	−1.4893	−0.9783	89.60
indyr	1	−0.5715	0.2019	−0.9672	−0.1758	**8.01**
surfyr	1	−0.2464	0.1887	−0.6162	0.1233	**1.71**
Scale	0	1.0000	0.0000	1.0000	1.0000	

Analysis of Parameter Estimates

Parameter	Pr > ChiSq
Intercept	<0.0001
indyr	0.0046
surfyr	0.1914
Scale	

LR Statistics for Type 3 Analysis

Source	DF	Chi-Square	Pr > ChiSq
indyr	1	**8.18**	0.0042
surfyr	1	**1.71**	0.1909

Probit Link
  The GENMOD Procedure

Model Information

Data set	WORK.A
Distribution	Binomial
Link function	**Probit**
Dependent variable	death
Observations used	1040

PROC GENMOD is modeling the probability that death = '1'.

Criteria for Assessing Goodness of Fit

Criterion	DF	Value	Value/DF
Deviance	1037	**983.7354**	0.9486
Scaled deviance	1037	983.7354	0.9486
Pearson chi-square	1037	1040.0000	1.0029
Scaled Pearson X2	1037	1040.0000	1.0029
Log likelihood		**−491.8677**	

Analysis of Parameter Estimates

Parameter	DF	Estimate	Standard Error	Wald 95% Confidence Limits		Chi-Square
Intercept	1	−0.7537	0.0758	−0.9023	−0.6051	98.84
indyr	1	−0.3212	0.1128	−0.5423	−0.1002	**8.11**
surfyr	1	−0.1413	0.1081	−0.3532	0.0706	**1.71**
Scale	0	1.0000	0.0000	1.0000	1.0000	

Analysis of Parameter Estimates

Parameter	Pr > ChiSq
Intercept	<0.0001
indyr	0.0044
surfyr	0.1911
Scale	

LR Statistics for Type 3 Analysis

Source	DF	Chi-Square	Pr > ChiSq
indyr	1	**8.18**	0.0042
surfyr	1	**1.71**	0.1909

Complementary Log–Log Link
The GENMOD Procedure

Model Information

Data set	WORK.A
Distribution	Binomial
Link function	**CLL**
Dependent variable	death
Observations used	1040

PROC GENMOD is modeling the probability that death = '1'.

Criteria for Assessing Goodness of Fit[a]

Criterion	DF	Value	Value/DF
Deviance	1037	**983.7354**	0.9486
Scaled deviance	1037	983.7354	0.9486
Pearson chi-square	1037	1039.9999	1.0029
Scaled Pearson X2	1037	1039.9999	1.0029
Log likelihood		**−491.8677**	

[a] Algorithm converged.

Analysis of Parameter Estimates

Parameter	DF	Estimate	Standard Error	Wald 95% Confidence Limits		Chi-Square
Intercept	1	−1.3643	0.1150	−1.5897	−1.1389	140.69
indyr	1	−0.5181	0.1835	−0.8777	−0.1584	**7.97**
surfyr	1	−0.2202	0.1686	−0.5507	0.1103	**1.71**
Scale	0	1.0000	0.0000	1.0000	1.0000	

Analysis of Parameter Estimates

Parameter	Pr > ChiSq
Intercept	<0.0001
indyr	0.0048
surfyr	0.1916
Scale	

LR Statistics for Type 3 Analysis

Source	DF	Chi-Square	Pr > ChiSq
indyr	1	**8.18**	0.0042
surfyr	1	**1.71**	0.1909

XIV.2. Models That Make Assumptions on Mean–Covariate Relationship

Fitting Different Link Functions to Binary Outcome
Logit Link with Birth Weight
  The GENMOD Procedure

Model Information

Data set	WORK.A
Distribution	Binomial
Link function	**Logit**
Dependent variable	death
Observations used	1040

Criteria for Assessing Goodness of Fit

Criterion	DF	Value	Value/DF
Deviance	1035	**806.6641**	0.7794
Scaled deviance	1035	806.6641	0.7794
Pearson chi-square	1035	1040.2302	1.0051
Scaled Pearson X2	1035	1040.2302	1.0051
Log likelihood		**−403.3320**	

Analysis of Parameter Estimates

Parameter	DF	Estimate	Standard Error	Wald 95% Confidence Limits		Chi-Square
Intercept	1	2.3158	0.3847	1.5618	3.0697	36.24
bw	1	−0.0038	0.0003	−0.0045	−0.0032	126.18
bwsq	1	0.0000	0.0000	0.0000	0.0000	9.52
indyr	1	**−0.6796**	0.2258	−1.1222	−0.2369	9.05
surfyr	1	**−0.4381**	0.2150	−0.8594	−0.0168	4.15
Scale	0	1.0000	0.0000	1.0000	1.0000	

Analysis of Parameter Estimates

Parameter	Pr > ChiSq
Intercept	<0.0001
bw	<0.0001
bwsq	0.0020
indyr	0.0026
surfyr	0.0416

LR Statistics for Type 3 Analysis

Source	DF	Chi-Square	Pr > ChiSq
bw	1	166.68	<0.0001
bwsq	1	9.52	0.0020
indyr	1	**9.23**	0.0024
surfyr	1	**4.18**	0.0409

Probit Link with Birth Weight
The GENMOD Procedure

Model Information

Data set	WORK.A
Distribution	Binomial
Link function	**Probit**
Dependent variable	death
Observations used	1040

Criteria for Assessing Goodness of Fit

Criterion	DF	Value	Value/DF
Deviance	1035	**806.9772**	0.7797
Scaled deviance	1035	806.9772	0.7797
Pearson chi-square	1035	1045.6487	1.0103
Scaled Pearson X2	1035	1045.6487	1.0103
Log likelihood		**−403.4886**	

Analysis of Parameter Estimates

Parameter	DF	Estimate	Standard Error	Wald 95% Confidence Limits		Chi-Square
Intercept	1	1.2518	0.2074	0.8453	1.6583	36.42
bw	1	−0.0022	0.0002	−0.0025	−0.0018	145.12
bwsq	1	0.0000	0.0000	0.0000	0.0000	13.77
indyr	1	**−0.3697**	0.1240	−0.6128	−0.1266	8.88
surfyr	1	**−0.2417**	0.1200	−0.4769	−0.0066	4.06
Scale	0	1.0000	0.0000	1.0000	1.0000	

Analysis of Parameter Estimates

Parameter	Pr > ChiSq
Intercept	<0.0001
bw	<0.0001
bwsq	0.0002
indyr	0.0029
surfyr	0.0439
Scale	

LR Statistics for Type 3 Analysis

Source	DF	Chi-Square	Pr > ChiSq
bw	1	166.83	<0.0001
bwsq	1	13.80	0.0002
indyr	1	**8.99**	0.0027
surfyr	1	4.08	0.0435

Complementary Log–Log Link with Birth Weight
   The GENMOD Procedure

Model Information

Data set	WORK.A
Distribution	Binomial
Link function	**CLL**
Dependent variable	death
Observations used	1040

Criteria for Assessing Goodness of Fit

Criterion	DF	Value	Value/DF
Deviance	1035	**808.4619**	0.7811
Scaled deviance	1035	808.4619	0.7811
Pearson chi-square	1035	1053.6994	1.0181
Scaled Pearson X2	1035	1053.6994	1.0181
Log likelihood		**−404.2310**	

Analysis of Parameter Estimates

Parameter	DF	Estimate	Standard Error	Wald 95% Confidence Limits		Chi-Square
Intercept	1	1.6788	0.3388	1.0148	2.3428	24.55
bw	1	−0.0033	0.0003	−0.0039	−0.0027	114.26
bwsq	1	0.0000	0.0000	0.0000	0.0000	4.14
indyr	1	**−0.5443**	0.1884	−0.9136	−0.1750	8.34
surfyr	1	**−0.3006**	0.1744	−0.6425	0.0413	2.97
Scale	0	1.0000	0.0000	1.0000	1.0000	

Analysis of Parameter Estimates

Parameter	Pr > ChiSq
Intercept	<0.0001
bw	<0.0001
bwsq	0.0418
indyr	0.0039
surfyr	0.0848
Scale	

LR Statistics for Type 3 Analysis

Source	DF	Chi-Square	Pr > ChiSq
bw	1	164.37	<0.0001
bwsq	1	3.96	0.0465
indyr	1	**8.52**	0.0035
surfyr	1	**2.97**	0.0847

CHAPTER FOURTEEN

Modeling Poisson Outcomes—The Analysis of Rates

Many investigations in population health are concerned with numbers of events (deaths, cases of disease, accidents, etc.) in the population. Under certain assumptions detailed below, the number of events follows the Poisson distribution described in Chapter 12 as one of the members of the exponential family of distributions. Usually, the interest of population health investigators lies in the rate of events, calculated as the number of events per person year of exposure. The rate is the parameter λ of the Poisson distribution as given in Chapter 12. In this case, as we see in Table 12.1, the canonical link is log. Other links are very rarely used with the Poisson distribution, although sometimes rates may be just assumed normally distributed, and the identity link used. Hence, the usual regression analysis of the number of events or the rate falls neatly into the framework of generalized linear models with canonical link.

14.1 REVIEW OF RATES

The observed rate of an event is defined as

$$r = \frac{\# \text{ events}}{\text{person time units at risk}}$$

or

$$r = \frac{\# \text{ events}}{\text{time unit}}$$

In the following discussion makes no conceptual difference what is chosen as the denominator for the rate. The important thing to remember is that the quantity t

Quantitative Methods in Population Health, by Mari Palta
ISBN 0-471-45505-9   Copyright © 2003 John Wiley & Sons, Inc.

in the Poisson distribution formula should be in the same units. Often, the person time units (say, person years) of exposure cannot be exactly obtained. In a geographic area, for example, people move in and out. It is then common to make the "stable population assumption" that holds when people who move spend on average half the year in the community, and that events occur uniformly through the time interval. With these assumptions, the number of person years of exposure equals the midyear population in the community, so that

$$r = \frac{\text{\# events}}{\text{person years at risk}} = \frac{\text{\# events}}{\text{mid year population}}$$

This is how most population-based rates are computed. For example, there were 405 cancer deaths among men aged 45–54 years in Wisconsin in 1996, with a midyear estimated population in the age group of 309,972. This led to a cancer mortality rate of 130.65 per 100,000, or 130.65 per 100,000 person-years.

As rates are often calculated for whole geographic areas, the argument can be made that they are then not estimators with sampling distributions, but actually observed parameters. Depending on the use of the rate, this can be a valid argument. (In addition, even if sampling variability is considered, it is often small because of the large sample size.) Assume that we are looking at nationwide, vital statistics based infant mortality rates for the United States and Canada for 1995. An example of the use of observed rates that would lend itself to comparison without consideration of sampling variation would be: "Was infant mortality in the United States in 1995 higher than infant mortality in Canada in 1995." Notice that generalization from the observed data to a larger population does not apply here. The populations of interest are represented in their entirety in the data. To answer the question, we only need to look at the two rates and see which is higher. On the other hand, questions such as "Is infant mortality in the United States higher than infant mortality in Canada?" and "Was infant mortality in 1995 higher in countries without a single payer system of health insurance?" imply possible generalization. In the first case, it is implied that although we have data from only 1995, we wish to infer something for other years. In the second case, we want to infer something for other countries with the same type of insurance system.

When we want to do inferences on rates, we need to consider from what type of distribution of events the rates may have arisen, so that we can compute sampling errors of the estimators. The basic assumptions underlying the Poisson distribution is that events occur independently—that is, that the occurrence of one event does not lead to higher probability of another event close in time and that the rate λ of events stays constant across time and individuals. Clearly, these assumption can be violated quite easily. Perhaps for population-wide total mortality, even if an accident or disaster killed a group of people within a certain time interval, this may be evened out by a time period of special caution, or simply have little impact on deaths from all causes. However, in a study of accident-related mortality in a smaller group of people (say), it may be that events are clustered by being caused either by accidents that killed more than one person or by subpopulations at higher risk. If accident occurrence rather than death was studied, events will be additionally clustered as there are accident-prone individuals. We will deal with these situations under the heading overdispersion.

If we persist in making the Poisson assumption and wish to take sampling variation into account, we recall that for the Poisson distribution the variance equals the mean. Hence, if we have observed y events in a year with a midyear population n, we have the rate $r = \frac{y}{n}$ with variance $\text{Var}(r) = \frac{1}{n^2}\text{Var}(y) = \frac{y}{n^2} = \frac{r}{n}$. There are some exact methods and tables available for forming tests and confidence intervals based on the Poisson distribution when the number of events is small. For reasonably large numbers of events, however, the distribution of the number of events (and the estimated rate) can be approximated by the normal. Hence we would obtain a 95% confidence interval for the true population rate by $r \pm 1.96\sqrt{\frac{r}{n}}$. The confidence interval for the cancer mortality rate of 45- to 54-year-old men in Wisconsin (note the implied generalization across years) is

$$130.65 \pm 1.96\sqrt{\frac{130.65}{309,972}} \times 100,000 = 130.65 \pm 12.7 \quad \text{per } 100,000$$

It should be noted that this confidence interval takes into account only the variability predicted from the Poisson distribution, not variability between years caused by mortality trends or other changes in circumstances (e.g., age shift within the age group). If there is nonconstancy of the rate between years due to other factors, the interval will be too narrow to capture the true rate 95% of the time. Comparing mortality across 19 years, we found that after adjusting for a downward trend in mortality in the age and sex group, the above standard error was fairly similar to estimated year-to-year variability.

Tests for comparing two rates can be based on the same types of standard errors.

14.1.1 Relationship Between Rate and Risk

It is useful to consider how rate is related to the risk of a person having an event in a given time period. We can start by constructing the probability that a person will not have an event during time period t. When the assumptions of the Poisson distribution holds, the probability of no events during t person time units (i.e. for duration t for one person) is

$$\text{Prob}(0) = \frac{(\lambda t)^0 \exp(-\lambda t)}{0!} = \exp(-\lambda t)$$

This is the probability of no event, or "event-free survival" to time t, so the complementary probability of at least one event (the risk) is

$$1 - \text{Prob}(0) = 1 - \exp(-\lambda t) \tag{14.1}$$

Expression (14.1) provides the connection between rate and risk in the situation when the assumptions of the Poisson distribution hold. The function $S(t) = \exp(-\lambda t)$ describing the probability of no events until time t is often referred to as an exponential survival function. It can be used in analyses where one compares survival of patients receiving treatments, or in studying the longevity of equipment, as long as the rate λ is constant. This assumption rarely holds for a long time period, but can be a good approximation for short subintervals.

With the cancer rate for men aged 45–54 in 1996 being 130.65 per 100,000, the probability for a person to die from cancer within 10 years is with the above assumption

$$1 - \exp(-10 \times 130.65/100{,}000) = 1.30\%$$

As the cancer mortality rate is 1.31%, per 10 years, we again see how risks are similar to rates when they are low.

Both the binomial and the Poisson distribution deal with counts of events. When the sample size giving rise to the events is large compared to the number of events, the two are almost indistinguishable. We see that, for example, the binomial variance for the number of events $m\pi(1 - \pi)$ is then $\approx m\pi \approx mr$, which is the Poisson variance, leading to very similar confidence intervals for the rate and risk.

From (14.1) we see that $-\log(1 - \pi) = \lambda$, so $\log(-\log(1 - \pi)) = \log(\lambda)$. Hence, when the assumptions hold and follow-up time does not vary between subjects, the log link for the rate and the complementary $\log(-\log)$ for the binary outcome give identical regression coefficients. This is true regardless of whether the risk is small. When π is small, in addition $\log(\frac{\pi}{1-\pi}) \approx \log(\pi)$, so that the link for the risk also yields similar results as the log link for the corresponding rate. We found already in Chapter 13 that for low π, logit and $\log(-\log)$ links are similar.

14.2 REGRESSION ANALYSIS

As the Poisson distribution is in the exponential family of distributions, we can rely on the framework of Chapter 12 to construct likelihoods. We see in Table 12.1 that $b(\theta) = \exp(\theta)$. It then follows that $b'(\theta) = \exp(\theta)$ and that $b''(\theta) = \exp(\theta)$ as well. Since the dispersion parameter ϕ equals 1, (as indicated in Table 12.1), $\mu = \exp(\theta)$ and $\text{Var}(y) = \mu$. The canonical link $b'^{-1}(\mu)$ equals $\log(\mu)$.

For the Poisson distribution there is a happy coincidence that the logarithmic function is the canonical link and that investigators are usually interested in ratios of rates. We will see below that with the log link, the regression parameters will be logarithms of rate ratios (just as the logit link for binary data provided logarithms of odds ratios).

It follows from the log likelihood for the exponential family that for the Poisson distribution the part of the likelihood that depends on λ (and therefore contributes to the estimating equations) is

$$\log(L) = \sum \left(\{y_i\theta - b(\theta)\}/a(\phi) \right)$$
$$= \sum \{y_i \log(\lambda_i t_i) - \exp(\log(\lambda_i t_i))\}$$
$$= \sum \left(y_i \log(\lambda_i t_i) - (\lambda_i t_i) \right)$$

The deviance is the difference in $-2\log(L)\phi$ computed with an estimator of λ_i and with $\lambda_i t_i$ replaced by the "perfectly fitting" observed values y_i. Hence

$$2\log(L_{\text{perfect}}) - 2\log(L_{\text{fitted}})$$
$$= 2\sum \left(y_i \log(y_i) - y_i \right) - 2\sum \left(y_i \log(\hat{\lambda}_i t_i) - (\hat{\lambda}_i t_i) \right)$$
$$= 2\sum \left(y_i \log \left(\frac{y_i}{\hat{\lambda}_i t_i} \right) - (y_i - \hat{\lambda}_i t_i) \right)$$

Just as in the binomial case, the deviance can be used to check the fit of the model, if the observations are in subsets that do not increase in number with the total number of events or follow-up time. Alternatively, the classical Pearson chi-square can be used:

$$\chi^2(n - k) = \sum \frac{(y_i - \hat{\lambda}_i t_i)^2}{\hat{\lambda}_i t_i}$$

where k is the number of parameters in the model. Similarly to the binomial case, this test compares the observed and expected (under Poisson) variability in counts.

Let the link function $h(\mu_i)$ be expressed as

$$h(\mu_i) = h(\lambda_i t) = \log(\lambda_i t) = \beta_0 + \beta_1 x_{1i} + \cdots \qquad (14.2)$$

This implies that

$$\mu_i = \lambda_i t = h^{-1}(\beta_0 + \beta_1 x_{1i} + \cdots) = \exp(\beta_0 + \beta_1 x_{1i} + \cdots)$$

However, in practice it is often the case that t is not the same for all observations. Typically, the geographic areas in the analysis may have unequal population sizes, or individuals being followed are in the study for varying lengths of time. It is therefore common to model λ instead of μ and replace (13.2) by

$$h(\mu_i) = h(\lambda t_i) = \log(\lambda t_i) = \log(\lambda) + \log(t_i) \quad \text{so}$$

$$\log(\lambda_i) = -\log(t_i) + \beta_0 + \beta_1 x_{1i} + \cdots$$

The quantity $\log(t_i)$ is referred to as an *off-set*. It can be viewed as an observed predictor with known regression coefficient $= 1$.

Following the development for canonical links, the estimating (score) equations for the Poisson are given by the matrix equation

$$\begin{pmatrix} 1 & 1 & \cdots & 1 \\ x_{11} & x_{12} & \cdots & x_{1n} \\ \cdots & \cdots & \cdots & \cdots \end{pmatrix} \left(\begin{pmatrix} y_1 \\ \vdots \\ y_n \end{pmatrix} - \begin{pmatrix} \exp(\log(t_1) + \beta_0 + \beta_1 x_{11} \cdots) \\ \vdots \\ \exp(\log(t_n) + \beta_0 + \beta_1 x_{1n} \cdots) \end{pmatrix} \right) = 0$$

14.3   EXAMPLE WITH CANCER MORTALITY RATES

We consider the relationship of total cancer-related mortality in Wisconsin in 1996 to age and sex. Data were obtained from CDC WONDER [75] in 10-year age groups starting at age 35 years. The variable AGEM was created to designate the age groups. We found that the relationship of log(rate) and log(age − 30) was nearly linear, as shown in the first plot in OUTPUT PACKET XV, and that there was an interaction effect between log(age − 30) and sex. This interaction is explained by breast cancers occurring at a young age among women, while men have higher rates of other cancers, such as lung cancer, later in life. An offset variable LPOP was created as the log of the population in the relevant age by sex group, and the following commands were run:

```
LAGE=LOG(MAGE-30);
RATE=100000*DTS/POP;
LRATE=LOG(RATE);
PROC PLOT; PLOT LRATE*LAGE=SEX;
PROC GENMOD; CLASS SEX;
MODEL DTS=LAGE SEX*LAGE SEX/DIST=POISSON OFFSET=LPOP;
OUT=PP P=PRED;
DATA C; SET PP;
PRED=100000*PRED/POP;
PROC PRINT; VAR AGEM RATE PRED
```

The last set of commands created a printout showing how observed and predicted rates agree. Coefficients and standard errors are in Table 14.1, and we see that predicted values are obtained by the formula

$$\text{pred} = \exp[-\log(\text{pop}) - 14.5 + (2.68 - 0.531(\text{female}))$$
$$\times \log(\text{age} - 30) + 1.52(\text{female}))]$$

Since the prediction is for the number of deaths, we convert it to a rate comparable with the observed rate. Rate ratios between genders and ages are obtained from the coefficients, and are somewhat complicated by the nonlinearity and interaction effects. For males we obtain, for example, that the rate ratio between ages 60 and 50 is given by

$$\exp[2.68(\log(30) - \log(20))] = \exp[2.68 \times 0.4055] = 2.97$$

We can also obtain rate ratios by the ESTIMATE command. For example, to obtain a rate ratio between ages 60 and 50, we can insert the multiplier 0.4055 and use the command

ESTIMATE 'RR BETWEEN AGES 60 AND 50' LAGE 0.4055/EXP;

SAS style in dealing with main effects that also have interaction effects involving class variable is to average the interaction effect in equal proportion across classes. This yields the rate ratio 2.66 [2.62, 2.72]. Often, the easiest way around these types of decisions by SAS is to bypass the CLASS feature and create one's own indicator variables.

Finally, we see that the model has significant deviance and Pearson $\chi^2(8)$ statistics, both with $p < 0.0001$. This can be due to lack of fit of the model for rate on age (nonlinearity) or due to the data not following the Poisson distribution. Since the observed and expected rates do not have systematic differences, we conjecture that the reason for lack of fit is variability beyond Poisson at the different ages or between genders. We will further examine the effect of such variability in Section 14.3.

14.3.1 Example with Hospitalization of Infants

We look at the rehospitalization rate of very-low-birth-weight infants in the first year of life. The number of hospitalizations (not counting the initial NICU stay) is given in OUTPUT PACKET XV. We see that while the majority of infants do not get rehospitalized, up to seven rehospitalizations took place. The subsequent analysis shows the fraction of the first year that the infant was at risk. Differences between infants arose, because they could not, by definition, become rehospitalized before they were discharged from the initial stay. The third analysis shows the results of Poisson regression. The commands run were

LTIME=LOG(TIME);
BWC=BW-1000; PROC CHART; HBAR NHOSP/DISCRETE;
PROC UNIVARIATE PLOT; VAR TIME;
PROC GENMOD;
MODEL NHOSP=BWC/DIST=POISSON OFFSET=LTIME;
ESTIMATE 'RATE RATIO' BW 100/EXP;

LINK=LOG could be specified, but is the default for the Poisson. Here, the variable TIME is used to create the offset (in this case the unit is years) as discussed above. We see from the output that birth weight in grams was predictive of the number of hospitalizations. To interpret the regression coefficient, we exponentiate it (either by hand or by using the ESTIMATE command). We see that for a 100 g increase in birth weight, the rate ratio is $\exp(100 \times (-0.0018)) = 0.84$. This means that the rate of rehospitalization is 0.84 times less for every 100 g increase in birth weight. The confidence interval for this ratio is given $[\exp(100 \times (-0.0025)) = 0.78, \exp(100 * (-0.0010)) = 0.90]$ or $[0.78, 0.90]$. These were obtained by the last statement with greater precision.

As usual, the fitting of a link function with a continuous predictor involves a linearity assumption. In this case, the assumption implies that the difference in the log rate stays constant with every unit increase in the predictor, or, equivalently, that the rate ratio stays constant. Because the predictor BW is continuous, we cannot assign p-values to the deviance and Pearson statistics in this case. The assumption can instead be checked in a few other ways. A plot similar to the one for cancer mortality can be generated for the log rate by birth weight groups. Other approaches are to fit indicator variables for birth-weight groups and look at the coefficient and fitting additional polynomial terms. Various residual plots can also be generated. For example, adding the commands

OUTPUT OUT=RR STDRESDEV=RESID P=PRED
PLOT RESID*PRED;

generates a residual plot of "deviance residuals" (the individual pieces in the deviance). As can be seen in OUTPUT PACKET XV, these residuals tend to be more difficult to interpret than those from ordinary regression.

14.4 OVERDISPERSION

It is very often the case with Poisson data, such as those in the above examples, that the assumption of independence of events leading to the mean equals variance property of the Poisson distribution is hardly believable. For example, there are many factors both known and unknown that make one infant be hospitalized repeatedly, while another is hospitalized once or not at all. It is even possible that one hospitalization may lead to another due to iatrogenic complications. Similarly, there may be unknown factors that influence cancer rate variation between age groups. For example, different types of cancer predominate at different ages. These types of circumstances lead to the variance of the counts being greater than expected based on the Poisson distribution. It is therefore known as overdispersion. The consequence of overdispersion is that standard errors of regression coefficients are underestimated, and significance over estimated by assuming that the Poisson mean-variance relationship holds.

Several approaches are available for dealing with overdispersion. First of all, it is advisable to avoid aggregation of data as far as possible. Retaining the smallest possible units with their individual covariates tends to reduce the problem of overdispersion. We discuss three other approaches and apply them to our data sets.

14.4.1 Fitting a Dispersion Parameter

One solution to the problem of overdispersion is to fit a dispersion parameter in the generalized linear model. This is achieved by the SCALE options in PROC GENMOD. Specifying a different scale does not change parameter estimates. However, because it is now assumed that the variance function is $\phi\mu$ (in the case of Poisson), standard errors of the parameters are multiplied by $\sqrt{\phi}$ (i.e., the SCALE parameter in the GENMOD output). Scaled χ^2 statistics are divided by ϕ. With overdispersion, taking ϕ into account can lead to sharply increased standard errors and reduce the significance of coefficients.

There are several methods for estimating the dispersion parameter. Perhaps the most popular is estimation by Pearson residuals. This is the Pearson chi-square divided by degrees of freedom or

$$\hat{\phi} = \sum \frac{(y_i - \hat{\mu}_i)^2}{\hat{\mu}_i}/(n-k)$$

where k is the number of parameters fit. As you can see, this quantity is almost like the mean square error from the residuals of the model, except each squared residual is divided by the mean, which equals the variance under the Poisson assumptions. Because we then have a quantity based on the ratio of observed to assumed variance, overdispersion is a fitting name if the estimated $\hat{\phi}$ is greater than 1.

The Pearson dispersion parameter estimate is obtained by

PROC GENMOD;
MODEL y = **VAR1....... / DIST=POISSON PSCALE;**

PSCALE can be replaced by DSCALE to obtain the deviance-based dispersion parameter adjustments.

14.4.2 Fitting a Different Distribution

Sometimes, a distribution can be found that would be expected to fit the data and that has an increase in variance as the mean increases. The negative binomial distribution is such an alternative. PROC GENMOD can fit a version of the negative binomial where the variance depends on the mean through a quadratic relationship, that is,

$$\text{Var}(y) = \mu + \nu\mu^2$$

The parameter ν is called the "dispersion", but as we can see, it is not equivalent to ϕ. The negative binomial is not in the exponential family, but PROC GENMOD fits the model by maximum likelihood. The default link is still the log, so the offset and the interpretation of parameters is the same as for the Poisson. The negative binomial is available as a choice in SAS version 8 as DIST=NB by using the commands

PROC GENMOD;
MODEL y = **VAR1....... / DIST=NB;**

14.4.3 Using Robust Standard Errors

Just as we did in the ordinary regression case by PROC MIXED, we can use PROC GENMOD to implement empirical-type standard errors based on ordinary residuals, instead of using model-based standard errors. We do not derive the formula here, because it involves Taylor expansion and demonstrating that the approximation becomes increasingly accurate for large n. For the canonical link (log for Poisson) the empirical or "robust" variance of the regression coefficient estimators is given by

$$\text{Var}(\hat{\boldsymbol{\beta}}) = (X'X)^{-1}(X'\hat{\boldsymbol{\epsilon}}\hat{\boldsymbol{\epsilon}}'X)(X'X)^{-1}$$

where $\hat{\boldsymbol{\epsilon}}$ is a diagonal matrix with residuals $(y_i - \exp(\hat{\beta}_0 + \hat{\beta}_1 x_{1i} \cdots))$ on diagonal. In SAS, GENMOD can be "tricked" similarly to PROC MIXED by the statements

PROC GENMOD; CLASS ID;
MODEL y = **VAR1....... / DIST=POISSON;**
REPEATED SUBJECT=ID;

PROC GENMOD differs from PROC MIXED in not having a "/" in front of the "SUBJECT" option. The desired standard errors are found in the second half of the resulting output under "Analysis of GEE Parameter Estimates—Empirical Standard Error Estimates."

14.4.4 Applying Adjustments for Over Dispersion to the Examples

Table 14.1 displays the coefficients and various standard errors for the cancer mortality example. The regression coefficient estimates are identical for all cases except the negative binomial, but they were very close even in this case and are not separately provided below (they are in OUTPUT PACKET XV).

There is definitely evidence of overdispersion in the data set. The standard error estimates are quite similar with all methods that take overdispersion into account. This is because the data are grouped, and the sample size is very large. We note, however, that the negative binomial does not seem to appropriately model the variance structure in these data.

A similar table (Table 14.2) is provided below for the infant hospitalization model.

Results of the adjustments are similar, with the exception of the DSCALE approach. Our preference is the empirical option, but we are not aware of studies that have systematically compared the different options for adjusting for overdispersion.

Finally, overdispersion is often reduced when additional variables are added to the model. In the infant hospitalization example, improvements were not dramatic because a full model (not shown) including many clinical conditions of the neonate estimated the scale to be 1.42 by the Pearson method and 1.16 by the deviance method.

Table 14.1   Standard Errors for Wisconsin Cancer Mortality in 1996 Model, Taking Overdispersion into Account

Predictor	$\hat{\beta}$	Poisson	dscale	pscale	nb	Empirical
Intercept	−14.5	0.140	0.324	0.324	0.240	0.314
log(age − 30)	2.68	0.0378	0.0878	0.0878	0.0670	0.0823
female	1.53	0.193	0.449	0.449	0.321	0.448
log(age − 30) × female	−0.531	0.0522	0.121	0.121	0.0899	0.117
scale/dispersion	1		2.32	2.32	0.048	

Table 14.2   Standard Errors for Infant Hospitalization Model, Taking Overdispersion into Account

Predictor	$\hat{\beta}$	Poisson	dscale	pscale	nb	Empirical
Intercept	−0.268	0.0721	0.113	0.0913	0.119	0.112
Birth weight	−0.0018	0.0003	0.0004	0.0004	0.0005	0.004
Scale/dispersion	1		1.27	1.57	2.55	

OUTPUT PACKET XV: POISSON REGRESSION

XV.1. Analysis of Cancer Mortality, Wisconsin 1996

Analysis of Wisconsin Cancer Mortality in 1996

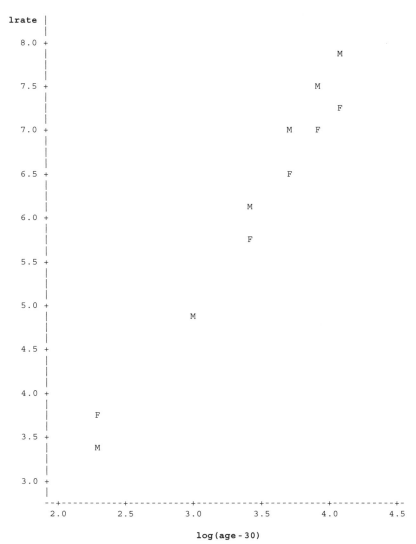

Note: 1 obs hidden.

Plot of lrate*lage: log of rate per 10000 versus log(age − 30). Symbol is value of sex.

Poisson Regression
  The GENMOD Procedure

Model Information

Data set	WORK.B
Distribution	Poisson
Link function	Log
Dependent variable	dts Number of cancer deaths
Offset variable	lpop
Observations used	12

Class Level Information

Class	Levels	Values
sex	2	F M

Criteria for Assessing Goodness of Fit[a]

Criterion	DF	Value	Value/DF
Deviance	8	43.1814	5.3977
Scaled deviance	8	43.1814	5.3977
Pearson chi-square	8	43.2141	5.4018
Scaled Pearson X2	8	43.2141	5.4018
Log likelihood		62701.4074	

[a] Algorithm converged.

Analysis of Parameter Estimates

Parameter		DF	Estimate	Standard Error	Wald 95% Confidence Limits		Chi-Square
Intercept		1	−14.5184	0.1395	−14.7918	−14.2450	10833.4
lage		1	2.6826	0.0378	2.6086	2.7566	5043.01
sex	F	1	1.5275	0.1933	1.1488	1.9063	62.48
sex	M	0	0.0000	0.0000	0.0000	0.0000	.
lage*sex	F	1	−0.5313	0.0522	−0.6337	−0.4290	103.53
lage*sex	M	0	0.0000	0.0000	0.0000	0.0000	.
Scale		0	1.0000	0.0000	1.0000	1.0000	

Analysis of Parameter Estimates

Parameter		Pr > ChiSq
Intercept		<.0001
lage		<.0001
sex	F	<.0001
sex	M	.
lage*sex	F	<.0001
lage*sex	M	.
Scale		

Note: The scale parameter was held fixed.

Contrast Estimate Results

Label	Estimate	Standard Error	Alpha	Confidence	Limits
RR age 60 vs. 50	0.9801	0.0106	0.05	0.9593	1.0008
Exp(RR age 60 vs. 50)	2.6646	0.0282	0.05	2.6099	2.7205

Contrast Estimate Results

Label	Chi-Square	Pr > ChiSq
RR age 60 vs. 50	8569.2	<0.0001
Exp(RR age 60 vs. 50)		

Rate Observed Versus Rate Predicted by Poisson Regression

Observed	Sex	agem	Rate	Predicted
1	M	40	29.02	23.84
2	M	50	130.65	153.07
3	M	60	457.02	454.21
4	M	70	1036.21	982.69
5	M	80	1768.68	1788.09
6	M	90	2799.60	2916.08
7	F	40	40.03	32.32
8	F	50	124.37	143.55
9	F	60	328.47	343.43
10	F	70	667.61	637.70
11	F	80	1055.09	1030.61
12	F	90	1470.87	1525.58

XV.2. Hospitalization of VLBW Infants—Newborn Lung Project

Rehospitalization of VLBW Infants—Newborn Lung Project
Distribution of Number of Hospitalizations per Infant

```
 nhosp                                        Cum.              Cum.
                                      Freq.   Freq.  Percent   Percent
        |
   0    |*************************      245     245    71.01     71.01
        |
   1    |*****                           54     299    15.65     86.67
        |
   2    |***                             25     324     7.25     93.91
        |
   3    |*                               10     334     2.90     96.81
        |
   4    |                                 3     337     0.87     97.68
        |
   5    |                                 4     341     1.16     98.84
        |
   6    |                                 1     342     0.29     99.13
        |
   7    |                                 3     345     0.87    100.00
        |
        -----+----+----+----+----+
            50  100  150  200  250

                  Frequency
```

Distribution of Time at Risk (unit = year)
  The UNIVARIATE Procedure

Variable: time

Moments

N	345	Sum of weights	345
Mean	0.82533254	Sum of observations	284.739726
Std deviation	0.08101985	Variance	0.00656422
Skewness	−1.4165375	Kurtosis	3.87385908
Uncorrected SS	237.263051	Corrected SS	2.25809013
Coeff variation	9.81663057	Standard error of mean	0.00436196

Basic Statistical Measures

Location		Variability	
Mean	0.825333	Standard deviation	0.08102
Median	0.841096	Variance	0.00656
Mode	0.849315	Range	0.58630
		Interquartile range	0.09589

Quantile	Estimate
100% Max	1.000000
99%	0.950685
95%	0.928767
90%	0.909589
75% Q3	0.879452
50% Median	0.841096
25% Q1	0.783562
10%	0.720548
5%	0.687671
1%	0.490411
0% Min	0.413699

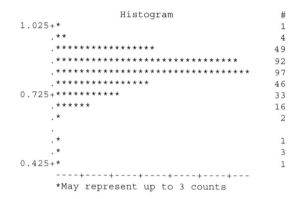

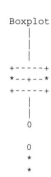

```
          Histogram                         #          Boxplot
1.025+*                                      1           |
     .**                                     4           |
     .*****************                      49          |
     .*****************************          92       +-----+
     .********************************       97       *--+--*
     .****************                       46       +-----+
0.725+***********                            33          |
     .******                                 16          |
     .*                                       2          0
     .
     .*                                        1         0
     .*                                        3         *
0.425+*                                        1         *
     ----+----+----+----+----+----+---
     *May represent up to 3 counts
```

Poisson Regression
The GENMOD Procedure

Model Information

Data set	WORK.A
Distribution	**Poisson**
Link function	**Log**
Dependent variable	nhosp
Offset variable	ltime
Observations used	345

Criteria for Assessing Goodness of Fit

Criterion	DF	Value	Value/DF
Deviance	343	550.8603	1.6060
Scaled deviance	343	550.8603	1.6060
Pearson chi-square	343	841.5825	2.4536
Scaled Pearson X2	343	841.5825	2.4536
Log likelihood		−300.3755	

Analysis of Parameter Estimates

Parameter	DF	Estimate	Standard Error	Wald 95% Confidence Limits		Chi-Square
Intercept	1	−0.2678	0.0721	−0.4091	−0.1266	13.81
bwc	1	−0.0018	0.0003	−0.0023	−0.0012	37.75
Scale	0	1.0000	0.0000	1.0000	1.0000	

Analysis of Parameter Estimates

Parameter	Pr > ChiSq
Intercept	0.0002
bw	<0.0001
Scale	

Contrast Estimate Results

Label	Estimate	Standard Error	Alpha	Confidence Limits	
RATE RATIO	−0.1762	0.0287	0.05	−0.2324	−0.1200
Exp(RATE RATIO)	**0.8385**	**0.0240**	**0.05**	**0.7926**	**0.8869**
RATE at 1000 g	−0.2678	0.0721	0.05	−0.4091	−0.1266
Exp(RATE at 1000 g)	**0.7650**	**0.0551**	**0.05**	**0.6642**	**0.8811**

Contrast Estimate Results

Label	Chi-Square	Pr > ChiSq
RATE RATIO	37.75	<0.0001
Exp(RATE RATIO)		
RATE at 1000 g	13.81	0.0002
Exp(RATE at 1000 g)		

Deviance Residuals Versus Predicted Values

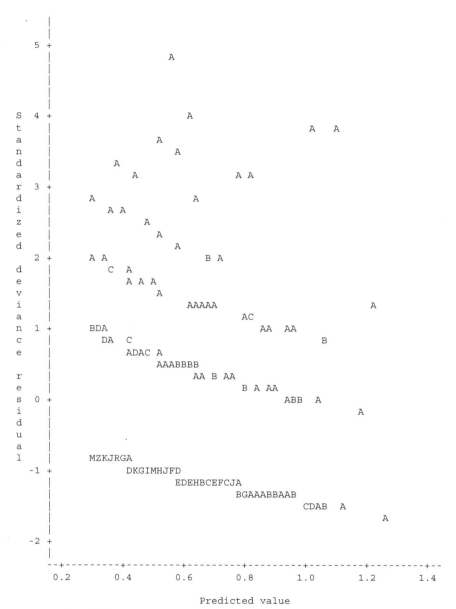

Note: 1 obs hidden.

Plot of resid*pred. Legend: A = 1 obs, B = 2 obs, and so on.

OUTPUT PACKET XVI: DEALING WITH OVERDISPERSION IN RATES

XVI.1. Four Methods Applied to Wisconsin Cancer Mortality in 1996

Overdispersion in Wisconsin Cancer Mortality in 1996
Poisson Regression with Deviance Overdispersion
   The GENMOD Procedure

Model Information

Data set	WORK.B	
Distribution	Poisson	
Link function	Log	
Dependent variable	dts	Number of cancer deaths
Offset variable	lpop	
Observations used	12	

Criteria for Assessing Goodness of Fit

Criterion	DF	Value	Value/DF
Deviance	**8**	**43.1814**	**5.3977**
Scaled deviance	8	8.0000	1.0000
Pearson chi-square	8	43.2141	5.4018
Scaled Pearson X2	8	8.0061	1.0008
Log likelihood		11616.3719	

Analysis of Parameter Estimates

Parameter		DF	Estimate	Standard Error	Wald 95% Confidence Limits		Chi-Square
Intercept		1	−14.5184	0.3241	−15.1536	−13.8832	2007.05
lage		1	2.6826	0.0878	2.5106	2.8546	934.29
sex	F	1	1.5275	0.4490	0.6475	2.4075	11.57
sex	M	0	0.0000	0.0000	0.0000	0.0000	.
lage*sex	F	1	−0.5313	0.1213	−0.7691	−0.2935	19.18
lage*sex	M	0	0.0000	0.0000	0.0000	0.0000	.
Scale		**0**	**2.3233**	**0.0000**	**2.3233**	**2.3233**	

Analysis of Parameter Estimates

Parameter		Pr > ChiSq
Intercept		<.0001
lage		<.0001
sex	F	0.0007
sex	M	.
lage*sex	F	<.0001

Note: The scale parameter was estimated by the square root of DEVIANCE/DOF.

Poisson Regression with Pearson Overdispersion
The GENMOD Procedure

Model Information

Data set	WORK.B	
Distribution	Poisson	
Link function	Log	
Dependent variable	dts	Number of cancer deaths
Offset variable	lpop	
Observations used	12	

Criteria for Assessing Goodness of Fit

Criterion	DF	Value	Value/DF
Deviance	8	43.1814	5.3977
Scaled deviance	8	7.9939	0.9992
Pearson Chi-square	**8**	**43.2141**	**5.4018**
Scaled Pearson X2	8	8.0000	1.0000
Log likelihood		11607.5850	

Analysis of Parameter Estimates

Parameter	DF		Estimate	Standard Error	Wald 95% Confidence Limits		Chi-Square
Intercept		1	−14.5184	0.3242	−15.1538	−13.8830	2005.53
lage		1	2.6826	0.0878	2.5105	2.8547	933.59
sex	F	1	1.5275	0.4492	0.6472	2.4078	11.57
sex	M	0	0.0000	0.0000	0.0000	0.0000	.
lage*sex	F	1	−0.5313	0.1214	−0.7692	−0.2934	19.17
lage*sex	M	0	0.0000	0.0000	0.0000	0.0000	.
Scale		**0**	**2.3242**	**0.0000**	**2.3242**	**2.3242**	

Analysis of Parameter Estimates

Parameter		Pr > ChiSq
Intercept		<0.0001
lage		<0.0001
sex	F	0.0007
sex	M	.
lage*sex	F	<0.0001

Note: The scale parameter was estimated by the square root of Pearson's chi-square/DOF.

Negative Binomial Regression
The GENMOD Procedure

Model Information

Data set	WORK.B	
Distribution	**Negative binomial**	
Link function	Log	
Dependent variable	dts	Number of cancer deaths
Offset variable	lpop	
Observations used	12	

Criteria for Assessing Goodness of Fit

Criterion	DF	Value	Value/DF
Deviance	8	14.0236	1.7530
Scaled deviance	8	14.0236	1.7530
Pearson chi-square	8	13.6014	1.7002
Scaled Pearson X2	8	13.6014	1.7002
Log likelihood		62706.9634	

Analysis of Parameter Estimates

Parameter		DF	Estimate	Standard Error	Wald 95% Confidence Limits		Chi-Square
Intercept		1	−14.3718	0.2398	−14.8418	−13.9018	3591.55
lage		1	2.6400	0.0670	2.5087	2.7714	1551.16
sex	F	1	1.5640	0.3209	0.9351	2.1930	23.75
sex	M	0	0.0000	0.0000	0.0000	0.0000	.
lage*sex	F	1	−0.5407	0.0899	−0.7168	−0.3645	36.20
lage*sex	M	0	0.0000	0.0000	0.0000	0.0000	.
Dispersion		**1**	**0.0048**	**0.0032**	**0.0013**	**0.0177**	

Analysis of Parameter Estimates

Parameter		Pr > ChiSq
Intercept		<0.0001
lage		<0.0001
sex	F	<0.0001
sex	M	.
lage*sex	F	<.0001

Note: The negative binomial dispersion parameter was estimated by maximum likelihood.

Robust Variance
  The GENMOD Procedure

Model Information

Data set	WORK.B	
Distribution	Poisson	
Link function	Log	
Dependent variable	dts	Number of cancer deaths
Offset variable	lpop	
Observations used	12	

Criteria For Assessing Goodness of Fit

Criterion	DF	Value	Value/DF
Deviance	8	43.1814	5.3977
Scaled deviance	8	43.1814	5.3977
Pearson chi-square	8	43.2141	5.4018
Scaled Pearson X2	8	43.2141	5.4018
Log likelihood		62701.4074	

Analysis of Initial Parameter Estimates

Parameter		DF	Estimate	Standard Error	Wald 95% Confidence Limits		Chi-Square
Intercept		1	−14.5184	0.1395	−14.7918	−14.2450	10833.4
lage		1	2.6826	0.0378	2.6086	2.7566	5043.01
sex	F	1	1.5275	0.1933	1.1488	1.9063	62.48
sex	M	0	0.0000	0.0000	0.0000	0.0000	.
lage*sex	F	1	−0.5313	0.0522	−0.6337	−0.4290	103.53
lage*sex	M	0	0.0000	0.0000	0.0000	0.0000	.
Scale		0	1.0000	0.0000	1.0000	1.0000	

Analysis of GEE Parameter Estimates
Empirical Standard Error Estimates

Parameter		Estimate	Standard Error	95% Confidence Limits		Z	Pr > |Z|
Intercept		−14.5184	0.3141	−15.1340	−13.9028	−46.23	<0.0001
lage		2.6826	0.0823	2.5212	2.8440	32.58	<0.0001
sex	F	1.5275	0.4483	0.6489	2.4061	3.41	0.0007
sex	M	0.0000	0.0000	0.0000	0.0000	.	.
lage*sex	F	−0.5313	0.1173	−0.7613	−0.3014	−4.53	<0.0001
lage*sex	M	0.0000	0.0000	0.0000	0.0000	.	.

XVI.1 Four Methods Applied to Rehospitalization of VLBW Infants

Overdispersion in Rehospitalization of VLBW Infants
Deviance-Based Overdispersion Correction
   The GENMOD Procedure

Model Information

Data set	WORK.A
Distribution	Poisson
Link Function	Log
Dependent variable	nhosp
Offset variable	ltime
Observations used	345

Criteria for Assessing Goodness of Fit[a]

Criterion	DF	Value	Value/DF
Deviance	**343**	**550.8603**	**1.6060**
Scaled deviance	343	343.0000	1.0000
Pearson chi-square	343	841.5825	2.4536
Scaled Pearson X2	343	524.0218	1.5278
Log likelihood		−187.0325	

[a] Algorithm converged.

Analysis of Parameter Estimates

Parameter	DF	Estimate	Standard Error	Wald 95% Confidence Limits		Chi-Square
Intercept	1	−0.2678	0.0913	−0.4469	−0.0888	8.60
bwc	1	−0.0018	0.0004	−0.0025	−0.0010	23.50
Scale	**0**	**1.2673**	**0.0000**	**1.2673**	**1.2673**	

Analysis of Parameter Estimates

Parameter	Pr > ChiSq
Intercept	0.0034
bwc	< 0.0001
Scale	

Note: The scale parameter was estimated by the square root of DEVIANCE/DOF.

Pearson Based Overdispersion Correction
The GENMOD Procedure

Model Information

Data set	WORK.A
Distribution	Poisson
Link function	Log
Dependent variable	nhosp
Offset variable	ltime
Observations used	345

Criteria for Assessing Goodness of Fit[a]

Criterion	DF	Value	Value/DF
Deviance	343	550.8603	1.6060
Scaled deviance	343	224.5116	0.6546
Pearson chi-square	**343**	**841.5825**	**2.4536**
Scaled Pearson X2	343	343.0000	1.0000
Log likelihood		−122.4227	

[a] Algorithm converged.

Analysis of Parameter Estimates

Parameter	DF	Estimate	Standard Error	Wald 95% Confidence Limits		Chi-Square
Intercept	1	−0.2678	0.1129	−0.4891	−0.0465	5.63
bwc	1	−0.0018	0.0004	−0.0026	−0.0009	15.38
Scale	0	1.5664	0.0000	1.5664	1.5664	

Analysis of Parameter Estimates

Parameter	Pr > ChiSq
Intercept	0.0177
bwc	<0.0001
Scale	

Note: The scale parameter was estimated by the square root of Pearson's chi-square/DOF.

Fitting Negative Binomial Distribution
  The GENMOD Procedure

Model Information

Data set	WORK.A
Distribution	**Negative Binomial**
Link function	**Log**
Dependent variable	nhosp
Offset variable	ltime
Observations used	345

Criteria for Assessing Goodness of Fit[a]

Criterion	DF	Value	Value/DF
Deviance	343	243.7728	0.7107
Scaled deviance	343	243.7728	0.7107
Pearson chi-square	343	354.6229	1.0339
Scaled Pearson X2	343	354.6229	1.0339
Log likelihood		−243.6425	

[a] Algorithm converged.

Analysis of Parameter Estimates

Parameter	DF	Estimate	Standard Error	Wald 95% Confidence Limits		Chi-Square
Intercept	1	−0.2391	0.1187	−0.4717	−0.0065	4.06
bwc	1	−0.0017	0.0005	−0.0026	−0.0008	14.33
Dispersion	**1**	**2.5537**	**0.5054**	**1.7327**	**3.7638**	

Analysis of Parameter Estimates

Parameter	Pr > ChiSq
Intercept	0.0440
bwc	0.0002
Dispersion	

Note: The negative binomial dispersion parameter was estimated by maximum likelihood.

Robust (Empirical) Standard Errors
  The GENMOD Procedure

Model Information

Data set	WORK.A
Distribution	Poisson
Link function	Log
Dependent variable	nhosp
Offset variable	ltime
Observations used	345

Criteria for Assessing Goodness of Fit

Criterion	DF	Value	Value/DF
Deviance	343	550.8603	1.6060
Scaled deviance	343	550.8603	1.6060
Pearson chi-square	343	841.5825	2.4536
Scaled Pearson X2	343	841.5825	2.4536
Log likelihood		−300.3755	

Analysis of Initial Parameter Estimates

Parameter	DF	Estimate	Standard Error	Wald 95% Confidence Limits		Chi-Square
Intercept	1	−0.2678	0.0721	−0.4091	−0.1266	13.81
bwc	1	−0.0018	0.0003	−0.0023	−0.0012	37.75
Scale	0	1.0000	0.0000	1.0000	1.0000	

Analysis of Initial Parameter Estimates

Parameter	Pr > ChiSq
Intercept	0.0002
bwc	<0.0001
Scale	

GEE Model Information

Correlation structure	Independent
Subject effect	id (345 levels)
Number of clusters	345
Correlation matrix dimension	1
Maximum cluster size	1
Minimum cluster size	1

Analysis of GEE Parameter Estimates
Empirical Standard Error Estimates

Parameter	Estimate	Standard Error	95% Confidence Limits		Z	Pr > |Z|
Intercept	−0.2678	0.1118	−0.4870	−0.0487	−2.40	0.0166
bwc	−0.0018	0.0004	−0.0026	−0.0009	−4.11	<0.0001

CHAPTER FIFTEEN

Modeling Correlated Outcomes with Generalized Estimating Equations

It is now time to bring two streams of development in this text together. Starting from Chapter 8, we dealt with correlated data, but only when the residuals could be assumed normally distributed. More recently, starting with Chapter 12, we dealt with non-normally distributed data, but only in the situation where the observations were independent. Obviously, it is very common to have both situation simultaneously. In the sleep cohort study, we may wish to model not only systolic blood pressure, but also hypertensive medication use over time. In the very-low-birthweight cohort, we may wish to study how the rate of hospitalization changes with age. These two are examples of longitudinal binary and Poisson data, respectively.

15.1 A BRIEF REVIEW AND REFORMULATION OF THE NORMAL DISTRIBUTION, LEAST SQUARES AND LIKELIHOOD

When we encountered correlated normally distributed data, two approaches presented themselves. The first was a linear transformation allowing extension of least-squares linear regression to correlated residuals. The theory of this approach was delineated in Chapters 8 and 9. It works when we specify and estimate a variance matrix for the data. We showed that even if the variance matrix is not correctly specified, the estimator β is still *unbiased*, and we had a fix-up called the *empirical variance* to still obtain correct standard errors for the regression coefficients. If the variance matrix is correct, the estimators are also *minimum variance* among those that are unbiased linear transformations of Y, although we did not prove this formally. In statistics there is a long history in working with least-squares estimators and proving their properties.

Quantitative Methods in Population Health, by Mari Palta
ISBN 0-471-45505-9   Copyright © 2003 John Wiley & Sons, Inc.

The second approach for normally distributed data is the *maximum likelihood approach*. It can be applied even to correlated data, because the so-called "joint" distribution generating all the data points can be specified as the *multivariate normal* distribution. Whenever we have a distribution for all the data points, we can specify a likelihood function and proceed along well-established lines constructing *score equations* and obtaining standard errors of the estimators from the *information matrix*. Maximum likelihood estimators have the most desirable properties of all (such as efficiency), but only in *large samples*, and test statistics become χ^2-distributed. For example, we can't usually say that maximum likelihood estimators are unbiased (which is a small sample property), only that they are *consistent*. This means that they will converge to the parameter value as the sample size n goes to infinity. We also, in most cases, don't know the sampling distributions of maximum likelihood estimators in small samples, only that they and test statistics become approximately normally or chi-square distributed in large samples. With normally distributed residuals we can often do better than likelihood theory in small samples by relying on special developments, such as unbiased estimators for variance components, t- and F-tests.

The multivariate normal distribution was given in Chapter 8 as

$$f_Y(Y) = \frac{1}{(2\pi)^{\frac{k}{2}}\sqrt{det\,V}}\exp\left[-\frac{1}{2}(Y-\mu)'V^{-1}(Y-\mu)\right]$$

In Chapter 8 we did not write the score equations arising from the multivariate normal distribution. However, because we already know that the estimator is [equation (8.2), replacing R by V to move away from PROC MIXED, REPEATED statement notation]

$$\hat{\beta} = \left(\sum_i X_i' V_i^{-1} X_i\right)^{-1}\sum_i X_i' V_i^{-1} Y_i$$

we can infer (backwards) that the score equations are

$$\sum_i X_i' V_i^{-1}(Y_i - X_i\hat{\beta}) = 0$$

Because (in line with what we have seen in Chapter 12) the derivatives of each element of $X_i\hat{\beta}$ with respect to the elements of $\hat{\beta}$ are $(1, x_{1i}, x_{2i}, \ldots)$, the matrix X_i is actually the matrix of derivatives from each data point for person i, and we can write the score equations in the notation similar to that of Chapter 12 as

$$\sum_i D_i' V_i^{-1}(Y_i - X_i\hat{\beta}) = \sum_i D_i' V_i^{-1}(Y_i - \hat{\mu}_i) \qquad (15.1)$$

15.2 FURTHER DEVELOPMENTS FOR THE EXPONENTIAL FAMILY

The basic problem in generalizing developments such as the above is that there are few convenient multivariate distributions corresponding to non-normal members of the exponential family. There are some, of course, and new formulations of distributions are continually proposed in the literature. However, the mainstream of analysis has moved away from the pure maximum likelihood approach and looked at other options.

The first step in further development of Chapter 12 without specifying new multivariate distributions is taking a close look at equation (12.6):

$$D'V^{-1}(Y - \hat{\mu}) = 0 \qquad (15.2)$$

Equation (15.2), as we recall, contains the score equations for the exponential family with arbitrary link function (i.e., when h is not necessarily the canonical link). When we solve the equations, we, of course, obtain maximum likelihood estimators for the regression parameters lurking inside the inverse link function. The difference between equations (15.2) and (15.1) is that in (15.2) the data points were assumed independent, so that V^{-1} is diagonal, and that μ contains the inverse of the link function h so D' contains s derivatives of that inverse besides the x's.

The beauty of (15.2) is that the only traces that are left of the original distribution used to construct the likelihood equation in the first place are its mean structure and its variance. All other quantities (e.g., its skewness and kurtosis) do not matter for obtaining the maximum likelihood estimators. This is a rather remarkable feature of the exponential family. Based on this observation, people started thinking that if they had the two functions needed—h describing the link between the mean and the regression equation, and g describing how the variance depends on the mean—they could just *assume* that (15.2) is a score equation from a likelihood. One can even integrate (15.2) and come up with a likelihood from a supposed distribution from the exponential family. Sometimes it turns out to be a known distribution. The method of starting from (15.2) assuming that the formula arose from a likelihood is referred to as *quasi-likelihood* [64]. When people use that approach they take second derivatives to obtain standard errors etc. Quasi-likelihood serves the purpose of taking us away from thinking we have to *know* the distribution. It is closely related to least squares because we have similar weighted estimating equations and have not made specific distributional assumptions. As long as we think we are dealing with some type of likelihood, we can form tests and obtain standard errors for large samples based on likelihood theory.

Quasi-likelihood as usually developed still only deals with independent data. However, looking at equation (15.1) and comparing it to (15.2), statisticians came up with the further idea that they could be combined. After all, quasi-likelihood had freed them from the need to specify distributions. Why not expand (15.2) to look like (15.1) by making the variance be a matrix containing both variances and covariances and then letting D have elements $h^{-1'}(\beta_0 + \beta_1 x_{1ij} + \cdots) \times x_{1ij}$. Note that a subscript j has been added to indicate that there are now several observations for each i. Assuming that observations from different individuals are independent (as we have done), we obtain

$$\sum_i D_i' V_i^{-1} (Y_i - \mu_i) = 0 \tag{15.3}$$

In these situations, it is common to separate the contributions of the correlation and the variance to V_i by writing

$$V_i = A_i^{\frac{1}{2}} R_i A_i^{\frac{1}{2}}$$

$$= \begin{pmatrix} \sigma_1 & 0 & 0 & \cdots \\ 0 & \sigma_2 & 0 & \cdots \\ 0 & 0 & \sigma_3 & \cdots \\ \cdots & \cdots & \cdots & \cdots \end{pmatrix} \begin{pmatrix} 1 & \rho_{12} & \rho_{13} & \cdots \\ \rho_{12} & 1 & \rho_{23} & \cdots \\ \rho_{13} & \rho_{23} & 1 & \cdots \\ \cdots & \cdots & \cdots & \cdots \end{pmatrix} \begin{pmatrix} \sigma_1 & 0 & 0 & \cdots \\ 0 & \sigma_2 & 0 & \cdots \\ 0 & 0 & \sigma_3 & \cdots \\ \cdots & \cdots & \cdots & \cdots \end{pmatrix}$$

We see that A_i is the matrix that has the variances of ϵ_{ij} in the diagonal and $A^{\frac{1}{2}i}$ has the square root of those variances (i.e., the standard deviations). The variances on the diagonal of A_i are based on the relationship between the mean and the variance. For example, if we are dealing with Poisson data, we have

$$\sigma_j^2 = \mu_{ij} = \exp(\beta_0 + \beta_1 x_{1i} + \cdots)$$

Because of the uncertainty about variances in the situation with correlated data, overdispersion is always taken into account in these situations. It happens automatically with the equations used in estimating the standard errors (see below). The equations contained in (15.3) in the case of correlated data are referred to as *generalized estimating equations (GEE)*. Also, because we don't know that R_i is the true correlation matrix, whatever we specify for the estimation is referred to as a *working correlation* matrix.

15.3 HOW ARE THE GENERALIZED ESTIMATING EQUATIONS JUSTIFIED?

The above development is intuitively appealing, but somewhat ad hoc. Of course it could not be used unless people had proven that the resulting estimators are reasonable. We obviously can no longer depend on maximum likelihood to assure us that things are OK. No distribution that gave rise to the estimating equations in the correlated case may exist. Nor do we necessarily know that we have specified the correct variance structure, even if a distribution with that structure existed and lead to score equations that depended only on the mean and variance. Because of this, the papers that originally introduced the above framework (the most well known and most often cited being by Liang and Zeger [76]) proved that:

1. The estimators obtained by solving (15.3) are *consistent* as long as the mean structure is correctly specified, and reasonable (converging as n becomes large) estimators are plugged in for the variance parameters. However, it is not necessary that the variance structure be correctly specified.

2. In large samples the variance matrix of estimators obtained from (15.3) can be estimated by

$$\hat{V}_\beta = \hat{\text{Var}}(\hat{\beta})$$

$$= \left(\sum D_i' W_i D_i\right)^{-1} \left(\sum D_i' W_i \hat{\epsilon}_i \hat{\epsilon}' W_i D_i\right) \left(\sum D_i' W_i D_i\right)^{-1} \quad (15.4)$$

where W_i is V_i^{-1} with the working correlation.

Formula (15.4) is very similar to that of the **empirical variance** (8.5) used by PROC MIXED and the one we used to adjust for overdispersion in Chapter 14. When h is the identity link function, the empirical variance from PROC MIXED and (15.4) are indeed the same. For other cases, X_i is replaced by D_i that contains the derivatives of the inverse link function, besides x. In this general case, $\hat{\epsilon}$ consists of the elements

$$\epsilon_{ij} = y_{ij} - h^{-1}(\beta_0 + \beta_1 x_{1i} + \cdots)$$

Note that equation (15.4) does not explicitly include the dispersion parameter. Rather, the "variance" is empirically obtained for each observation. In other words, $\sum \hat{\epsilon}_i \hat{\epsilon}'_i$ is not obtained as a single estimator ϕ (and ϵ_i are the ordinary, not Pearson or deviance, residuals).

It is important to note that although the results here look similar to those for the multivariate normal distribution, all statements about the properties of the estimators are prefaced *in large samples.* Instead of unbiasedness in the face of misspecification of the variance structure, we have *consistency*; and the variance of the regression parameters also holds only in large samples. Its derivation, in addition to the formulas for variances for linear transformations we used before, contains Taylor approximations that hold only in large samples. The actual way the parameters are estimated is beyond the scope here. As usual, an iterative least-squares solution is employed.

We demonstrate the application and results of the above procedures in our longitudinal data sets with systolic blood pressure as an example of a variable with normally distributed residuals, hypertension as an example of binary outcome, and the number of hospitalizations at each age up to 5 years as an example of count data.

15.3.1 Analysis of Longitudinal Systolic Blood Pressure by PROC MIXED and GENMOD

We start with a comparison of PROC MIXED and PROC GENMOD for fitting the longitudinal (continuous) data on systolic blood pressure from the Wisconsin Sleep Cohort. This is a normally distributed residual case with identity link function, and we fit a compound symmetry correlation structure. (Although the AR(1) structure fits better, the compound symmetry option makes the comparison of the procedures more transparent.) In the context of generalized estimating equations, the compound symmetry is often referred to as "exchangeable," but GENMOD accepts either name in its REPEATED statement. *Not* specifying a correlation structure for GENMOD in SAS version 8 leads to the independence option just as it does in PROC MIXED. The commands we used for PROC MIXED were as usual, except that we requested the ML method for greater comparability with GENMOD:

PROC MIXED NOCLPRINT EMPIRICAL METHOD=ML;
CLASSES ID SEX;
MODEL SBP=SEX AGEM AGED BMIC AGEM*BMIC/S;
REPEATED/SUBJECT=ID TYPE=CS RCORR;

For PROC GENMOD the commands were

PROC GENMOD; CLASSES ID SEX;
MODEL SBP=SEX AGEM AGED BMIC AGEM*BMIC;
REPEATED SUBJECT=ID/TYPE=CS CORRW;

In each case we requested the correlation matrix to be printed by the RCORR and CORRW options, respectively. The output is in OUTPUT PACKET XVII. It is important to notice that GENMOD has given two sets of analyses. The first assumes that the data are independent. The likelihood, and so on, refer to that case, and they are markedly different from the likelihood given by MIXED that is based on the multivariate normal distribution with nonzero correlation between residuals. The second part of the GENMOD output is based on the generalized estimating equation (GEE) approach. For the normal case, the estimating equations are actually (14.1) from the likelihood, but GENMOD does not acknowledge this. Because GEE is generalized beyond the likelihood situation, no likelihood related statistics are provided for the correlated analysis. We compare coefficients with the CS option, empirical standard errors, and some other statistics in Table 15.1.

Comparing parameter estimates and standard errors from the second part of GENMOD and MIXED, one sees that they are very similar, but not identical. This is due to differences in algorithms used in fitting and of little consequence. The $-2\log(L)$ from GENMOD ($=19,397$) is comparable to the $-2\log(REML)$

Table 15.1   Comparing Results from PROC MIXED and PROC GENMOD for SBP

	MIXED	GENMOD
Intercept	126 (0.459)	126 (0.458)
Female	-5.82 (0.659)	-5.83 (0.659)
Age between (centered at 50)	0.419 (0.0451)	0.421 (0.0450)
Age within (centering cancels)	-0.710 (0.104)	-0.710 (0.104)
BMI (centered at 27)	0.678 (0.0551)	0.679 (0.0550)
Age between *BMI (centered)	-0.0124 (0.00695)	-0.0126 (0.0069)
within individual correlation	0.378	0.354
Total variance	$71.0570 + 116.74 = 188$	$13.6742^2 = 187$
Residual variance	116.74	
$-2\log(L)$ for CS model	19230.7	
$-2\log(L)$ with independence		2(9698.822)

from PROC MIXED in Section 8.5.3 of 19,491.5. The SCALE parameter from GENMOD and the residual from MIXED are fundamentally different as GENMOD estimates the SCALE for the independence situation, and they do not separate out the variance parameters. Rather the SCALE from GENMOD corresponds to the square root of the total variance from PROC MIXED. It is clear that for the special case of normally distributed residuals, PROC MIXED provides more information than does PROC GENMOD.

15.3.2 Analysis of Longitudinal Hypertension Data by PROC GENMOD

Throughout this text, we have alluded to the fact that differences in the between- and within-individual coefficients when regressing systolic blood pressure on age were caused by an increase in taking hypertensive medications. We are now finally in a position to analyze data on hypertension that take into account medication use. Readers who might have thought all along that we could somehow have "adjusted" analyses of SBP for medication use are referred to Heitjan and Landis [77] for a discussion of the difficulties.

Hypertension status was determined by blood pressure (SBP $\geq$ 140 or DBP $\geq$ 90) for individuals not taking hypertensive medication. All individuals on hyper- tensive medication at a given visit were classified as hypertensive at that visit. The longitudinal hypertension data were analyzed as hypertensive (HBP $= 1$) or not (HBP $= 0$) by PROC GENMOD. We first confirm that the difference in within- and between-individual coefficients is gone, by a procedure that is parallel to the one we recommended in Chapter 9 (Chao, Palta, and Young [78] generalized the approach to binary outcome data).

PROC GENMOD DESCENDING; CLASS ID SEX;
MODEL HBP=SEX AGEM AGED BMIC AGEM*BMIC/DIST=BINOMIAL;
REPEATED SUBJECT=ID/TYPE=CS;

Outputs are in OUTPUT PACKET XVII. The results show that both the coef- ficient of mean age and the coefficient of the age by BMI interaction are now far from significance and are also small in size compared to the main effects. Pos- sibly, the interaction we found with continuous outcome was generated by more obese older persons being more likely to receive hypertensive medication. The longitudinal model for hypertension was therefore fit without these effects by the commands:

PROC GENMOD DESCENDING; CLASS ID SEX;
MODEL HBP= SEX AGEC BMIC/DIST=BINOMIAL;
REPEATED SUBJECT=ID/TYPE=CS CORRW;

Again our attention will be directed to the second part of the output that uses the empirical standard errors. Table 15.2 shows the independence-based and correlation-corrected regression coefficients and standard errors.

We see that the standard errors are uniformly larger from the correlated analysis than those assuming independence of observations. If the model fits well, we expect

Table 15.2 $\hat{\beta}$(Model se) for Independence and $\hat{\beta}$ (Empirical se) for Compound Symmetry

	Independence		Compound Symmetry	
Intercept (age 50, BMI 27)	−0.846	(0.637)	−0.846	(0.0723)
Female	−0.688	(0.0997)	−0.633	(0.112)
Age (per year)	0.0506	(0.0059)	0.0529	(0.0065)
BMI	0.0965	(0.0075)	0.0923	(0.0085)

little difference in the estimates of the regression coefficients whether independence (as in the first part of the output) or compound symmetry (second part) is used. Finally, we see in the output that the correlation between the binary observations for an individual is estimated at 0.322. It is common for binary outcomes to yield lower correlation than the corresponding continuous outcomes.

15.3.2.1   Some Additional Adjustments

There is still a slight difference between coefficients based on the independence and compound symmetry models, and we may want to make sure there is not bias due to some individuals completing a larger number of visits.

We demonstrate one way to adjust for the number of visits by a so-called pattern mixture approach [79,80]. We ran the following commands where the variable NOBS is the number of visits completed by an individual centered at 1.77 (i.e., $k_i - 1.77$ in our usual notation). The centering was chosen, because 2 is the average number of visits. We ran

PROC GENMOD DESCENDING; CLASS ID SEX;
MODEL HBP= SEX AGEC BMIC NOBS NOBS*SEX/DIST=BINOMIAL;
REPEATED SUBJECT=ID/TYPE=CS;

These commands have the effect of "adjusting" the effect of gender to the "level of follow-up for the average person." We have shown this to be an acceptable procedure for adjusting for dropout in many situations [80]. Table 15.3 provides adjusted coefficients for the independence and compound symmetry models. Finally, we also reapplied the survey weights discussed in Chapter 7. This is done by a WEIGHT statement in GENMOD. Although GENMOD refers to the weights

Table 15.3   Adjusting for Number of Follow-up Visits and for Survey Weights

	IN Adjusted		CS Adjusted		CS Adjusted with Survey Weights	
Intercept (age 50, BMI27)	−0.883	(0.0747)	−0.863	(0.0744)	−0.943	(0.0844)
Female	−0.602	(0.116)	−0.587	(0.115)	−0.491	(0.129)
Age (per year)	0.0503	(0.0059)	0.0530	(0.0065)	0.0578	(0.0073)
BMI	0.0961	(0.0075)	0.0921	(0.0085)	0.0901	(0.0097)

as "scale weights," their application leads to the desirable end result, as long as the empirical GEE standard errors are chosen. (In fact the weights we applied in PROC REG and PROC MIXED were also internally treated as scale weights.)

The coefficients of NOBS and its interaction hold no subject matter importance, and they cannot be generalized to other situations. They just serve to adjust for study dropout. We see that the adjustment for the number of visits has little effect on odd analysis. Survey weights affect the coefficient of sex in the hypertension analysis, although the effect of applying weights in the systolic blood pressure analysis in Chapter 7 was moderate disguised the weight effect.

The regression coefficients are as always with the logit link interpreted as log(odds ratios). The commands

ESTIMATE 'PER DECADE' AGEC 10/EXP;
ESTIMATE 'PER UNIT BMI' BMIC 1/EXP;
ESTIMATE 'FEMALE' SEX 1 -1/EXP;

were added to the run. These produce odds ratios and confidence intervals for the associations of hypertension with a 10-year increase in age, with a unit increase in BMI, and between females and males. Note how the last ESTIMATE statement accommodates the fact that the variable SEX was declared in the CLASS statement.

We provide the odds ratios, 95% confidence intervals, and risk of hypertension at age 50 and BMI 27 in Table 15.4. The odds ratios were obtained by ESTIMATE commands, and the risk was obtain by

$$\hat{\pi}_0 = \exp(\hat{\beta}_0)/(1 + \exp(\hat{\beta}_0)) = \exp(-0.943)/(1 + \exp(-0.943)) = 0.280$$

The confidence intervals for this risk were obtained by the formula from Chapter 6 (also cf. formulas in Section 13.2),

$$\mathrm{Var}[f(y)] \approx [f'(\mu_y)]^2 \mathrm{Var}(y) = [0.280(1 - 0.280)]^2 \times (0.0844)^2 = 0.000240$$

where the last quantity is the standard error of $\hat{\beta}_0$. Then $\mathrm{se}(\hat{\pi}_0) = \sqrt{0.00301} = 0.0174$, and the confidence interval for the risk follows.

15.3.3 Analysis of Hospitalizations Among VLBW Children Up to Age 5

In the data set on very-low-birth-weight children, medical records were obtained up to age 5, and all hospitalizations were recorded. Turning to a longitudinal analysis of

Table 15.4 Risk, Odds Ratios, and 95% Confidence Intervals from Final Model

Hypertension risk (age 50, BMI 27)	0.280 [0.247, 0.313]
Odds ratio: female vs. male	0.612 [0.476, 0.788]
Odds ratio: for age (per decade)	1.783 [1.545, 2.058]
Odds ratio: for BMI (per unit)	1.094 [1.074, 1.115]

the hospitalization data, OUTPUT PACKET XVIII first shows the total number of hospitalizations at each age. It is clear that the majority of hospitalizations occurred in infancy. A regression was fit to all years of follow-up by the commands

AGESQ=AGE**2;
BWC=BW-1000;
LTIME=LOG(TIME);
PROC GENMOD; CLASS ID;
MODEL NHOSP=AGE AGESQ BWC/DIST=POISSON OFFSET=LTIME;
REPEATED SUBJECT=ID/TYPE=CS CORRW;
ESTIMATE 'BW/100G' BW 100/EXP;
ESTIMATE 'AGE 2 VS. 0' AGE 2 AGESQ 4/EXP;
ESTIMATE 'RATE AGE 0 1000G' INTERCEPT/EXP;

This run tells GENMOD to use the compound symmetry correlation option. The CORRW options asks GENMOD to print out the estimated correlation matrix. Output is in OUTPUT PACKET XVIII. Again, the "initial estimates" do not take correlation into account, and attention should be directed toward the second set "GEE Parameter Estimates." Table 15.5 shows a comparison of the longitudinal results with those of modeling hospitalization only during the first year of life. In both cases, we show the empirical standard errors produced by GENMOD.

Not much power was gained by the longitudinal analysis over using just the first-year observations. This is because the number of hospitalization decreased drastically with age. Of course, GEE has the unique advantage of allowing us to include age as a covariate in the first place. We see that the hospitalization rate decreased with age, but then flattened out. We used the ESTIMATE commands to translate the model into the rate at age 0 and 1000 g birth weight, the rate ratio with 100 g increase in birth weight and the rate ratio between ages 2 and 0 (Table 15.6). This used the commands

ESTIMATE 'RR/100G' BWC 100/EXP;
ESTIMATE 'RR age 0 vs 2' AGE 2 AGESQ 4/EXP;
ESTIMATE ' AGE 0, 1000 G' INTERCEPT 1/EXP;

The 95% confidence intervals are automatically based on the empirical standard errors. A point to be noted is that because all children are observed at the same ages in the above analyses and since birth weight is a non-time-varying covariate,

Table 15.5   Regression Coefficients (Empirical se) for Hospitalization of VLBW Children

	First Year Only	Up to Age 5
Intercept	−0.268 (0.112)	−0.278 (0.112)
Age		−1.40 (0.166)
Age squared		0.246 (0.397)
Birth weight (g)	−0.0018 (0.0004)	−0.0015 (0.0004)

Table 15.6   Rate and Rate Ratios (Empirical se) for Hospitalization of VLBW Children

Rate at age 0, 1000 g	0.758 [0.609, 0.943]
Rate ratio age 2 vs. 0	0.162 [0.111, 0.236]
Rate ratio per 100 g birth weight	0.859 [0.797, 0.927]

the issue of between- and within-individual effects does not enter. All age effects are automatically within-individual effects.

The CORRW option estimates a correlation of 0.386 between years, but it should be noted that the correlation matrix is not estimated very reliably by GEE. In addition, the correlation between binary or count variables is not the most interpretable measure of association. There are alternative approaches that yield more meaningful parameters of association between measurements.

15.4   ANOTHER WAY TO DEAL WITH CORRELATED BINARY DATA

A pure within-individual (i.e., pure longitudinal) analysis can be performed by so-called conditional likelihood. With this approach, all comparisons are within-individual, and non-time-varying covariates can only enter as interaction effects with time-varying covariates. Conditional logistic regression is well known in epidemiologic applications with matched cases and controls [65]. PROC PHREG in SAS can be tricked into doing conditional logistic regression. As an illustration, a conditional logistic regression for the hypertension data can be run by

```
AGE10=AGE/10;
STATUS=2-HBP;
PROC PHREG NOSUMMARY;
MODEL STATUS*HBP(0)= AGE10 BMIC/TIES=DISCRETE RL;
STRATA ID;
```

The explanation of what this program does is beyond the scope here. Basically, it just happens that the likelihood for grouped, stratified survival data coincides with that for conditional logistic regression. The NOSUMMARY option prevents the printing of all the IDs, much like the NOCLPRINT option in PROC MIXED. The RL option leads to the printing of confidence intervals.

The odds ratios as computed by this procedure are compared with the corresponding odds ratios from GENMOD based on Table 15.2. The conditional logistic odds ratio for age was obtained by the above rescaling of age to be measured in decades. Note the labeling "hazard ratio," which implies that the exponentiated coefficient is in fact a rate ratio. This is not the case, however, with "discrete" outcomes as here, where the odds ratio is used as an approximation to the hazard ratio.

The results are in OUTPUT PACKET XIX. Table 15.7 illustrates the substantial loss in power when cross-sectional information (e.g., comparison of people at different ages and BMI's) is discarded. This leads to individuals who did not change

Table 15.7 Odds Ratios [95% CI] from GEE and from Conditional Logistic Regression

	GEE	Conditional Logistic
Age (per decade)	1.71 [1.50, 1.95]	3.16 [1.82, 5.48]
BMI	1.10 [1.08, 1.12]	1.04 [0.952, 1.14]

hypertension status not entering the analysis at all. In fact, BMI is no longer significant. We note the much higher odds ratio for age with the conditional logistic procedure. This partly due to the known discrepancy [65] that matched odds ratios are higher than unmatched ones. This difference is difficult to operationalize, but can be best understood in terms of the latent variable concept [81]. In this context, conditional ratios, sometimes known as "subject-specific" odds ratios, are regression coefficients standardized to the within-individual standard deviation of the outcome. GEE, also known as "marginal" or "population-averaged" coefficients, are standardized to the standard deviation that includes between-individual variation. Neuhaus et al. [82] performed an extensive comparison of subject-specific and population-averaged coefficients.

Finally, we have not covered here a whole host of procedures based on random effects for generalized linear models. Such models differ quite fundamentally from the GENMOD approach outlined above. Random effects models for binary data, in fact, are closely related to the latent variable approach briefly introduced in Chapter 12, because a continuous random effect will serve as a latent variable. When independence of random effects from the covariates is satisfied, coefficients from random effects models for binary data produce regression coefficients that are, in principle, the same as those from conditional logistic regression. However, between-individual information is not discarded, and within- and between-individual coefficients can differ just as with a marginal analysis [83].

Random effects models for generalized linear models with normally distributed random effects can be fit in SAS by PROC NLMIXED. Pendergast et al. [84] provides a broad review of the methods of this chapter and others.

OUTPUT PACKET XVII: MIXED VERSUS GENMOD FOR LONGITUDINAL SBP AND HYPERTENSION DATA

XVII.1. Longitudinal Analysis with ML and Compound Symmetry

Analysis of sbp-MIXED vs. GENMOD—All Visits Wisconsin Sleep Cohort
Compound Symmetry with PROC MIXED
  The Mixed Procedure

Model Information

Data set	WORK.AB
Dependent variable	SBP
Covariance structure	Compound symmetry
Subject effect	id
Estimation method	**ML**
Residual variance method	Profile
Fixed effects SE method	**Empirical**
Degrees-of-freedom method	Between–within

Dimensions

Covariance parameters	2
Columns in X	7
Columns in Z	0
Subjects	1370
Maximum observations per subject	3
Observations used	2404
Observations not used	33
Total observations	2437

Estimated R Correlation: Matrix for id S0001

Row	Col1	Col2	Col3
1	1.0000	**0.3784**	**0.3784**
2	0.3784	1.0000	**0.3784**
3	0.3784	0.3784	1.0000

Covariance Parameter Estimates

Covariance Parameter	Subject	Estimate
CS	id	**71.0570**
Residual		**116.74**

Fit Statistics

−2 Log likelihood	**19230.7**
AIC (smaller is better)	19246.7
AICC (smaller is better)	19246.8
BIC (smaller is better)	19288.5

Solution for Fixed Effects

Effect	Sex	Estimate	Standard Error	DF	t Value	$Pr > |t|$
Intercept		125.55	0.4588	1367	273.67	<0.0001
sex	F	−5.8227	0.6590	1367	−8.84	<0.0001
sex	M	0	.	.	.	.
agem		0.4191	0.04508	1367	9.30	<0.0001
aged		−0.7100	0.1044	1031	−6.80	<0.0001
bmic		0.6776	0.05509	1031	12.30	<0.0001
agem*bmic		−0.01242	0.006953	1031	−1.79	0.0743

Type 3 Tests of Fixed Effects

Effect	Num DF	Den DF	F Value	$Pr > F$
sex	1	1367	78.06	<0.0001
agem	1	1367	86.43	<0.0001
aged	1	1031	46.24	<0.0001
bmic	1	1031	151.26	<0.0001
agem*bmic	1	1031	3.19	0.0743

Compound Symmetry with PROC GENMOD
   The GENMOD Procedure

Model Information

Data set	WORK.AB	
Distribution	**Normal**	
Link function	**Identity**	
Dependent variable	SBP	(Systolic blood pressure in mmHg)
Observations used	2404	
Missing values	33	

Class Level Information

Class	Levels	Values							
id	1374	S0001	S0003	S0005	S0007	S0008	S0009	S0012	S0013
		S0014	S0017	S0018	S0019	S0020	S0021	S0022	S0023
		S0027	S0028	S0031	S0032	S0035	S0036	S0037	S0038
		S0039	S0040	S0042	S0046	S0049	S0050	S0051	S0053
		S0054	S0055	S0057	S0061	S0062	S0065	S0066	S0067
		S0071	S0072	...					
sex	2	F M							

Parameter Information

Parameter	Effect	Sex
Prm1	Intercept	
Prm2	sex	F
Prm3	sex	M
Prm4	agem	
Prm5	aged	
Prm6	bmic	
Prm7	agem*bmic	

Criteria for Assessing Goodness of Fit[a]

Criterion	DF	Value	Value/DF
Deviance	2398	449511.3477	**187.4526**
Scaled deviance	2398	2404.0000	1.0025
Pearson chi-square	2398	449511.3477	187.4526
Scaled Pearson X2	2398	2404.0000	1.0025
Log likelihood		−9698.8228	

[a] Algorithm converged.

Analysis of Initial Parameter Estimates

Parameter		DF	Estimate	Standard Error	Wald 95% Confidence Limits		Chi-Square
Intercept		1	125.5403	0.3935	124.7690	126.3115	101772
sex	F	1	−5.9850	0.5674	−7.0971	−4.8729	111.26
sex	M	0	0.0000	0.0000	0.0000	0.0000	.
agem		1	0.4387	0.0397	0.3609	0.5164	122.37
aged		1	−0.7079	0.1195	−0.9422	−0.4737	35.08
bmic		1	0.7048	0.0455	0.6157	0.7938	240.45
agem*bmic		1	−0.0143	0.0057	−0.0255	−0.0031	6.25
Scale		1	13.6742	0.1972	13.2931	14.0663	

Analysis of Initial Parameter Estimates

Parameter		Pr > ChiSq
Intercept		<0.0001
sex	F	<0.0001
sex	M	.
agem		<0.0001
aged		<0.0001
bmic		<0.0001
agem*bmic		0.0124
Scale		

Note: The scale parameter was estimated by maximum likelihood.

GEE Model Information[a]

Correlation structure	Exchangeable
Subject effect	id (1370 levels)
Number of clusters	1370
Clusters with missing values	33
Correlation matrix dimension	3
Maximum cluster size	3
Minimum cluster size	0

[a] Algorithm converged.

Working Correlation Matrix

	Col1	Col2	Col3
Row1	1.0000	**0.3542**	**0.3542**
Row2	0.3542	1.0000	**0.3542**
Row3	0.3542	0.3542	1.0000

Analysis of GEE Parameter Estimates
Empirical Standard Error Estimates

Parameter		Estimate	Standard Error	95% Confidence Limits		Z	Pr > |Z|
Intercept		125.5499	0.4584	124.6515	126.4482	273.91	<0.0001
sex	F	−5.8303	0.6589	−7.1216	−4.5389	−8.85	<0.0001
sex	M	0.0000	0.0000	0.0000	0.0000	.	.
agem		0.4205	0.0450	0.3322	0.5088	9.34	<0.0001
aged		−0.7100	0.1044	−0.9147	−0.5053	−6.80	<0.0001
bmic		0.6791	0.0550	0.5713	0.7869	12.35	<0.0001
agem*bmic		−0.0126	0.0069	−0.0262	0.0010	−1.81	0.0703

XVII.2. Analysis of Longitudinal Hypertension Data (Binary Outcome)

Analysis of Longitudinal Hypertension Data with GENMOD
Checking Model Fit by Including Mean Age
   The GENMOD Procedure

Model Information

Data set	WORK.AB
Distribution	**Binomial**
Link function	**Logit**
Dependent variable	HBP
Observations used	2404
Missing values	1

Class Level Information

Class	Levels	Values							
id	1370	S0001	S0003	S0005	S0007	S0008	S0009	S0012	S0013
		S0014	S0017	S0018	S0019	S0020	S0021	S0022	S0023
		S0027	S0028	S0031	S0032	S0035	S0036	S0037	S0038
		S0039	S0040	S0042	S0046	S0049	S0050	S0051	S0053
		S0054	S0055	S0057	S0061	S0062	S0065	S0066	S0067
		S0071	S0072	...					
sex	2	F M							

Response Profile[a]

Ordered Value	HBP	Total Frequency
1	1	752
2	0	1652

[a]PROC GENMOD is modeling the probability that hbp = '1'.

Criteria for Assessing Goodness of Fit

Criterion	DF	Value	Value/DF
Deviance	2398	2677.8374	1.1167
Scaled deviance	2398	2677.8374	1.1167
Pearson chi-square	2398	2367.4793	0.9873
Scaled Pearson X2	2398	2367.4793	0.9873
Log likelihood		−1338.9187	

Analysis of Initial Parameter Estimates

Parameter		DF	Estimate	Standard Error	Wald 95% Confidence Limits		Chi-Square
Intercept		1	−0.8352	0.0642	−0.9611	−0.7094	169.29
sex	F	1	−0.6958	0.0998	−0.8914	−0.5001	48.58
sex	M	0	0.0000	0.0000	0.0000	0.0000	.
agec		1	0.0591	0.0200	0.0200	0.0982	8.78
agem		1	−0.0027	0.0211	−0.0441	0.0386	0.02
bmic		1	0.0935	0.0077	0.0783	0.1086	146.55
agem*bmic		1	−0.0016	0.0010	−0.0036	0.0004	2.53
Scale		0	1.0000	0.0000	1.0000	1.0000	

GEE Model Information

Correlation structure	Exchangeable
Subject effect	id (1370 levels)
Number of clusters	1370
Clusters with missing values	1
Correlation matrix dimension	3
Maximum cluster size	3
Minimum cluster size	1

Analysis of GEE Parameter Estimates
Empirical Standard Error Estimates

Parameter		Estimate	Standard Error	95% Confidence Limits		Z	Pr > |Z|
Intercept		−0.8361	0.0729	−0.9790	−0.6933	−11.47	<0.0001
sex	F	−0.6379	0.1119	−0.8573	−0.4185	−5.70	<0.0001
sex	M	0.0000	0.0000	0.0000	0.0000	.	.
agec		0.0589	0.0172	0.0252	0.0926	3.43	0.0006
agem		**−0.0015**	**0.0189**	**−0.0386**	**0.0357**	**−0.08**	**0.9388**
bmic		0.0893	0.0088	0.0721	0.1065	10.19	<0.0001
agem*bmic		**−0.0014**	**0.0012**	**−0.0037**	**0.0009**	**−1.15**	**0.2485**

Initial Model for Hypertension
  The GENMOD Procedure

Model Information

Data set	WORK.AB
Distribution	**Binomial**
Link function	**Logit**
Dependent variable	HBP
Observations used	2404
Missing values	1

Criteria for Assessing Goodness of Fit

Criterion	DF	Value	Value/DF
Deviance	2400	2680.5704	1.1169
Scaled deviance	2400	2680.5704	1.1169
Pearson chi-square	2400	2360.3061	0.9835
Scaled Pearson X2	2400	2360.3061	0.9835
Log likelihood		−1340.2852	

Analysis of Initial Parameter Estimates

Parameter		DF	Estimate	Standard Error	Wald 95% Confidence Limits		Chi-Square
Intercept		1	−0.8464	0.0637	−0.9713	−0.7215	176.32
sex	F	1	−0.6878	0.0997	−0.8832	−0.4924	47.59
sex	M	0	0.0000	0.0000	0.0000	0.0000	.
agec		1	0.0506	0.0059	0.0391	0.0620	74.53
bmic		1	0.0965	0.0075	0.0817	0.1112	164.81
Scale		0	1.0000	0.0000	1.0000	1.0000	

Analysis of Initial Parameter Estimates

Parameter		Pr > ChiSq
Intercept		<0.0001
sex	F	<0.0001
sex	M	.
agec		<0.0001
bmic		<0.0001
Scale		

Note: The scale parameter was held fixed.

GEE Model Information

Correlation structure	Exchangeable
Subject effect	id (1370 levels)
Number of clusters	1370
Clusters with missing values	1
Correlation matrix dimension	3
Maximum cluster size	3
Minimum cluster size	1

Working Correlation Matrix

	Col1	Col2	Col3
Row1	1.0000	**0.3216**	**0.3216**
Row2	0.3216	1.0000	**0.3216**
Row3	0.3216	0.3216	1.0000

Analysis of GEE Parameter Estimates
Empirical Standard Error Estimates

Parameter		Estimate	Standard Error	95% Confidence Limits		Z	Pr > |Z|
Intercept		−0.8460	0.0723	−0.9877	−0.7043	−11.70	<0.0001
sex	F	−0.6328	0.1120	−0.8522	−0.4133	−5.65	<0.0001
sex	M	0.0000	0.0000	0.0000	0.0000	.	.
agec		0.0529	0.0065	0.0402	0.0656	8.18	<0.0001
bmic		0.0923	0.0085	0.0757	0.1090	10.90	<0.0001

XVII.3. Adjusting for Compliance and Survey Weights

Analysis of Longitudinal Hypertension Data with GENMOD
Adjusting for Number of Visits
   The GENMOD Procedure

Model Information

Data set	WORK.AB
Distribution	Binomial
Link function	Logit
Dependent variable	HBP
Observations used	2404
Missing values	1

Criteria for Assessing Goodness of Fit

Criterion	DF	Value	Value/DF
Deviance	2398	2676.0363	1.1159
Scaled deviance	2398	2676.0363	1.1159
Pearson chi-square	2398	2354.3237	0.9818
Scaled Pearson X2	2398	2354.3237	0.9818
Log likelihood		−1338.0182	

Analysis of Initial Parameter Estimates

Parameter		DF	Estimate	Standard Error	Wald 95% Confidence Limits		Chi-Square
Intercept		1	−0.8825	0.0695	−1.0186	−0.7463	161.37
sex	F	1	−0.6020	0.1071	−0.8120	−0.3921	31.58
sex	M	0	0.0000	0.0000	0.0000	0.0000	.
agec		1	0.0503	0.0059	0.0387	0.0619	72.40
bmic		1	0.0961	0.0075	0.0814	0.1109	163.42
nobs		1	0.1105	0.0818	−0.0499	0.2708	1.82
nobs*sex	F	1	−0.2894	0.1362	−0.5564	−0.0225	4.52
nobs*sex	M	0	0.0000	0.0000	0.0000	0.0000	.
Scale		0	1.0000	0.0000	1.0000	1.0000	

Analysis of GEE Parameter Estimates
Empirical Standard Error Estimates

Parameter		Estimate	Standard Error	95% Confidence Limits		Z	Pr > |Z|
Intercept		−0.8627	0.0744	−1.0085	−0.7169	−11.60	<0.0001
sex	F	−0.6586	0.1147	−0.8115	−0.3693	−5.11	<0.0001
sex	M	0.0000	0.0000	0.0000	0.0000	.	.
agec		0.0530	0.0065	0.0403	0.0658	8.14	<0.0001
bmic		0.0921	0.0085	0.0755	0.1088	10.83	<0.0001
nobs		**0.0867**	**0.0964**	**−0.1023**	**0.2757**	**0.90**	**0.3687**
nobs*sex	**F**	**−0.2823**	**0.1566**	**−0.5893**	**0.0246**	**−1.80**	**0.0714**
nobs*sex	M	0.0000	0.0000	0.0000	0.0000	.	.

The GENMOD Procedure

Model Information

Data set	WORK.AB
Distribution	Binomial
Link function	**Logit**
Dependent variable	**HBP**
Scale weight variable	**wgt**
Observations used	2404
Missing values	1

GEE Model Information

Correlation structure	Exchangeable
Subject effect	id (1370 levels)
Number of clusters	1370
Clusters with missing values	1
Correlation matrix dimension	3
Maximum cluster size	3
Minimum cluster size	1

Working Correlation Matrix

	Col1	Col2	Col3
Row1	1.0000	**0.3281**	**0.3281**
Row2	0.3281	1.0000	**0.3281**
Row3	0.3281	0.3281	1.0000

Analysis of GEE Parameter Estimates
Empirical Standard Error Estimates

Parameter		Estimate	Standard Error	95% Confidence Limits		Z	$\Pr > |Z|$
Intercept		−0.9427	0.0844	−1.1081	−0.7773	−11.17	<0.0001
sex	F	−0.4910	0.1238	−0.7434	−0.2385	−3.81	<0.0001
sex	M	0.0000	0.0000	0.0000	0.0000	.	.
agec		0.0578	0.0073	0.0435	0.0722	7.90	<0.0001
bmic		0.0901	0.0097	0.0710	0.1092	9.25	<0.0001
nobs		−0.0222	0.1101	−0.2379	0.1935	−0.20	0.8402
nobs*sex	F	−0.2535	0.1722	−0.5910	0.0839	−1.47	0.1409
nobs*sex	M	0.0000	0.0000	0.0000	0.0000	.	.

Contrast Estimate Results

Label	Estimate	Standard Error	Alpha	Confidence	Limits
per decade	0.5783	0.0732	0.05	0.4349	0.7218
Exp(per decade)	**1.7831**	**0.1305**	**0.05**	**1.5448**	**2.0581**
per unit bmi	0.0901	0.0097	0.05	0.0710	0.1092
Exp(per unit bmi)	**1.0943**	**0.0107**	**0.05**	**1.0736**	**1.1153**
female	−0.4910	0.1278	0.05	−0.8001	−0.2992
Exp(female)	**0.6120**	**0.0788**	**0.05**	**0.4755**	**0.7878**

OUTPUT PACKET XVIII: LONGITUDINAL ANALYSIS OF RATES

Rehospitalization of VLBW children—Newborn Lung Project
Number of Hospitalizations (Total) by Age

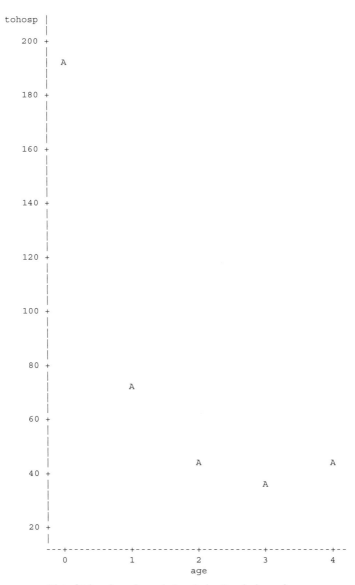

Plot of tohosp*age. Legend: A = 1 obs, B = 2 obs, and so on.

Poisson Regression with Rate Ratio per 100 g Birth Weight
  The GENMOD Procedure

Model Information

Data set	WORK.G
Distribution	**Poisson**
Link function	**Log**
Dependent variable	nhosp
Offset variable	ltime
Observations used	1725

Criteria for Assessing Goodness of Fit

Criterion	DF	Value	Value/DF
Deviance	1721	1488.1153	0.8647
Scaled deviance	1721	1488.1153	0.8647
Pearson chi-square	1721	3632.8425	2.1109
Scaled Pearson X2	1721	3632.8425	2.1109
Log likelihood		−864.0146	

Analysis of Initial Parameter Estimates

Parameter	DF	Estimate	Standard Error	Wald 95% Confidence Limits		Chi-Square
Intercept	1	−0.2878	0.0714	−0.4277	−0.1479	16.25
age	1	−1.3747	0.1262	−1.6220	−1.1274	118.73
agesq	1	0.2413	0.0334	0.1758	0.3067	52.22
bwc	1	−0.0014	0.0002	−0.0017	−0.0010	45.11
Scale	0	1.0000	0.0000	1.0000	1.0000	

Analysis of Initial Parameter Estimates

Parameter	Pr > ChiSq
Intercept	<0.0001
age	<0.0001
agesq	<0.0001
bwc	<0.0001
Scale	

Note: The scale parameter was held fixed.

GEE Model Information

Correlation structure	Exchangeable
Subject effect	id (345 levels)
Number of clusters	345
Correlation matrix dimension	5
Maximum cluster size	5
Minimum cluster size	5

Working Correlation Matrix

	Col1	Col2	Col3	Col4	Col5
Row1	1.0000	**0.3862**	**0.3862**	**0.3862**	**0.3862**
Row2	0.3862	1.0000	**0.3862**	**0.3862**	**0.3862**
Row3	0.3862	0.3862	1.0000	**0.3862**	**0.3862**
Row4	0.3862	0.3862	0.3862	1.0000	**0.3862**
Row5	0.3862	0.3862	0.3862	0.3862	1.0000

Analysis of GEE Parameter Estimates and Empirical Standard Error Estimates

Parameter	Estimate	Standard Error	95% Confidence Limits		Z	Pr > |Z|
Intercept	−0.2775	0.1117	−0.4963	−0.0587	−2.49	0.0129
age	−1.4021	0.1660	−1.7275	−1.0767	−8.45	<0.0001
agesq	0.2463	0.0397	0.1685	0.3241	6.21	<0.0001
bwc	−0.0015	0.0004	−0.0023	−0.0008	−3.92	<0.0001

Contrast Estimate Results

Label	Estimate	Standard Error	Alpha	Confidence	Limits
RR/100 g	−0.1517	0.0387	0.05	−0.2276	−0.0758
Exp(RR/100 g)	**0.8593**	**0.0333**	**0.05**	**0.7965**	**0.9270**
RR age 0 vs. 2	−1.8189	0.1919	0.05	−2.1950	−1.4429
Exp(RR age 0 vs. 2)	**0.1622**	**0.0311**	**0.05**	**0.1114**	**0.2362**
rate age 0, 1000 g	−0.2775	0.1117	0.05	−0.4963	−0.0587
Exp(age 0,1000 g)	**0.7577**	**0.0846**	**0.05**	**0.6088**	**0.9430**

OUTPUT PACKET XIX: CONDITIONAL LOGISTIC REGRESSION OF HYPERTENSION DATA

Conditional Logistic Regression of Hypertension
  The PHREG Procedure

Model Information

Data set	WORK.AB
Dependent variable	status
Censoring variable	hbp
Censoring value(s)	0
Ties handling	DISCRETE

Convergence Status

Convergence criterion (GCONV = 1E-8) satisfied.

Model Fit Statistics

Criterion	Without Covariates	With Covariates
−2 LOG L	378.988	354.951
AIC	378.988	358.951
SBC	378.988	368.138

Testing Global Null Hypothesis: BETA = 0

Test	Chi-Square	DF	Pr > ChiSq
Likelihood ratio	24.0365	2	<0.0001
Score	23.4913	2	<0.0001
Wald	22.5662	2	<0.0001

Analysis of Maximum Likelihood Estimates

Variable	DF	Parameter Estimate	Standard Error	Chi-Square	Pr > ChiSq
age10	1	1.14893	0.28182	16.6209	<0.0001
bmic	1	0.04166	0.04610	0.8166	0.3662

Analysis of Maximum Likelihood Estimates

Variable	Hazard Ratio	95% Hazard Confidence	Ratio Limits
age10	3.155	1.816	5.481
bmic	1.043	0.952	1.141

References

1. SAS Institute Inc., *SAS/STAT User's Guide. Version 8*, SAS Institute Inc., Cary, NC, 1999.

2. M. Palta, G. Shen, C. Allen, R. Klein, and D. D'Alessio, "Longitudinal Glycosylated Hemoglobin Patterns from Diagnosis in a Population Based Cohort with IDDM," *American Journal of Epidemiology*, **114**, 954–961 (1996).

3. D. L. DeMets, and M. Halperin, "Estimation of a Simple Regression Coefficient in Samples Arising from a Sub-sampling Procedure," *Biometrics*, **33**, 47–56 (1977).

4. R. J. Carroll, D. Ruppert, and L. A. Stefanski, *Measurement Error in Nonlinear Models*, Chapman and Hall, London, 1995.

5. C. E. McCullagh, and S. R. Searle, *Generalized, Linear, and Mixed Models*, Wiley-Interscience, Chichester, 2000.

6. P. Diggle, P. Heagerty, K.-Y. Liang, and S. Zeger, *Analysis of Longitudinal Data*, 2nd edition, Oxford University Press, New York, 2002.

7. J. A Rice, *Mathematical Statistics and Data Analysis,* Duxbury Press, Belmont, CA, 1995.

8. G. W. Snedecor and W. G. Cochran, *Statistical Methods*, 7th edition, Iowa State University Press, Ames, IA, 1980.

9. P. J. Huber, "The Behavior of Maximum Likelihood Estimates under Non-Standard conditions," *Proceedings of the Fifth Berkeley Symposium on Mathematical Statistics and Probability*, **1**, 221–233 (1967).

10. H. White, "A Heteroskedasticity Consistent Covariance Matrix Estimator and a Direct Test for Heteroskedasticity," *Econometrica*, **48**, 817–830 (1980).

11. D. G. Fryback, T. Young, M. Palta, L. Finn, and P. Meek, "Direct Outpatient Medical Costs of Sleep Apnea: A Population Study," *Medical Decision Making*, **18**, 466 (1998).

12. J. Mullahy, "Much Ado about Two: Reconsidering Retransformation and the Two-Part Model in Health Econometrics," *Journal of Health Economics*, **17**, 247–281 (1998).

13. W. Manning, and J. Mullahy, "Estimating Log Models: To Transform or Not to Transform?" *Journal of Health Economics*, **17**, 461–494 (2001).

14. N. W. Draper and H. Smith, *Applied Regression Analysis*, John Wiley & Sons, New York, 1998.

Quantitative Methods in Population Health, by Mari Palta
ISBN 0-471-45505-9   Copyright © 2003 John Wiley & Sons, Inc.

15. J. A. Hausman, "Specification Tests in Econometrics," *Econometrics*, **46**, 1251–1271 (1978).

16. T. Young, M. Palta, J. Dempsey, J. Skatrud, S. Weber, and S. Badr, "Occurrence of Sleep Disordered Breathing among Middle-Aged Adults," *New England Journal of Medicine*, **328**, 69–77 (1993).

17. E. L. Korn, and B. I. Graubard, *Analysis of Health Surveys*, Wiley-Interscience, Chichester, 1999.

18. L. C. Lazzeroni and R. J. A. Little, "Random-Effects Models for Smoothing Post-stratification Weights," *Journal of Official Statistics*, **14**, 61–78 (1998).

19. R. J. A. Little, and D. B. Rubin, *Statistical Analysis with Missing Data*, John Wiley, New York, 1987.

20. M. Palta, M. Sadek, M. Evans, M. R. Weinstein, and G. McGuinness, "Functional Assessment of a Multicenter VLBW Cohort at Age 5 Years," *Archives of Pediatrics and Adolescent Medicine*, **154**, 23–30 (2000).

21. S. M. Haley, W. J. Caster, L. H. Ludlow, J. T. Haltiwanger, and P. J. Andrellos, *Pediatric Evaluation of Disability Inventory (PEDI), Version 1, Development, Standardization and Administration Manual.* New England Medical Center-PEDI Research Group, Boston, 1992.

22. M. Palta, M. R. Weinstein, G. McGuinness, D. Gabbert, W. Brady, and M. E. Peters, "A Population Study: Mortality and Morbidity after Availability of Surfactant Therapy," *Archives of Pediatrics and Adolescent Medicine*, **148**, 1295–1301 (1994).

23. J. M. Wooldridge, *Introductory Econometrics: A Modern Approach*, 2nd edition, South-Western College Publishing, Mason, OH, 2002.

24. D. O. Scharfstein, A. Rotnitzky, and J. M. Robins, "Adjusting for Nonignorable Drop-Out Using Semiparametric Nonresponse Models (with discussion)," *Journal of the American Statistical Association*, **94**, 1096–1120 (1999).

25. G. E. P. Box, G. M. Jenkins, and G. C. Reinsel, *Time Series Analysis: Forecasting & Control*, 3rd edition, Prentice-Hall, Upper Saddle River, NJ, 1994.

26. S. Lipschutz, and M. L. Lipson, *Schaum's Outline of Linear Algebra*, 3rd edition, McGraw-Hill, New York, 2000.

27. T. W. Anderson, *An Introduction to Multivariate Statistical Analysis*, 2nd edition, John Wiley & Sons, New York, 1984.

28. H. Brown and R. Prescott, *Applied Mixed Models in Medicine*, Wiley-Interscience, Chichester, 1999.

29. R. V. Hogg and A. T. Craig, *Introduction to Mathematical Statistics*, 5th edition, Prentice-Hall, Upper Saddle River, NJ, 1994.

30. T. S. Lin and C. M. Dayton, "Model-Selection Information Criteria for Non-nested Latent Class Models," *Journal of Educational and Behavioral Statistics*, **22**, 249–264 (1997).

31. J. Wishart, "Growth-Rate Determinations in Nutrition Studies with the Bacon Pig, and Their Analysis," *Biometrika*, **30**, 16–28 (1938) .

32. M. Palta and T-J. Yao, "Analysis of Longitudinal Data with Unmeasured Confounders," *Biometrics* **47**, 1355–1369 (1991).

33. J. M. Neuhaus and J. D. Kalbfleisch, "Between and Within-Cluster Covariate Effects in the Analysis of Clustered Data," *Biometrics*, **54**, 638–645 (1998).

34. L. Shen, M. Palta, J. Shao, and S. Park S, "Model Misspecification and Different Between- and Within-Cluster Covariate Effects in the Analysis of Correlated Data,"

Proceedings of the Biometrics Section of the American Statistical Association, 219–224 (1999).

35. W. Pan, T. A., Louis, and J. E. Connett, "A Note on Marginal Linear Regression with Correlated Response Data," *The American Statistician*, **54**, 191–195 (2000).

36. J. A. Berlin, S. E. Kimmel, T. R. Ten Have, and M. D. Samuel, "Empirical Comparison of Several Clustered Data Approaches under Confounding Due to Cluster Effects in the Analysis of Complications of Coronary Angioplasty," *Biometrics*, **55**, 470–476 (1999).

37. W. M. Vollmer, L. R. Johnson, L. E. McCamant, and A. S. Buist, "Longitudinal Versus Cross-Sectional Estimation of Lung Function Decline—Further Insights," *Statistics in Medicine*, **7**, 685–696 (1988).

38. J. H. Ware, D. W. Dockery, T. A. Louis, X. Xu, B. J. Ferris, and F. E. Speizer, "Longitudinal and Cross-Sectional Estimates of Pulmonary Function Decline in Never-Smoking Adults," *American Journal of Epidemiology*, **132**, 685–700, (1990).

39. C. J. Newschaffer, T. L. Bush, T. L., and W. E. Hale, "Aging and Total Cholesterol Level: Cohort, Period and Survivorship Effect," *American Journal of Epidemiology*, **136**, 23–34 (1992).

40. G. S. Maddala, "The Use of Variance Components Models in Pooling Cross Sectional and Time Series Data," *Econometrica*, **39**, 341–358 (1971).

41. Y. Mundlak, "On the Pooling of Time Series and Cross-Sectional Data," *Econometrics*, **46**, 69–86 (1978).

42. J. A. Hausman and W. E. Taylor, "Panel Data and Unobservable Individual Effects," *Econometrics*, **49**, 1377–1398 (1981).

43. J. M. Wooldridge, *Econometric Analysis of Cross Section and Panel Data*, MIT Press, Boston, 2001.

44. B. H. Baltagi, *Econometric Analysis of Panel Data*, John Wiley & Sons, Chichester, 2001.

45. A. J. Scott and D. Holt, "The Effect of Two-Stage Sampling on Ordinary Least Squares Methods," *Journal of the American Statistical Association*, **77**, 848–854 (1982).

46. J. H. Dwyer, M. Feinleib, P. Lippert, and H. Hoffmeister, *Statistical Models for Longitudinal Studies of Health*, Chapter 1, Oxford University Press, New York, 1992.

47. T. T. Wansbeek and E. Meijer, *Measurement Error and Latent Variables in Econometrics, Advanced Textbooks in Economics* 37, C. J. Bliss and M. D. Intriligator, eds. North-Holland, Elsevier Science B.V., Amsterdam, The Netherlands, 2000.

48. L. Shen, M. Palta, J. Shao, and S. Park, "Consistent Estimation of Marginal Regression Parameters for Longitudinal Data with Covariate Measurement Error When Replicates Are Not Available," *Proceedings of the Biometrics Section of the American Statistical Association*, 2000.

49. T. A. Louis, J. Robins, D. W. Dockery, A. III. Spiro, and J. F. Ware, "Explaining Discrepancies Between Longitudinal and Cross-Sectional Models," *Journal of Chronic Diseases*, **39**, 831–839 (1986).

50. L. Shen, *Analyses of Longitudinal Data: Measurement Error, Confounding and Model Misspecification,* Ph.D. Dissertation, University of Wisconsin, Madison, 2001.

51. M. Palta and C. Seplaki, "Causes, Problems and Benefits of Different Between and Within Effects in the Analysis of Clustered Data," *Health Services and Outcomes Research*, in press (2003).

52. M. Nerlove, *Essays in Panel Data Econometrics*, Cambridge University Press, New York, 2002.

53. M. Palta, T. J. Yao, and R. Velu, "Testing for Omitted Variables and Non-linearity in Regression Models for Longitudinal Data," *Statistics in Medicine*, **13**, 2219–2231 (1994).

54. V. L. Burt, J. A. Cutler, M. Higgins, M. J. Horan, D. Labarthe, P. Whelton, C. Brown, and E. J. Roccella, "Trends in the Awareness, Treatment and Control of Hypertension in the Adult US Population," *Hypertension*, **26**, 60–69 (1995).

55. P. E. Peppard, T. Young T, M. Palta, and J. Skatrud, "Association Between Sleep Disordered Breathing and Hypertension," *New England J. of Medicine*, **342**, 1378–1384 (2000).

56. N. M. Laird and J. H. Ware, "Random Effects Models for Longitudinal Data," *Biometrics*, **38**, 963–974 (1982).

57. G. Verbeke and G. Molenberghs, *Linear Mixed Models in Practice: An Sas-Oriented Approach*, Lecture Notes in Statistics, Vol. 126, Springer-Verlag, New York, 1997.

58. S. W. Raudenbush and A. S. Bryk, *Hierarchical Linear Models: Applications and Data Analysis Methods, Advanced Quantitative Techniques in the Social Sciences*, 2nd edition, Sage Publications, Thousand Oaks, CA, 2002.

59. N. Blomquist, "On the Relation Between Change and Initial Value," *Journal of the American Statistical Association*, **72**, 746–749 (1977).

60. C. Morris, "Parametric Empirical Bayes Inference: Theory and Applications," *Journal of the American Statistical Association*, **78**, 47–55 (1983).

61. A. Hrobjartson and P. C. Gøtzsche, "Is the Placebo Powerless? An Analysis of Clinical Trials Comparing Placebo with No Treatment," *New England Journal of Medicine*, **344**, 1594–1602 (2001).

62. L. W. Pickle, M. N. Mungiole, G. K. Jones, and A. A. White, *Atlas of United States Mortality*, National Center for Health Statistics, Hyattsville, 1996.

63. T. A. Louis and E. Conlon, "Evaluating Region-Specific Geographic Risk Using Bayes and Empirical Bayes Methods," *BIOMED-WHO Workshop on Disease Mapping and Risk Assessment for Public Health Decision Making*, 1997.

64. P. McCullagh and J. A. Nelder, *Generalized Linear Models*, 2nd edition, CRC Press, Boca Raton, FL, 1989.

65. N. E. Breslow and N. E. Day, *Statistical Methods in Cancer Research*, Vol I. International Agency for Research on Cancer, Lyon 1980.

66. L. Harms, "Leading Diagnoses Associated with Pediatric Hospitalizations in Wisconsin, 1990," *Wisconsin Health Data Review*, **5(7)**, 1–7 (1991).

67. J. Grizzle, C. F. Starmer, and G. G. Koch, "Analysis of Categorical Data by Linear Models," *Biometrics*, **25**, 489–504 (1969).

68. D. W. Hosmer and S. Lemeshow, *Applied Logistic Regression*, 2nd edition, John Wiley & Sons, New York, 2000.

69. G. A. Milliken and D. E. Johnson, *Analysis of Messy Data. Volume 1: Designed Experiments,* Chapman & Hall, London, 1992.

70. S. Selvin, *Statistical Analysis if Epidemiologic Data*, 2nd edition, Oxford University Press, New York, 1996.

71. A. Hald, *Statistical Theory with Engineering Applications*, John Wiley & Sons, New York, 1952.

72. R. J. Tallarida and L. S. Jacob, *The Dose–Response Relation in Pharmacology*, Springer-Verlag, New York, 1979.

73. B. O. Muthen, "A Structural Probit Model with Latent Variables," *Journal of The American Statistical Association*, **74**, 807–881 (1979).

74. J. P. Klein and M. L. Moeschberger, *Survival Analysis, Techniques for Censored and Truncated Data*, Springer-Verlag, New York, 1997.

75. Centers for Disease Control. Wideranging ONline Data for Epidemiologic Research (WONDER). USPHS, DHSS.

76. K. Y. Liang and S. L. Zeger, "Longitudinal Data Analysis Using Generalized Linear Models," *Biometrika*, **73**, 13–22 (1986).

77. D. F. Heitjan, and J. R. Landis, "Assessing Secular Trends in Blood Pressure: A Multiple Imputation Approach," *Journal of the American Statistical Association*, **89**, 750–759 (1994).

78. W. Chao, M. Palta, and T. Young T, "Effect of Omitted Confounders on the Analysis of Correlated Binary Data," *Biometrics*, **53**, 678–689 (1997).

79. M. C. Wu and D. A. Follman, "Use of Summary Measures to Adjust for Informative Missingness in Repeated Measures Data with Random Effects" *Biometrics*, **55**, 75–84 (1999).

80. S. Park, M. Palta, J. Shao, and L. Shen, "Bias Adjustment in Analyzing Longitudinal Data with Informative Missingness," *Statistics in Medicine*, **21**, 277–291 (2002).

81. M. Palta and C-Y. Lin, "Latent Variables, Measurement Error and Methods for Analysing Longitudinal Binary and Ordinal Data," *Statistics in Medicine*, **18**, 385–396 (1999).

82. J. M. Neuhaus, J. D. Kalbfleisch, and W. W. Hauck, "A Comparison of Cluster-Specific and Population-Averaged Approaches for Analyzing Clustered Binary Data," *International Statistical review*, **59**, 25–31 (1991).

83. M. Palta, C-Y. Lin, and W. Chao, "Effect of Confounding and Other Misspecification in Models for Longitudinal Data," in *Modeling Longitudinal and Spatially Correlated Data*. Lecture Notes in Statistics Series, 122. Proceedings of the Nantucket Conference on Longitudinal and Correlated Data, Springer-Verlag, New York, 1997.

84. J. E. Pendergast, S. J. Gange, M. A. Newton, M. J. Lindstrom, M. Palta, and M. R. Fisher, "A Survey of Methods for Analyzing Clustered Binary Response Data," *International Statistical Review*, **64**, 1–30 (1996).

Appendix: Matrix Operations

Matrices are two-dimensional arrays of numbers that come with rules on how to combine and transform them in various ways by addition, multiplication, and inversion. The purpose of working with matrices is to be able to write, in shorthand, expressions where large sets of numbers are summed or form sums of cross products. The algebraic rules for matrices are designed so that most properties of ordinary numbers hold. Matrices are extensively used in a wide range of applications including statistics, population ecology, and physics.

A matrix is typically constructed when there are several sets of multiple numbers measuring a set of phenomena. For example, there may be a set of covariates measured on each person, or there may be percentages of a population in different age groups at given time points. To demonstrate matrix operations, we let these numbers be generic and chosen to be easy to add and multiply. Matrices are typically designated by bold uppercase letters. Let the matrix $\mathbf{A}$ be defined as

$$\mathbf{A} = \begin{pmatrix} 1 & 5 & 2 \\ 4 & 3 & 1 \end{pmatrix}$$

Typically, this means that one person or time point had measurements 1, 5, 2 and another had 4, 3, 1. These individual numbers are called *elements* of the matrix. We refer to the above matrix as having 2 rows and 3 columns, or as being of *dimension* 2 by 3 (written as 2×3). The special case of a 1×1 matrix consists of just one number. Generically, we will designate the number of rows as n and the number of columns as m, and write a matrix as

$$\mathbf{A} = \begin{pmatrix} a_{11} & a_{12} & \cdot & a_{1j} & \cdot & a_{1m} \\ a_{21} & a_{22} & \cdot & a_{2j} & \cdot & a_{2m} \\ \cdot & \cdot & \cdot & \cdot & \cdot & \cdot \\ a_{i1} & a_{i2} & \cdot & a_{ij} & \cdot & a_{im} \\ \cdot & \cdot & \cdot & \cdot & \cdot & \cdot \\ a_{n1} & a_{n2} & \cdot & a_{nj} & \cdot & a_{nm} \end{pmatrix}$$

Quantitative Methods in Population Health, by Mari Palta
ISBN 0-471-45505-9   Copyright © 2003 John Wiley & Sons, Inc.

Here the generic element is a_{ij}, with i denoting row and j column. A matrix with the same number of rows as columns (i.e., $n = m$) is called a *square matrix*. For example,

$$A = \begin{pmatrix} 1 & 5 \\ 4 & 3 \end{pmatrix}$$

is a square 2×2 matrix. An important type of square matrix is a *symmetric* matrix. In a symmetric matrix, the ith row is the same as the ith column, so that the upper right triangle is the "mirror image" of the lower left triangle. An example of a symmetric matrix is

$$A = \begin{pmatrix} 1 & 4 & 2 \\ 4 & 3 & 6 \\ 2 & 6 & 9 \end{pmatrix}$$

Clearly, a symmetric matrix can be specified by just its diagonal and the elements above it. The reader has probably seen computer outputs with correlation coefficients between a set of variables. These can be arranged into a symmetric matrix.

A special case of a symmetric (square) matrix is a *diagonal* matrix. In a diagonal matrix, all elements off the diagonal are 0. An example of a diagonal matrix is

$$A = \begin{pmatrix} 2 & 0 & 0 & 0 \\ 0 & 9 & 0 & 0 \\ 0 & 0 & 4 & 0 \\ 0 & 0 & 0 & 1 \end{pmatrix}$$

A.1 ADDING MATRICES

Matrices of the same dimension can be added. The sum is the matrix that contains the sum of all the corresponding elements in the matrices being added. If, for example,

$$A = \begin{pmatrix} 1 & 4 & 2 \\ 4 & 3 & 6 \\ 2 & 6 & 9 \end{pmatrix}$$

and

$$B = \begin{pmatrix} 3 & 1 & -4 \\ 4 & 1 & 6 \\ 7 & 2 & 1 \end{pmatrix}$$

then

$$A + B = \begin{pmatrix} 1+3 & 4+1 & 2-4 \\ 4+4 & 3+1 & 6+6 \\ 2+7 & 6+2 & 9+1 \end{pmatrix} = \begin{pmatrix} 4 & 5 & -2 \\ 8 & 4 & 12 \\ 9 & 8 & 10 \end{pmatrix}$$

Because addition of matrices involves only adding individual elements, all the usual rules of ordinary addition apply. For example, it does not matter what order the matrices are added, that is,

$$\mathbf{A} + \mathbf{B} = \mathbf{B} + \mathbf{A}$$

and subtraction involves adding the negative of an element. Naturally, any number of matrices can be added together.

A.2 MULTIPLYING MATRICES BY A NUMBER

In the matrix context, a number is often referred to as a *scalar* to differentiate it from a matrix. A matrix can be multiplied by a scalar by multiplying each element by it. For example,

$$0.5 \begin{pmatrix} 2 & 1 & 5 \\ 1 & 3 & 1 \end{pmatrix} = \begin{pmatrix} 1 & 0.5 & 2.5 \\ 0.5 & 1.5 & 0.5 \end{pmatrix}$$

The usual rules of arithmetic apply to multiplication of a matrix by a scalar.

A.3 MULTIPLYING MATRICES BY EACH OTHER

Multiplication of matrices with each other is a more complex operation. Matrices $\mathbf{A}$ and $\mathbf{B}$ can be multiplied $\mathbf{A} \times \mathbf{B}$ if they "match" in such a way that the number of columns in $\mathbf{A}$ equals the number of rows in $\mathbf{B}$. The general formula for matrix multiplication is

$$\mathbf{A} \times \mathbf{B} = \mathbf{AB}$$

$$= \begin{pmatrix} a_{11} & a_{12} & \cdot & a_{1j} & \cdot & a_{1m} \\ a_{21} & a_{22} & \cdot & a_{2j} & \cdot & a_{2m} \\ \cdot & \cdot & \cdot & \cdot & \cdot & \cdot \\ a_{i2} & a_{i2} & \cdot & a_{ij} & \cdot & a_{im} \\ \cdot & \cdot & \cdot & \cdot & \cdot & \cdot \\ a_{n1} & a_{n2} & \cdot & a_{nj} & \cdot & a_{nm} \end{pmatrix} \begin{pmatrix} b_{11} & b_{12} & \cdot & b_{1j} & \cdot & b_{1p} \\ b_{21} & b_{22} & \cdot & b_{2j} & \cdot & b_{2p} \\ \cdot & \cdot & \cdot & \cdot & \cdot & \cdot \\ b_{i2} & b_{i2} & \cdot & b_{ij} & \cdot & a_{ip} \\ \cdot & \cdot & \cdot & \cdot & \cdot & \cdot \\ b_{m1} & b_{m2} & \cdot & b_{mj} & \cdot & b_{mp} \end{pmatrix}$$

$$= \begin{pmatrix} \sum_{l=1}^{m} a_{1l}b_{l1} & \sum_{l=1}^{m} a_{1l}b_{l2} & \cdot & \sum_{l=1}^{m} a_{1l}b_{lj} & \cdot & \sum_{l=1}^{m} a_{1l}b_{lp} \\ \sum_{l=1}^{m} a_{2l}b_{l1} & \sum_{l=1}^{m} a_{2l}b_{l2} & \cdot & \sum_{l=1}^{m} a_{2l}b_{lj} & \cdot & \sum_{l=1}^{m} a_{2l}b_{lp} \\ \cdot & \cdot & \cdot & \cdot & \cdot & \cdot \\ \sum_{l=1}^{m} a_{il}b_{l1} & \sum_{l=1}^{m} a_{il}b_{l2} & \cdot & \sum_{l=1}^{m} a_{il}b_{lj} & \cdot & \sum_{l=1}^{m} a_{il}b_{lp} \\ \cdot & \cdot & \cdot & \cdot & \cdot & \cdot \\ \sum_{l=1}^{m} a_{nl}b_{l1} & \sum_{l=1}^{m} a_{nl}b_{l2} & \cdot & \sum_{l=1}^{m} a_{nl}b_{lj} & \cdot & \sum_{l=1}^{m} a_{nl}b_{lp} \end{pmatrix}$$

We see that each element in the product is constructed as the sum of cross products of rows of **A** with columns of **B**. Consider a simple example:

$$
\begin{pmatrix} 2 & 4 & 1 \\ 1 & 6 & 5 \end{pmatrix}
\begin{pmatrix} 1 & 3 & 2 & 1 & 4 \\ 2 & 1 & 5 & 6 & 2 \\ 4 & 3 & 1 & 6 & 5 \end{pmatrix}
$$

$$
= \begin{pmatrix} 2 \times 1 + 4 \times 2 + 1 \times 4 & 2 \times 3 + 4 \times 1 + 1 \times 3 & 25 & 32 & 21 \\ 1 \times 1 + 6 \times 2 + 5 \times 4 & 1 \times 3 + 6 \times 1 + 5 \times 3 & 37 & 67 & 41 \end{pmatrix}
$$

Another example shows how matrices can be used to calculate sums and sums of squares:

$$
\begin{pmatrix} 1 & 1 & 1 \\ x_1 & x_2 & x_3 \end{pmatrix}
\begin{pmatrix} 1 & x_1 \\ 1 & x_2 \\ 1 & x_3 \end{pmatrix}
= \begin{pmatrix} 3 & \sum_{i=1}^{3} x_i \\ \sum_{i=1}^{3} x_i & \sum_{i=1}^{3} x_i^2 \end{pmatrix}
$$

The above type of matrix operation is performed often in regression analysis.

A difference between ordinary multiplication and matrix multiplication is that the order matters. Usually, **AB** does not equal **BA**. However, it is very useful to know that $(\mathbf{AB})' = \mathbf{B}'\mathbf{A}'$. For example,

$$
\left[\begin{pmatrix} 2 & 4 \\ 3 & 1 \end{pmatrix} \begin{pmatrix} 7 & 1 \\ 4 & 2 \end{pmatrix} \right]' = \begin{pmatrix} 30 & 10 \\ 25 & 5 \end{pmatrix}' = \begin{pmatrix} 30 & 25 \\ 10 & 5 \end{pmatrix}
$$

which equals

$$
\begin{pmatrix} 7 & 4 \\ 1 & 2 \end{pmatrix} \begin{pmatrix} 2 & 3 \\ 4 & 1 \end{pmatrix} = \begin{pmatrix} 14 + 16 & 21 + 4 \\ 2 + 8 & 3 + 2 \end{pmatrix} = \begin{pmatrix} 30 & 25 \\ 10 & 5 \end{pmatrix}
$$

It follows from the above rule that $\mathbf{AA}'$ and $\mathbf{A}'\mathbf{A}$ are both (square) symmetric matrices. Note, however, that they are not equal. Even their dimensions are usually not the same, as $\mathbf{AA}'$ is a $n \times n$ matrix, while $\mathbf{A}'\mathbf{A}$ is a $m \times m$ matrix.

The *commutative* property $\mathbf{AB} = \mathbf{BA}$ is the only property of ordinary multiplication of numbers that does not hold for the multiplication of matrices. Both the *associative*

$$
\mathbf{A}(\mathbf{BC}) = (\mathbf{AB})\mathbf{C}
$$

and *distributive*

$$
\mathbf{A}(\mathbf{B} + \mathbf{C}) = \mathbf{AB} + \mathbf{AC}
$$

properties hold.

Diagonal matrices have especially simple properties in matrix multiplication. When multiplying by a diagonal matrix from the left, every row i in the matrix being multiplied is multiplied by the corresponding element d_{ii} in the diagonal matrix.

$$\begin{pmatrix} 1.5 & 0 & 0 \\ 0 & 2 & 0 \\ 0 & 0 & 0.5 \end{pmatrix} \begin{pmatrix} 6 & 2 \\ 2 & 3 \\ 1 & 5 \end{pmatrix} = \begin{pmatrix} 9 & 3 \\ 4 & 6 \\ 0.5 & 2.5 \end{pmatrix}$$

When multiplying with a diagonal matrix from the right, it is every column that gets multiplied. It follows that multiplication by a diagonal matrix with all the elements identical has the same effect as multiplication by a scalar. For example,

$$\begin{pmatrix} 2 & 0 & 0 \\ 0 & 2 & 0 \\ 0 & 0 & 2 \end{pmatrix} \begin{pmatrix} 3.5 \\ 2 \\ 4 \end{pmatrix} = \begin{pmatrix} 7 \\ 4 \\ 8 \end{pmatrix} = 2 \begin{pmatrix} 3.5 \\ 2 \\ 4 \end{pmatrix}$$

A diagonal matrix with 1's on the diagonal is called an *identity* matrix and is written as **I**. Multiplication by **I** does not change a matrix, that is,

$$\mathbf{IA} = \mathbf{AI} = \mathbf{A}$$

A.4   THE INVERSE OF A MATRIX

"Division" of matrices is accomplished via multiplication by an *inverse*. With ordinary numbers, we can write a/b or equivalently ab^{-1}. Here the inverse number b^{-1} has the property that $bb^{-1} = b^{-1}b = 1$. Similarly for matrices, the inverse of a square matrix **A** is defined as the matrix $\mathbf{A}^{-1}$ that has the property

$$\mathbf{AA}^{-1} = \mathbf{A}^{-1}\mathbf{A} = \mathbf{I}$$

The concept of inverses is practical only for square matrices. The inverse can be used to solve matrix equations, similarly to how ordinary equations of numbers are solved. For example, if we have the equation

$$\mathbf{AX} = \mathbf{B}$$

we can multiply each side by $\mathbf{A}^{-1}$ and obtain

$$\mathbf{A}^{-1}\mathbf{AX} = \mathbf{A}^{-1}\mathbf{B}$$

or

$$\mathbf{X} = \mathbf{A}^{-1}\mathbf{B}$$

Often in statistics, a matrix is changed into a square matrix by multiplication by the transpose so that the inverse can be constructed.

Actually obtaining the inverse of a matrix is not a trivial task in most cases. For a diagonal matrix, it is easy, because the inverse is just the matrix with the inverses of the individual elements on its diagonal, that is,

$$
\begin{pmatrix} a_1 & 0 & 0 \\ 0 & a_2 & 0 \\ 0 & 0 & a_3 \end{pmatrix}^{-1} = \begin{pmatrix} \frac{1}{a_1} & 0 & 0 \\ 0 & \frac{1}{a_2} & 0 \\ 0 & 0 & \frac{1}{a_3} \end{pmatrix}
$$

This can easily be verified by multiplying the two matrices.

For other matrices, the computation of an inverse is tied to the concept of a *determinant*. First of all, only matrices with nonzero determinants can be inverted. For a diagonal matrix the determinant is the product of all the diagonal elements. Clearly, if one of the elements is 0, the inverse of that element would entail division by 0, so the inverse of the matrix cannot be formed. For a 1×1 matrix the determinant equals the single element of the matrix. For a 2×2 matrix, the determinant can also be easily calculated. The determinant of is sometimes denoted by *det* of the matrix, or by slashes around the elements, as follows:

$$
det \begin{pmatrix} a & b \\ c & d \end{pmatrix} = \begin{vmatrix} a & b \\ c & d \end{vmatrix} = ad - bc
$$

For example

$$
\begin{vmatrix} 2 & 3 \\ 0 & 1 \end{vmatrix} = 2
$$

indicating that the matrix is invertible. A matrix with determinant >0 is referred to as *positive definite*. However,

$$
\begin{vmatrix} 3 & 2 \\ 6 & 4 \end{vmatrix} = 0
$$

indicating that the matrix is not invertible. A determinant is 0 when a row (or a column) is a multiple or linear combination of other rows or columns. We see that in the above matrix the second row is obtained by multiplying each corresponding element in the first row by 2. The determinant will also, more obviously, be 0 if an entire row or column consists of 0's.

The inverse of a 2×2 matrix is given by

$$
\begin{pmatrix} a & b \\ c & d \end{pmatrix}^{-1} = \frac{1}{ad - bc} \begin{pmatrix} d & -b \\ -c & a \end{pmatrix}
$$

Notice that the determinant is in the denominator, so the requirement that it not be 0 makes sense. On can easily verify that the above expression yields the inverse by carrying out the multiplication

$$\begin{pmatrix} a & b \\ c & d \end{pmatrix} \frac{1}{ad - bc} \begin{pmatrix} d & -b \\ -c & a \end{pmatrix} = \frac{1}{ad - bc} \begin{pmatrix} a & b \\ c & d \end{pmatrix} \begin{pmatrix} d & -b \\ -c & a \end{pmatrix}$$

$$= \frac{1}{ad - bc} \begin{pmatrix} ad - bc & -ab + ba \\ cd - dc & -cb + da \end{pmatrix} = \begin{pmatrix} 1 & 0 \\ 0 & 1 \end{pmatrix}$$

Notice how, in the first step, we made use of the fact that a scalar can be moved anywhere in the chain of multiplication (but obviously matrices have to stay in their positions).

As an example, the inverse of the matrix

$$\begin{pmatrix} 2 & 3 \\ 0 & 1 \end{pmatrix} \text{ is } \tfrac{1}{2} \begin{pmatrix} 1 & -3 \\ 0 & 2 \end{pmatrix} = \begin{pmatrix} 0.5 & -1.5 \\ 0 & 1 \end{pmatrix}$$

To be able to write determinants and inverses in general form requires the definition of the *cofactor*. The cofactor of a matrix element a_{ij} is defined in as the determinant of the smaller matrix obtained when row i and column j are deleted, multiplied by $(-1)^{i+j}$ of a matrix element a_{ij}. In the above 2×2 matrix,

$$\begin{pmatrix} a & b \\ c & d \end{pmatrix}$$

the cofactor of the element a is $(-1)^2 b = b$, and the cofactor of the element b is $(-1)^3 c = -c$. In a 3×3 matrix

$$\begin{pmatrix} a_{11} & a_{12} & a_{13} \\ a_{21} & a_{22} & a_{23} \\ a_{31} & a_{32} & a_{33} \end{pmatrix}$$

the cofactor of a_{11} is $(-1)^2 (a_{22}a_{33} - a_{23}a_{32})$ while the cofactor of a_{23} is $(-1)^5$ $(a_{11}a_{32} - a_{12}a_{31})$.

The definition of the cofactor allows one to build up determinants in a recursive manner, because the determinant of any $n \times n$ matrix is given by the formula

$$\sum_{i=1}^{n} a_{i1}(-1)^{i+1} A_{i1}{}'$$

where $(-1)^{i+1} A_{i1}$ is the cofactor of element a_{i1}. Note that the determinant of a 2×2 matrix $\begin{vmatrix} a & b \\ c & d \end{vmatrix} = ad - bc$ can be derived by the cofactor formula as $(-1)^2 ad + (-1)^3 cb$. For the 3×3 matrix above, the determinant formula means that we go down the first column and calculate the determinants of the corresponding 2×2 matrices that result when the first column and respective row i are deleted. We will not use the general formula for the determinant in practice because computer algorithms are available to invert matrices for us.

Finally, the determinant and cofactors are used to obtain the general formula for an inverse of a matrix as

$$
\mathbf{A}^{-1} = \frac{1}{det\mathbf{A}}
\begin{pmatrix}
(-1)^2 A_{11} & (-1)^3 A_{12} & \cdot & (-1)^{1+j} A_{1j} & \cdot & (-1)^{1+m} A_{1m} \\
(-1)^3 A_{21} & (-1)^4 A_{22} & & (-1)^{2+j} A_{2j} & \cdot & (-1)^{2+m} A_{2m} \\
\cdot & & \cdot & & \cdot & \\
(-1)^{i+1} A_{i1} & (-1)^{i+2} A_{i2} & \cdot & (-1)^{i+j} A_{ij} & \cdot & (-1)^{i+m} A_{im} \\
\cdot & \cdot & \cdot & \cdot & \cdot & \\
(-1)^{n+1} A_{n1} & (-1)^{n+2} A_{n2} & \cdot & (-1)^{n+j} A_{nj} & \cdot & (-1)^{n+m} A_{nm}
\end{pmatrix}^{'}
$$

This is the inverse of the determinant times the transpose of the matrix of cofactors. In examples we will only compute the inverse of a 2×2 matrix, explicitly. Applying the above formula to a 2×2 matrix, we again obtain

$$
\frac{1}{ad-bc}
\begin{pmatrix}
d & -c \\
-b & a
\end{pmatrix}^{'}
=
\frac{1}{ad-bc}
\begin{pmatrix}
d & -b \\
-c & a
\end{pmatrix}
$$

Index

Quantitative Methods in Population Health, by Mari Palta
ISBN 0-471-45505-9 Copyright © 2003 John Wiley & Sons, Inc.

WILEY SERIES IN PROBABILITY AND STATISTICS

ESTABLISHED BY WALTER A. SHEWHART AND SAMUEL S. WILKS

Editors

David J. Balding, Noel A. C. Cressie, Nicholas I. Fisher, Iain M. Johnstone, J. B. Kadane, Louise M. Ryan, David W. Scott, Adrian F. M. Smith, Jozef L. Teugels

Editors Emeriti: *Vic Barnett, J. Stuart Hunter David G. Kendall*

The *Wiley Series in Probability and Statistics* is well established and authoritative. It covers many topics of current research interest in both pure and applied statistics and probability theory. Written by leading statisticians and institutions, the titles span both state-of-the-art developments in the field and classical methods.

Reflecting the wide range of current research in statistics, the series encompasses applied, methodological and theoretical statistics, ranging from applications and new techniques made possible by advances in computerized practice to rigorous treatment of theoretical approaches.

This series provides essential and invaluable reading for all statisticians, whether in academia, industry, government, or research.

*Now available in a lower priced paperback edition in the Wiley Classics Library.

*Now available in a lower priced paperback edition in the Wiley Classics Library.

DAVID and NAGARAJA · Order Statistics, *Third Edition*

*DEGROOT, FIENBERG, and KADANE · Statistics and the Law

DEL CASTILLO · Statistical Process Adjustment for Quality Control

DETTE and STUDDEN · The Theory of Canonical Moments with Applications in
    Statistics, Probability, and Analysis

DEY and MUKERJEE · Fractional Factorial Plans

DILLON and GOLDSTEIN · Multivariate Analysis: Methods and Applications

DODGE · Alternative Methods of Regression

*DODGE and ROMIG · Sampling Inspection Tables, *Second Edition*

*DOOB · Stochastic Processes

DOWDY and WEARDEN · Statistics for Research, *Second Edition*

DRAPER and SMITH · Applied Regression Analysis, *Third Edition*

DRYDEN and MARDIA · Statistical Shape Analysis

DUDEWICZ and MISHRA · Modern Mathematical Statistics

DUNN and CLARK · Applied Statistics: Analysis of Variance and Regression, *Second Edition*

DUNN and CLARK · Basic Statistics: A Primer for the Biomedical Sciences,
    Third Edition

DUPUIS and ELLIS · A Weak Convergence Approach to the Theory of Large Deviations

*ELANDT-JOHNSON and JOHNSON · Survival Models and Data Analysis

ENDERS · Applied Econometric Time Series

ETHIER and KURTZ · Markov Processes: Characterization and Convergence

EVANS, HASTINGS, and PEACOCK · Statistical Distributions, *Third Edition*

FELLER · An Introduction to Probability Theory and Its Applications, Volume I,
    Third Edition, Revised; Volume II, *Second Edition*

FISHER and VAN BELLE · Biostatistics: A Methodology for the Health Sciences

*FLEISS · The Design and Analysis of Clinical Experiments

FLEISS · Statistical Methods for Rates and Proportions, *Second Edition*

FLEMING and HARRINGTON · Counting Processes and Survival Analysis

FULLER · Introduction to Statistical Time Series, *Second Edition*

FULLER · Measurement Error Models

GALLANT · Nonlinear Statistical Models

GHOSH, MUKHOPADHYAY, and SEN · Sequential Estimation

GIFI · Nonlinear Multivariate Analysis

GLASSERMAN and YAO · Monotone Structure in Discrete-Event Systems

GNANADESIKAN · Methods for Statistical Data Analysis of Multivariate Observations,
    Second Edition

GOLDSTEIN and LEWIS · Assessment: Problems, Development, and Statistical Issues

GREENWOOD and NIKULIN · A Guide to Chi-Squared Testing

GROSS and HARRIS · Fundamentals of Queueing Theory, *Third Edition*

*HAHN and SHAPIRO · Statistical Models in Engineering

HAHN and MEEKER · Statistical Intervals: A Guide for Practitioners

HALD · A History of Probability and Statistics and their Applications Before 1750

HALD · A History of Mathematical Statistics from 1750 to 1930

HAMPEL · Robust Statistics: The Approach Based on Influence Functions

HANNAN and DEISTLER · The Statistical Theory of Linear Systems

HEIBERGER · Computation for the Analysis of Designed Experiments

HEDAYAT and SINHA · Design and Inference in Finite Population Sampling

HELLER · MACSYMA for Statisticians

HINKELMAN and KEMPTHORNE: · Design and Analysis of Experiments, Volume 1:
    Introduction to Experimental Design

HOAGLIN, MOSTELLER, and TUKEY · Exploratory Approach to Analysis
    of Variance

HOAGLIN, MOSTELLER, and TUKEY · Exploring Data Tables, Trends and Shapes

*HOAGLIN, MOSTELLER, and TUKEY · Understanding Robust and Exploratory Data Analysis

*Now available in a lower priced paperback edition in the Wiley Classics Library.

KOTZ and JOHNSON (editors) · Encyclopedia of Statistical Sciences: Supplement Volume

KOTZ, READ, and BANKS (editors) · Encyclopedia of Statistical Sciences: Update Volume 1

KOTZ, READ, and BANKS (editors) · Encyclopedia of Statistical Sciences: Update Volume 2

KOVALENKO, KUZNETZOV, and PEGG · Mathematical Theory of Reliability of Time-Dependent Systems with Practical Applications

LACHIN · Biostatistical Methods: The Assessment of Relative Risks

LAD · Operational Subjective Statistical Methods: A Mathematical, Philosophical, and Historical Introduction

LAMPERTI · Probability: A Survey of the Mathematical Theory, *Second Edition*

LANGE, RYAN, BILLARD, BRILLINGER, CONQUEST, and GREENHOUSE · Case Studies in Biometry

LARSON · Introduction to Probability Theory and Statistical Inference, *Third Edition*

LAWLESS · Statistical Models and Methods for Lifetime Data, *Second Edition*

LAWSON · Statistical Methods in Spatial Epidemiology

LE · Applied Categorical Data Analysis

LE · Applied Survival Analysis

LEE and WANG · Statistical Methods for Survival Data Analysis, *Third Edition*

LePAGE and BILLARD · Exploring the Limits of Bootstrap

LEYLAND and GOLDSTEIN (editors) · Multilevel Modelling of Health Statistics

LIAO · Statistical Group Comparison

LINDVALL · Lectures on the Coupling Method

LINHART and ZUCCHINI · Model Selection

LITTLE and RUBIN · Statistical Analysis with Missing Data, *Second Edition*

LLOYD · The Statistical Analysis of Categorical Data

MAGNUS and NEUDECKER · Matrix Differential Calculus with Applications in Statistics and Econometrics, *Revised Edition*

MALLER and ZHOU · Survival Analysis with Long Term Survivors

MALLOWS · Design, Data, and Analysis by Some Friends of Cuthbert Daniel

MANN, SCHAFER, and SINGPURWALLA · Methods for Statistical Analysis of Reliability and Life Data

MANTON, WOODBURY, and TOLLEY · Statistical Applications Using Fuzzy Sets

MARDIA and JUPP · Directional Statistics

MASON, GUNST, and HESS · Statistical Design and Analysis of Experiments with Applications to Engineering and Science, *Second Edition*

McCULLOCH and SEARLE · Generalized, Linear, and Mixed Models

McFADDEN · Management of Data in Clinical Trials

McLACHLAN · Discriminant Analysis and Statistical Pattern Recognition

McLACHLAN and KRISHNAN · The EM Algorithm and Extensions

McLACHLAN and PEEL · Finite Mixture Models

McNEIL · Epidemiological Research Methods

MEEKER and ESCOBAR · Statistical Methods for Reliability Data

MEERSCHAERT and SCHEFFLER · Limit Distributions for Sums of Independent Random Vectors: Heavy Tails in Theory and Practice

*MILLER · Survival Analysis, *Second Edition*

MONTGOMERY, PECK, and VINING · Introduction to Linear Regression Analysis, *Third Edition*

MORGENTHALER and TUKEY · Configural Polysampling: A Route to Practical Robustness

MUIRHEAD · Aspects of Multivariate Statistical Theory

MURRAY · X-STAT 2.0 Statistical Experimentation, Design Data Analysis, and Nonlinear Optimization

---

*Now available in a lower priced paperback edition in the Wiley Classics Library.

*Now available in a lower priced paperback edition in the Wiley Classics Library.